Challenging Concepts in Congenital and Acquired Heart Disease in the Young

Published and forthcoming titles in the Challenging Concepts in series

Anaesthesia (Edited by Dr Phoebe Syme, Dr Robert Jackson, and Professor Tim Cook)

Cardiovascular Medicine (Edited by Dr Aung Myat, Dr Shouvik Haldar, and Professor Simon Redwood)

Emergency Medicine (Edited by Dr Sam Thenabadu, Dr Fleur Cantle, and Dr Chris Lacy)

Infectious Disease and Clinical Microbiology (Edited by Dr Amber Arnold and Professor George Griffin)

Interventional Radiology (Edited by Dr Irfan Ahmed, Dr Miltiadis Krokidis, and Dr Tarun Sabharwal)

Neurology (Edited by Dr Krishna Chinthapalli, Dr Nadia Magdalinou, and Professor Nicholas Wood)

Neurosurgery (Edited by Mr Robin Bhatia and Mr Ian Sabin)

Obstetrics and Gynaecology (Edited by Dr Natasha Hezelgrave, Dr Danielle Abbott, and Professor Andrew Shennan)

Oncology (Edited by Dr Madhumita Bhattacharyya, Dr Sarah Payne, and Professor Iain McNeish)

Oral and Maxillofacial Surgery (Edited by Mr Matthew Idle and Mr Andrew Monaghan)

Respiratory Medicine (Edited by Dr Lucy Schomberg and Dr Elizabeth Sage)

Challenging Concepts in Congenital and Acquired Heart Disease in the Young

Cases with Expert Commentary

Edited by

Dr Salim G M Jivanji
Consultant Congenital Interventional Cardiologist
Alder Hey Children's NHS Foundation Trust Hospital & Liverpool Heart and Chest Hospital, Liverpool, UK

Dr Michael L Rigby
Consultant Cardiologist
Royal Brompton and Harefield NHS Foundation Trust, London, UK

Series editors

Dr Aung Myat
NIHR Academic Clinical Lecturer in Interventional Cardiology, Brighton and Sussex Medical School, Brighton, UK

Dr Shouvik Haldar
Consultant Cardiologist and Electrophysiologist, Heart Rhythm Centre, Royal Brompton and Harefield NHS Foundation Trust, Honorary Clinical Senior Lecturer, Imperial College London, London, UK

Professor Simon Redwood
Professor of Interventional Cardiology and Honorary Consultant Cardiologist, King's College London and St Thomas' Hospital, London, UK

OXFORD
UNIVERSITY PRESS

OXFORD
UNIVERSITY PRESS

Great Clarendon Street, Oxford, OX2 6DP,
United Kingdom

Oxford University Press is a department of the University of Oxford. It furthers the University's objective of excellence in research, scholarship, and education by publishing worldwide. Oxford is a registered trade mark of Oxford University Press in the UK and in certain other countries

First Edition published in 2020

Impression: 1

Published in the United States of America by Oxford University Press
198 Madison Avenue, New York, NY 10016, United States of America

British Library Cataloguing in Publication Data
Data available

Library of Congress Control Number: 2019957406

ISBN 978–0–19–875944–7

Printed and bound by
CPI Group (UK) Ltd, Croydon, CR0 4YY

To my mum and dad - thank you for always believing in me.

To my beautiful wife – Rubya – I would not have been able to do this without your encouragement and support. We can finally do something else!

To my left and right heart – Hafiz and Saarah. I love you both for making me really late in completing this project!

To Farida, Khuzema, Alifyah, Taher, Hatim, Naeem and Kumail – yes I actually did this!

To the rest of my family and friends.
I am indebted that you are part of my life.

Finally to all those who have inspired me through the years, made me learn and continue to learn, to give me the chance to be a part of the best medical specialty there is.

Thank you and
I hope you enjoy this book!

Salim G M Jivanji
Liverpool, January 2020

I want to acknowledge the many friends who have challenged me and contributed to my learning and continuing education during my professional life.

I feel particularly indebted to many role models and teachers including Olive Scott and Fergus Macartney from Killingbeck Hospital Leeds, Dick Rowe and Bob Freedom from The Hospital for Sick Children Toronto, Vera Aiello from The Heart Institute, Sao Paulo Brazil, Anton Becker from The Academic Medical Centre Amsterdam and Derek Gibson, Graham Miller, Elliot Shinebourne, Bob Anderson, Jane Sommerville, Chris Lincoln, Darryl Shore, Jan Till, Yen Ho, Sabine Ernst, Michael Gatzoulis, Piers Daubeney and Julene Carvalho from the Royal Brompton Hospital London.

Thank you to the many cardiologists, surgeons and fellows not only from the UK, but also from Brazil, Argentina, Chile, USA, Canada, Europe, Australia and Asia who have spent time at the Royal Brompton and stimulated me to continue to learn and to teach.

Finally, I have been lucky enough to have a wonderful family and 3 fabulous and supportive daughters to whom I owe a great deal. Thank you to you all and to those many others who have influenced my life in a positive way.

Michael Rigby
London, January 2020

PREFACE

Just over 70 years ago, Eileen Saxon was operated on as a result of the illustrious and controversial collaboration between Alfred Blalock, Helen Taussig, and Vivien Thomas. This resulted in a child going to sleep 'blue' and waking up 'pink'. The 'blue baby' operation required no clinical trials but rather resulted in propelling an era for paediatric cardiovascular medicine and surgery.

Since then, there have been several important milestones in the treatment of congenital heart disease. Among these, Walton Lillehei's development of not-always-successful 'inside the heart' operations using 'crossed circulation' in 1954 and the culmination of decades of work by John Gibbons in the creation of the bypass machine in 1953 were the springboards for the development of open heart surgery. Survival was further improved by William Rashkind carrying out the first balloon atrial septostomy in 1966, Coceani's and Olley's report of the significance of prostaglandin E1 in keeping the arterial duct open in lambs in 1973, and Adib Jatene's development of the arterial switch operation in 1976. Diagnosis accuracy soared after the collaborative effort between the Americans, Europeans, and Japanese in the rise of echocardiography and Doppler in the 1970s and 1980s. Finally the late Kurt Amplatz's work in the creation of various devices to close atrial and ventricular septal defects in the late 1990s and most recently, Philip Bonhoeffer's work in the conception and delivery of a percutaneous valve have each transformed the scope of interventional cardiac catheterizations.

Extending the boundaries of treatment has always been accompanied by the common goal of bettering outcomes for individuals with congenital heart disease. Improvements in clinical practice in paediatric cardiology has been achieved as a result of not only ingenuity, but also incorporating experience from other branches of medicine and surgery, particularly adult cardiology.

The lack of large studies and trials in the paediatric population is a difficult predicament. As such, managing congenital heart disease is often a delicate balance between experience and evidence base. Hence there is often subtle variation in practice between various centres across the world.

The format of this book tries to address these conundrums. The contributors are from all across the congenital centres in the United Kingdom, but also from the United States, Canada, Ireland, Hong Kong, parts of Europe, Australia and New Zealand. Importantly, the experience of the experts is vital, as a number of them have not only been formative in the history of congenital heart disease, but also garnered experience in various parts of the world. Their experience places valuable insight and addresses the pitfalls of managing patients in centres with a wide variety of skill sets.

The text is aimed primarily at trainees and newly qualified consultants, but we hope that there will be several aspects which may appeal to senior clinicians alike. The chapters also attempt to cover most aspects of congenital heart disease in the young. As such, allied professionals, including specialist nurses, echocardiographers, and cardiac physiologists, will hopefully find this book useful as well.

This original text adheres to the principle of the Challenging Concept series and presents 24 chapters covering all aspects of congenital heart disease. The format allows the reader to experience examples of conditions that may present in day-to-day practice and provide various management options. 'Learning points', 'Clinical tips', and the 'Expert comments' emphasize the management and accompany the main body of the text. This will allow the reader to experience the nuances of managing a patient with congenital heart disease.

While we have tried to achieve a uniformity of approach from the authors, for the most part, opinions expressed are exclusively those of the contributors, and not necessarily our own. Readers may well find themselves disagreeing with some of the opinions expressed. However, in mirroring how cardiologists practice, the chapters' focus is on the patient who remain the centre of the decision-making process.

Finally we would like to take the opportunity to thank all the contributors for this book. As will be noted, the experience is worldwide and, as such, we are indebted to all the contributors for their patience in allowing this book to take shape. Additionally, we are grateful for the support and guidance of OUP in the entire process of getting this book published.

We hope you enjoy the work of our many contributors.

SGMJ
MLR

TABLE OF CONTENTS

EXPERTS

Tara Bharucha
Counsultant Paediatric Cardiologist
University Hospital Southampton NHS Foundation Trust
Southampton
UK

Roberta Bini
Consultant in Paediatric Cardiology and Pulmonary Hypertension
Great Ormond Street Hospital
London
UK

Michael Burch
Professor of Paediatric Cardiology
Director of Heart and Lung Transplant Services
Great Ormond Street Hospital
London
UK

Michael Cheung
Director & Associate Professor
Department of Cardiology
Royal Children's Hospital

Heart Research Group Leader
Murdoch Children's Research Institute
Melbourne

Principal Fellow
University of Melbourne
Melbourne
Australia

Piers Daubeney
Consultant in Paediatric and Fetal Cardiology
Royal Brompton & Harefield NHS Foundation Trust

Professor of Practice in Paediatric Cardiology
Imperial College London
London
UK

Catherine Head
Consultant ACHD Cardiologist
Norfolk and Norwich Hospital
Norwich
UK

Lindsey E Hunter
Consultant Paediatric & Fetal Cardiologist
Royal Hospital for Children
Glasgow

Honorary Senior Clinical Lecturer
Glasgow University
Glasgow
Scotland

Juan Pablo Kaski
Consultant Paediatric Cardiologist
Centre for Inherited Cardiovascular Diseases

Great Ormond Street Hospital
Honorary Associate Professor
University College London
UK

Damien Kenny
Consultant Paediatric Cardiologist Children's Health Ireland at Crumlin

Clinical Associate Professor of Paediatrics
Royal College of Surgeons in Ireland
Ireland

Sachin Khambadkone
Consultant Paediatric Interventional Cardiologist
Clinical Lead for Transitioning
Great Ormond Street Hospital
London
UK

Jasveer Mangat
Consultant Paediatric Cardiologist and Electrophysiologist
Great Ormond Street Hospital
London
UK

Robin P Martin
Past Consultant Paediatric and Adult
Congenital Cardiologist
Bristol Royal Hospital for Children and
Bristol Heart Institute

Past President of the British Congenital
Cardiac Association

Brian A McCrossan
Consultant Paediatric Cardiologist
Royal Belfast Hospital for Sick Children
Belfast
Northern Ireland

Krishnakumar Nair
Consultant Cardiologist and Electrophysiologist
Toronto General Hospital
University Health Network
Toronto
Canada

Reza Razavi
Honorary Consultant Paediatric Cardiologist
Evelina London Children's Hospital

Professor of Paediatric Cardiovascular Science
Vice President and Vice Principal (Research)
Kings College London

Director of the King's Wellcome Trust
EPSRC Centre For Medical Engineering
London
UK

Andrew N Redington
Chief of Cardiology
Professor of Paediatrics
Heart Institute
Cincinnati Children's Hospital Medical Center
Cincinnati OH
USA

Michael Rigby
Consultant Cardiologist
Royal Brompton & Harefield NHS Foundation Trust
London
UK

Eric Rosenthal
Professor of Paediatric and Adult Congenital Cardiology
Evelina London Children's Hospital
London
UK

Gurleen Sharland
Professor of Fetal Cardiology
Evelina London Children's Hospital
London
UK

John M Simpson
Professor of Paediatric and Fetal Cardiology
Evelina London Children's Hospital
London
UK

Oliver Stumper
Consultant Paediatric Cardiologist
Birmingham Women's and Children's NHS Trust
Birmingham
UK

Nidhy P Varghese
Medical Director – Pulmonary Hypertension Program
Texas Children's Hospital

Assistant Professor of Pediatrics
Section of Pulmonary Medicine
Baylor College of Medicine
USA

Vita Zidere
Consultant in Paediatric and Fetal Cardiology
Evelina London Children's Hospital
London
UK

CONTRIBUTORS

Mohammad Ryan Abumehdi
Paediatric Cardiology SpR
Birmingham Women's and Children's NHS Trust
Birmingham
UK

Rubya Adamji
Post CCST StR in Paediatric Dentistry
Royal National ENT & Eastman Dental Hospitals
University College London Hospitals NHS
Foundation Trust
London
UK

Tarek Alsaeid
Paediatric Cardiologist
Assistant Professor of Paediatrics
Heart Institute
Cincinnati Children's Hospital Medical Center
Cincinnati OH
USA

Aaron Bell
Consultant Paediatric Cardiologist
Evelina London Children's Hospital
London
UK

Hannah Belsham-Revell
Consultant Paediatric Cardiologist
Evelina London Children's Hospital
London
UK

Colm Breatnach
Paediatric Cardiology SpR
Children's Health Ireland at Crumlin
Crumlin
Ireland

Alexander Van De Bruaene
Assistant Professor
University Hospitals Leuven
Leuven
Belgium

Corey A Chartan
Pediatric Critical Care/Pulmonary Hypertension
Associate Medical Director – Right Ventricular
Failure Program
Texas Children's Hospital

Assistant Professor of Pediatrics
Sections of Critical Care Medicine and Pulmonary
Medicine
Baylor College of Medicine
USA

Robin HS Chen
Consultant
Department of Paediatric Cardiology
Queen Mary Hospital

Honorary Clinical Associate Professor
Department of Paediatrics and Adolescent Medicine
University of Hong Kong
Hong Kong SAR

Ryan D Coleman
Pediatric Critical Care/Pulmonary Hypertension
Medical Director – Right Ventricular Failure Program
Clinical Quality Lead – ECMO
Texas Children's Hospital

Assistant Professor of Pediatrics and Medical Ethics
Sections of Critical Care Medicine and Pulmonary
Medicine
Center for Medical Ethics and Health Policy
Baylor College of Medicine
USA

Thomas Day
Post-CCT Clinical Research Fellow
Evelina London Children's Hospital
London
UK

Grazia Delle Donne
Locum Consultant Paediatric Cardiologist
Leeds Children's Hospital
Leeds
UK

Sophie Duignan
Paediatric Cardiology SpR
Children's Health Ireland at Crumlin
Crumlin
Ireland

Shouvik Haldar
Consultant Cardiologist and Electrophysiologist
Royal Brompton & Harefield NHS Foundation Trust
London
UK

Michael Harris
Consultant in Paediatric and Fetal Cardiology
Birmingham Women's and Children's NHS Trust
Birmingham
UK

Andrew Ho
Consultant Paediatric Cardiologist
University Hospital Southampton NHS
Foundation Trust
Southampton
UK

Salim Jivanji
Consultant Congenital Interventional Cardiologist
Alder Hey Children's Hospital & Liverpool Heart and
Chest Hospital
Liverpool
UK

Sok-Leng Kang
Consultant Congenital Interventional Cardiologist
Alder Hey Children's Hospital & Liverpool Heart
and Chest Hospital
Liverpool
UK

Filip Kucera
Locum Consultant Paediatric Cardiologist
Great Ormond Street Hospital
London
UK

David Lloyd
Locum Consultant in Paediatric and Fetal Cardiology
Evelina London Children's Hospital
London
UK

Louise Morrison
Consultant Paediatric Cardiologist
Royal Belfast Hospital for Sick Children
Belfast
Northern Ireland

Gabrielle Norrish
Clinical Research Fellow in Inherited Cardiovascular
Diseases
Centre for Inherited Cardiovascular Diseases
Great Ormond Street Hospital
London
UK

Gemma Penford
Consultant Paediatric Cardiologist
Starship Hospital
Auckland
New Zealand

Will Regan
Paediatric Cardiology Registrar
Evelina London Children's Hospital
London
UK

Paraskevi Theocharis
Consultant Paediatric Cardiologist
Evelina London Children's Hospital
London
UK

Justin T Tretter
Paediatric Cardiologist
Assistant Professor of Paediatrics
Heart Institute
Cincinnati Children's Hospital Medical Center
Cincinnati OH
USA

Laura Vazquez-Garcia
Locum Consultant Paediatric Cardiologist
Royal Brompton & Harefield NHS Foundation Trust
London
UK

James Wong
Consultant Paediatric Cardiologist
Evelina London Children's Hospital
London
UK

ABBREVIATIONS

A & E	accident and emergency
6MWD	6-minute walking distance
ACA	aborted cardiac arrest
ACE	angiotensin-converting enzyme
AEPC	Association for European Pediatric and Congenital Cardiology
AET	atrial ectopic tachycardia
AF	atrial fibrillation
AHA	American Heart Association
ALCAPA	anomalous left coronary artery arising from the pulmonary artery
AP	accessory pathway
APC	antigen-presenting cell
APLS	Advanced Paediatric Life Support
ARSCA	aberrant right subclavian artery
AS	aortic stenosis
ASA	acetyl salicylic acid
ATP	anti-tachycardia pacing
AV	atrioventricular
AVA	aortic valve area
AVCTI	atrioventricular contraction time interval
AVNRT	atrioventricular nodal re-entry tachycardia
AVRT	atrioventricular re-entry tachycardia
AVSD	atrioventricular septal defect
AVT	acute vasodilation testing
AWI	aortic wall injury
AZA	azathioprine
BAS	balloon atrial septostomy
bd	twice daily
BE	base excess
BiVAD	biventricular assist device
BJV	bovine jugular vein
BMPR2	bone morphogenetic protein receptor 2
BNF	British National Formulary
BNP	brain natriuretic peptide, B-type natriuretic peptide
bpm	beats per minute
BPV	bioprosthetic pulmonary valve
BT	Blalock–Taussig
BV	balloon valvuloplasty
CAF	coronary artery fistula
CATS	Children's Acute Transport Service
CAV	cardiac allograft vasculopathy
CBP SIRS	cardiac bypass systemic inflammatory response syndrome
CCB	calcium channel blocker
CCISC	Congenital Cardiovascular Interventional Study Consortium
CCPS	covered CP stent
CGA	corrected gestational age
cGMP	cyclic guanosine monophosphate
CHB	complete heart block
CHD	congenital heart disease
CHSS	Congenital Heart Surgeons' Society
CI	confidence interval
CLD	chronic lung disease
cm	centimetre
CMR	cardiac magnetic resonance
CMV	cytomegalovirus
CO	cardiac output
CO2	carbon dioxide
CoAFU	Coarctation Repair in Long-term Follow-Up (study)
COAST	Coarctation of the Aorta Stent Trial
CP	Cheatham Platinum (stent)
CPAP	continuous positive airway pressure
CPET	cardiopulmonary exercise testing
CPVT	catecholaminergic polymorphic ventricular tachycardia
CRP	C-reactive protein
CRT	cardiac resynchronization therapy
CRT-D	cardiac resynchronization therapy defibrillator
CSA	cross-sectional area
CT	computed tomography
CTPA	computed tomography pulmonary angiography
CW	continuous-wave
Cx	circumflex
CXR	chest X-ray
DC	direct current
DCDA	dichorionic diamniotic
DKS	Damus–Kaye–Stansel
DNA	deoxyribonucleic acid
DORV	double outlet right ventricle
EA	Ebstein's anomaly

EBV	Ebstein–Barr virus
ECG	electrocardiogram
ECMO	extracorporeal membrane oxygenation
ED	emergency department
EHRA	European Heart Rhythm Association
EMB	endomyocardial biopsy
ENT	ear, nose, and throat
EPC	endothelial progenitor cell
EPS	electrophysiological study
ERA	endothelin receptor antagonist
ERS	European Respiratory Society
ESC	European Society of Cardiology
ESM	ejection systolic murmur
ESR	erythrocyte sedimentation rate
ET	endothelin
FBC	full blood count
FDA	Food and Drug Administration
fECG	fetal electrocardiography
fMCG	fetal magnetocardiography
Fr	French
g	gram
GP	general practitioner
GUCH	grown-up congenital heart
HCM	hypertrophic cardiomyopathy
HFOV	high-frequency oscillatory ventilation
HIV	human immunodeficiency virus
HLA	human leucocyte antigen
HLHS	hypoplastic left heart syndrome
HPAH	hereditary pulmonary arterial hypertension
HRS	Heart Rhythm Society
HSV	herpes simplex virus
IART	intra-atrial re-entry tachycardia
ICD	implantable cardioverter–defibrillator
ICU	intensive care unit
IE	infective endocarditis
IL-1	interleukin-1
IL-2	interleukin 2
INR	international normalized ratio
IP3	inositol-1,4,5-trisphosphate
IPAH	idiopathic pulmonary arterial hypertension
IV	intravenous
IVC	inferior vena cava
IVH	intraventricular haemorrhage
IVIG	intravenous immunoglobulin
IVS	intact ventricular septum
IVUS	intravascular ultrasound
JET	junctional ectopic tachycardia
KD	Kawasaki disease
kg	kilogram
kPa	kilopascal
l	litre
LA:Ao	left atrial:aortic root (ratio)
LAD	left anterior descending
LAO	left anterior oblique
LCA	left coronary artery
LCSD	left cardiac sympathetic denervation
LLSE	left lower sternal edge
LPA	left pulmonary artery
LQTS	long QT syndrome
LSCA	left subclavian artery
LUSE	left upper sternal edge
LV	left ventricular
LVAD	left ventricular assist device
LVEF	left ventricular ejection fraction
LVEI	left ventricular eccentricity index
LV-EI(D)	left ventricular eccentricity index in diastole
LV-EI(S)	left ventricular eccentricity index in systole
LVOT	left ventricular outflow tract
LVOTO	left ventricular outflow tract obstruction
LVSVI	Left ventricular systolic volume indexed
m	metre
MAPCA	major aortopulmonary collateral artery
mcg	microgram
MDT	multidisciplinary team
min	minute
ml	millilitre
MLB	microlaryngoscopy and bronchoscopy
MMF	mycophenolate mofetil
mmHg	millimetre of mercury
MPA	main pulmonary artery
mPAP	mean pulmonary artery pressure
MR	magnetic resonance
MRI	magnetic resonance imaging
MSF	Melody® valve stent fracture
mTOR	mammalian target of rapamycin
NACCS	National Australian Childhood Cardiomyopathy Study
NEC	necrotizing enterocolitis
ng	nanogram
NICE	National Institute for Health and Care Excellence
NICU	neonatal intensive care unit

NIRS	near infrared spectroscopy
NO	nitric oxide
NSAID	non-steroidal anti-inflammatory drug
NT-pro-BNP	N-terminal pro-b-type natriuretic peptide
NYHA	New York Heart Association
od	once daily
OR	odds ratio
PA	pulmonary atresia; pulmonary artery
PAAT	pulmonary artery acceleration time
PACES	Pediatric and Congenital Electrophysiology Society
PAH	pulmonary arterial hypertension
PAH-CHD	pulmonary arterial hypertension associated with congenital heart disease
PAPCA	Prospective Assessment after Pediatric Cardiac Ablation (study)
PAWP	pulmonary arterial wedge pressure
PCH	pulmonary capillary haemangiomatosis
PCMR	Pediatric Cardiomyopathy Registry
PCR	polymerase chain reaction
PDA	patent ductus arteriosus
PDE	phosphodiesterase
PDE5	phosphodiesterase type 5
PEC	Paediatricians with Expertise in Cardiology
PFO	patent foramen ovale
PGE1	prostaglandin E1
PGI2	prostaglandin 2
PH	pulmonary hypertension
PH-CHD	patients with pulmonary hypertension associated with congenital heart disease
PICU	paediatric intensive care unit
PJRT	permanent junctional reciprocating tachycardia
PLE	protein-losing enteropathy
PPHN	persistent pulmonary hypertension of the newborn
PPM	permanent pacemaker
PPVI	percutaneous pulmonary valve implantation
PR	pulmonary regurgitation
PRA	panel reactive antibody
PTFE	polytetrafluoroethylene
PVA	pulmonary venous atrium
PVG	primary graft failure
PVOD	pulmonary vascular occlusive disease
PVR	pulmonary vascular resistance; pulmonary valve replacement
PVRi	pulmonary vascular resistance indexed
PW	pulsed-wave
RA	right atrial; right atrium
RCA	right coronary artery
RD	risk difference
REV	réparation à l'étage ventriculaire
RFA	right femoral artery
RIMP	right ventricular index of myocardial performance
ROP	retinopathy of prematurity
RPA	right pulmonary artery
RR	relative risk; risk ratio
RV	right ventricle; right ventricular
RVEDP	right ventricular end-diastolic pressure
RVEDV	right ventricular end-diastolic volume
RVEDVi	right ventricular end-diastolic volume indexed
RVEF	right ventricular ejection fraction
RVESV	right ventricular end-systolic volume
RVFAC	right ventricular fractional area change
RVOT	right ventricular outflow tract
RVOT AT	right ventricular outflow tract acceleration time
RVOTO	right ventricular outflow tract obstruction
RVSP	right ventricular systemic pressure
RVSVI	Right ventricular systolic volume indexed
s	second
SAD	sudden arrhythmic death
SCBU	special care baby unit
SDCEP	Scottish Dental Clinical Effectiveness Programme
SIDS	sudden infant death syndrome
SLE	systemic lupus erythematosus
SPECT	single-photon emission computed tomography
SSFP	steady-state free precession
SVC	superior vena cava
SVT	supraventricular tachycardia
TAPSE	tricuspid annular plane systolic excursion
TAVI	transcatheter aortic valve implantation
TCPC	total cavo-pulmonary connection
tds	three times daily
TGA	transposition of the great arteries
TNF	tumour necrosis factor
TOE	transoesophageal echocardiography
TOPP	Tracking Outcomes and Practice in Paediatric Pulmonary Hypertension (study)
TR	tricuspid regurgitation

TV	tricuspid valve
UK	United Kingdom
URTI	upper respiratory tract infection
US IDE	US Investigational Device Exemption (study)
VA	veno-arterial
VACTERL	vertebral defects, anal atresia, cardiac defects, tracheo-oesophageal fistula, renal anomalies, and limb abnormalities
VAD	ventricular assist device
VATS	video-assisted thoracoscopy
VF	ventricular fibrillation
VO_2	peak oxygen consumption
VRT	volume-rendering technique
VSD	ventricular septal defect
VT	ventricular tachycardia
VTI	velocity time integral
VZV	varicella-zoster virus
WCC	white cell count
WHO	World Health Organization
WPW	Wolff–Parkinson–White
WU	Wood unit

CASE

1 Back from the brink: a reversible cardiac cause of fetal hydrops

David Lloyd

Expert commentary John Simpson and Vita Zidere

Case history

A 32-year-old woman presented for fetal cardiology assessment after fetal hydrops was detected at 29 weeks' gestation. Maternal history was positive for type 2 diabetes and mild asthma. This was her third pregnancy, having previously delivered live dichorionic diamniotic (DCDA) twins and a singleton pregnancy (G3 P2), each by caesarean section. All her children were healthy, and there was no family history of congenital heart disease (CHD).

Nuchal translucency was measured at 1.2 mm (within normal range) in early pregnancy, and routine mid-trimester screening ultrasound, performed at 20 weeks, had detected no abnormalities. Repeat assessment at 29 weeks showed a new finding of ascites, with bilateral pleural effusions, and a diagnosis of fetal hydrops was made. No other abnormalities were detected, and the fetus was referred for urgent fetal cardiology assessment in an attempt to establish an underlying cause.

Learning point Fetal hydrops

Fetal hydrops is defined by the presence of excessive fluid in at least two serous body cavities (the abdomen, pleural space, or pericardium) or in body tissue (subcutaneous oedema) [1]. The phenomenon is unique to the physiology of the fetal lymphatic system, owing to increased capillary permeability, a highly compliant interstitial compartment, and a more marked influence of venous pressure on lymphatic return [2]. A disturbance at any point in the lymphatic system can lead to hydrops, which should be seen as a symptom of an underlying fetal disease, rather than a disorder in itself (Figure 1.1).

Historically, fetal hydrops was divided into two categories: immune (generally related to rhesus D haemolytic disease of the newborn) and non-immune causes. However, the immune form has diminished significantly since the introduction of rhesus isoimmunization prophylaxis, now accounting for <10% of cases in the developed world. Before 20 weeks, chromosomal abnormalities make up almost two-thirds of cases. However, attrition of these pregnancies in the second trimester leads to a gradual predominance of other aetiologies, with cardiac diseases responsible for almost one in four cases of fetal hydrops after 24 weeks (Table 1.1).

Important non-cardiac causes of fetal hydrops include fetal anaemia, associated not only with rhesus D haemolytic disease, but also with fetal haemorrhage, infection (particularly parvovirus B19), twin-to-twin transfusion syndrome, red cell or platelet defects, and inborn errors of metabolism. Thyrotoxicosis is another important cause to exclude. Excessive volume loading leading to cardiac failure can be caused by agenesis of the ductus venosus, which leads to a direct umbilical vein-to-cardiac connection (associated with Noonan syndrome), and fetal or placental arteriovenous malformations. Vascular tumours, such as sacrococcygeal tumours, haemangioendotheliomas, teratomas, and placental chorangiomas, can lead to hydrops via a combination of both fetal anaemia and volume loading, the latter due to arteriovenous shunting [3].

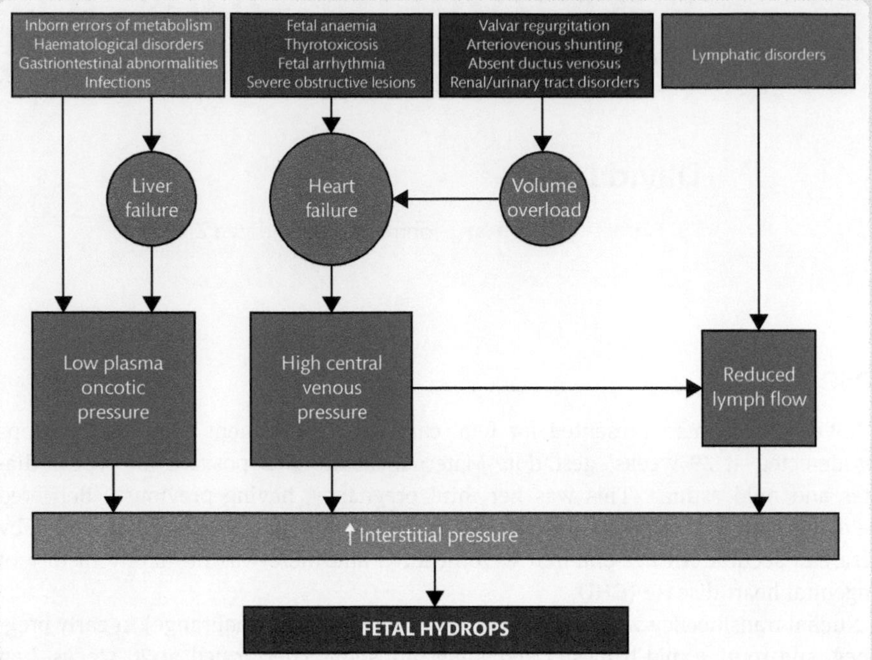

Figure 1.1 Physiological pathways leading to fetal hydrops.

Table 1.1 Proportion of causes of hydrops by gestational age [3]

Cause	<24–28 weeks' gestation	>24–28 weeks' gestation
Chromosomal	34.5%	5.4%
Cardiovascular	**9.0%**	**24.2%**
Genetic or syndromal	8.8%	8.2%
Infective	4.8%	5.8%
Pulmonary	7.4%	13.2%
Unknown	15.0%	22.1%

Source data from Anne Marie Coady, SB. *Twining's Textbook of Fetal Abnormalities* (3rd Edition). Churchill Williams, 2014.

Clinical tip Echocardiographic assessment of fetal hydrops

The most frequent cardiac causes of hydrops are listed in Box 1.1. All share the common final pathway of increased central venous pressure, due to either primary ('pump') or secondary heart failure (Figure 1.2). It should be noted that whilst structural CHD may be seen in hydrops (e.g. in association with genetic abnormalities), it is rarely the primary cause. Fetal heart failure is suggested by various means of echocardiographic findings [4], such as enlargement of the cardiac chambers (increased cardiothoracic ratio) and reduced 'eyeball' systolic function. A monophasic ventricular inflow pattern may be an early sign of diastolic dysfunction and can precede obvious systolic impairment.

Box 1.1 Cardiac causes of fetal hydrops

- Fetal tachyarrhythmias
- Fetal bradyarrhythmias
- Severe valvular regurgitation
- Other structural congenital heart disease (rare)
- Primary myocardial disease (very rare)

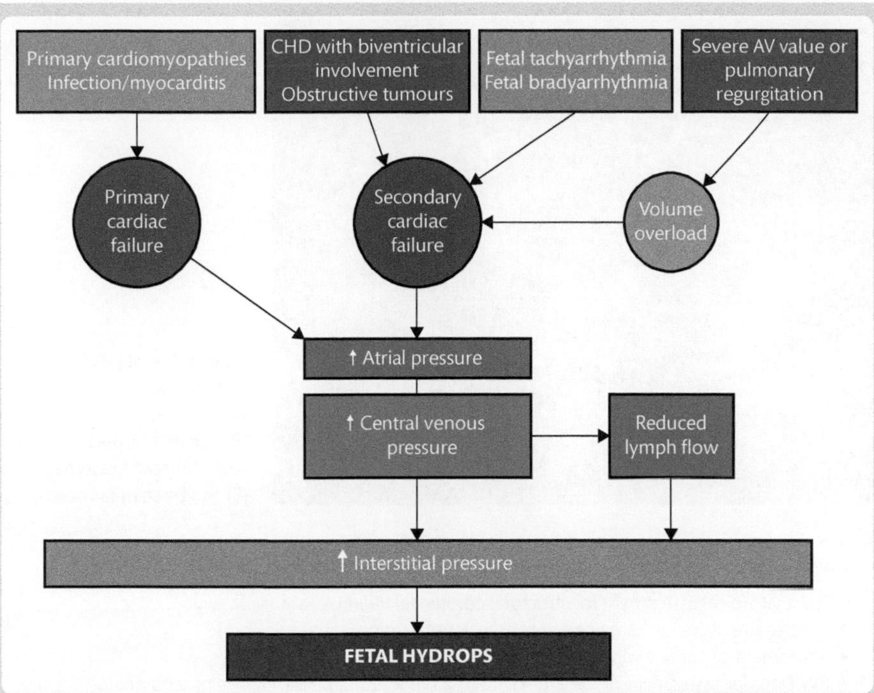

Figure 1.2 Physiological pathways relating to the primary cardiac causes of fetal hydrops. CHD, congenital heart disease; AD, arterial duct; FO, foramen ovale; AV, atrioventricular.

Pulsed-wave (PW) Doppler 'a-wave' reversal in either pulmonary vein or the ductus venosus may also be seen as diastolic function deteriorates, although it is crucial to ensure that the fetus is in sinus rhythm as any degree of atrioventricular dyssynchrony will produce the same effect. Mitral valve regurgitation is rare in the fetus and strongly suggests cardiac involvement. Holosystolic tricuspid valve regurgitation is also a poor prognostic marker (Figure 1.3). Pericardial effusion is common [5]. Pleural effusions, ascites, and subcutaneous oedema may also be observed (Figure 1.4). A suggested approach to echocardiographic assessment is shown in Box 1.2.

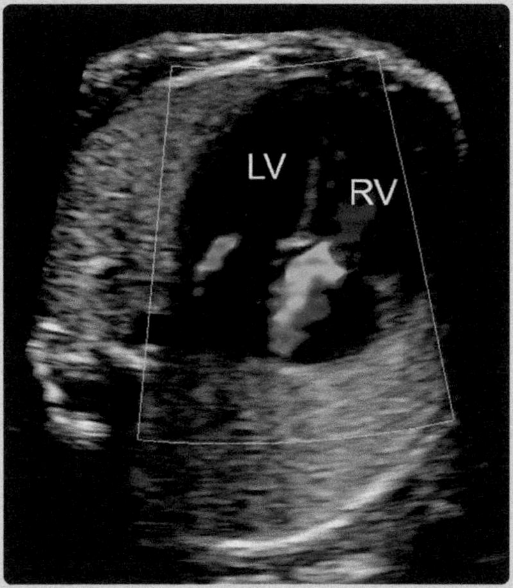

Figure 1.3 AV valve regurgitation in a 31-week fetus with fetal hydrops secondary to persistent atrial flutter. The heart was otherwise structurally normal. The presence of mitral regurgitation in this case is particularly indicative of cardiac involvement. LV, left ventricle; RV, right ventricle.

Expert comment

There is good evidence that the fetal heart size (and therefore the cardiothoracic ratio) correlates well with increasing central venous pressure, derived from fetal lamb studies using invasive measurements of umbilical vein pressure [6]. The absence of cardiomegaly therefore strongly militates against a primary cardiac cause of fetal hydrops, a useful initial observation during echocardiographic assessment.

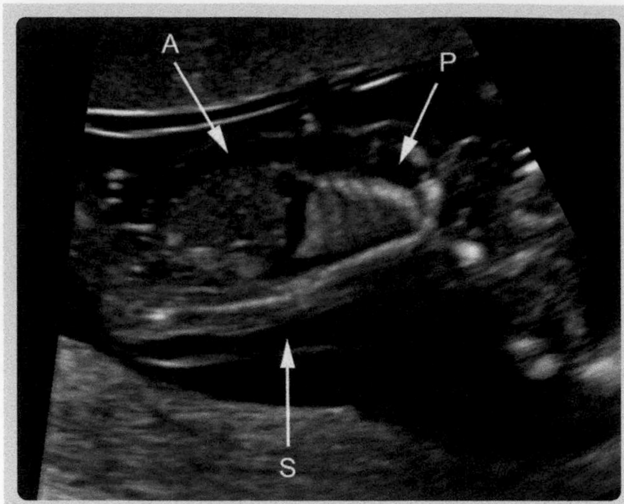

Figure 1.4 Sagittal view of a hydropic fetus at 14 weeks. Pleural effusions (P), ascites (A), and subcutaneous oedema (S) can be seen (arrowed).

Box 1.2 Structured approach to echocardiographic assessment of the fetus with hydrops

- Full anatomical assessment for structural congenital heart disease
- Cardiac size, function ± evidence of associated cardiomyopathy/tumours
- Assessment of cardiac valves for stenosis or regurgitation
- PW Doppler assessment of the arterial duct, atrial septum, pulmonary veins, and ductus venosus
- Assessment of heart rhythm using M-mode and Doppler

Fetal cardiology assessment confirmed the maternal history as mentioned. Echocardiography was performed, showing the heart and stomach on the left, with normal position of the aorta and inferior caval vein. There were concordant atrioventricular and ventriculoarterial connections. The fetal heart rate throughout the scan was noted to be around 260 bpm. The heart was enlarged, with a small pericardial effusion noted. Biventricular systolic function appeared to be reduced. There was normal offsetting of the mitral and tricuspid valves, with no regurgitation. There was no evidence of left or right ventricular outflow tract obstruction. The aortic and ductal arches passed to the left of the trachea, with no evidence of coarctation.

Learning point Structural CHD and hydrops

The nature of the fetal circulation means that the vast majority of congenital cardiac defects are well tolerated in the fetus and do not lead to haemodynamic compromise. When important cardiac malformations are seen with hydrops [for e.g. atrioventricular septal defects (AVSDs)] in the majority, this is likely due to parallel associations with chromosomal abnormalities (e.g. 45XO, trisomies 21 and 18), and not necessarily as the underlying cause [5]. In the rare cases in which CHD is the primary cause of hydrops, the final common pathway is a marked increase in atrial (and thus systemic venous) pressure (Box 1.3). This is most commonly due to severe atrioventricular valve insufficiency, although this can also be seen in severe hydrops from other causes [3].

Box 1.3 Structural abnormalities associated with development of fetal hydrops

- Volume overload with biventricular heart failure (severe atrioventricular valve regurgitation, Ebstein anomaly/severe tricuspid valve dysplasia, severe pulmonary regurgitation)
- Biventricular obstruction (e.g. bilateral valvular disease, common arterial trunk with stenotic truncal valve, bilateral cardiac tumours)

Expert comment

Most congenital malformations have limited haemodynamic impact in fetal life due to the parallel nature of the fetal circulation, and even when CHD is seen in this context, it is still important to rule out other causes (such as coexisting cardiac arrhythmias or genetic abnormalities). In order for structural defects to cause fetal cardiac failure, a degree of biventricular dysfunction must be present. An obvious example of this would be a common arterial trunk with severe truncal valve stenosis and/or regurgitation, effectively impeding cardiac output from both ventricles. A similar picture may be seen in severe unilateral lesions which lead to important biventricular interactions, such as Ebstein anomaly, or severe aortic stenosis with mitral regurgitation (± atrial restriction).

Treatment options may be very limited. Fetal interventions to relieve critical obstruction—particularly at atrial level—have seen limited success in some units. However, these are not practised widely [7]. Premature delivery and postnatal management may be technically feasible, but this can be extremely precarious and needs to be weighed against the risks of continuing pregnancy.

Learning point Fetal tachyarrhythmias

Fetal tachyarrhythmia (>180–200 bpm) is arguably the most important cause of hydrops to the fetal cardiologist, as it carries the best potential for successful treatment. In general, the incidence of fetal tachyarrhythmias mirrors the neonatal population, with accessory pathway-mediated **atrioventricular re-entry tachycardia** (AVRT) the most common cause. Atrial ectopic beats can be a marker of an accessory pathway, but such ectopics can be seen in 1–2% of normal pregnancies. Accessory conduction pathways are also occasionally seen in Ebstein anomaly and rhabdomyomas, an important consideration if either is seen in a hydropic fetus. In AVRT, the atrial and ventricular rates are identical. In the fetus with tachycardia in whom the atrial rate exceeds the ventricular rate, **atrial flutter** is the most likely diagnosis, accounting for around 30% of fetal tachyarrhythmias. It tends to present later than AVRT; however, the incidence of hydrops is similar in both conditions. The atrial rate is usually sustained at >400 bpm, an important diagnostic factor, with variable degrees of AV block (usually 2:1). There is an association between atrial flutter and accessory conduction pathways, and therefore, this may be the presenting rhythm in patients who go on to develop AVRT before or after birth. Flutter can be associated with Ebstein anomaly of the tricuspid valve; however, the prognosis in this scenario is poor [8]. **Ventricular tachycardia** is extremely rare in the fetus and may be suspected where the ventricular rate exceeds the atrial rate. This may be observed in fetal long QT syndrome. Other potential signs of fetal long QT syndrome include a slow sinus bradycardia. Permanent junctional reciprocating tachycardia (PJRT) and atrial ectopic tachycardia (AET) are less common and can be more difficult to treat. Atrioventricular nodal re-entry tachycardia (AVNRT) and atrial fibrillation (AF) are rare in the fetus.

Treatment

If there are only very brief episodes of fetal tachycardia, without hydrops, it may be reasonable to observe without instituting therapy. However, intermittent tachycardia may also lead to fetal hydrops and control of tachycardias is more difficult once hydrops develops. Thus, there is generally a low threshold for transplacental fetal therapy. These treatments are not without risk and should only be undertaken with a cardiologist's oversight and close maternal follow-up to assess both mother and fetus (Table 1.2). If cardioversion is successful, anti-arrhythmic therapy is generally continued after birth for 6–12 months until continuous sinus rhythm can be proven. The recurrence rate after successful cardioversion of atrial flutter is low (around 10%). In the case of the hydropic fetus refractory to transplacental therapy, direct fetal injection may be considered after maternal loading with the same drug (to prevent reverse transplacental distribution to the maternal circulation). Potential drugs that can be deliver in this way include adenosine, amiodarone, digoxin, and propafenone. This invasive treatment carries significant additional risk and should only be performed in specialist units after careful assessment [9].

Table 1.2 Anti-arrhythmic drugs used in fetal tachyarrhythmias

Drug	Dose	Notes	Side effects	Monitoring
Flecainide	100 mg tds	Class Ic Rapid response	Paraesthesiae, blurred vision, conduction defects, oedema, fatigue, fever	Maternal ECG: prolonged QRS
Digoxin	0.25 mg tds	Class V	Nausea, vomiting, conduction disturbance, dizziness	Maternal serum levels
Amiodarone	200–400 mg once daily (od) (after loading)	Class III (features of Ia, II, IV) Oral loading in hospital with ECG	Nausea, vomiting, taste disturbance Potentially thyrotoxic to fetus	Maternal ECG: prolonged QTc
Sotalol	80 mg twice daily (bd) (max 240 mg)	Class III	Bradycardia, conduction disturbances, vasoconstriction, bronchospasm	Maternal ECG: prolonged QTc

Expert comment

The key aim of intrauterine treatment of fetal arrhythmias is to allow for delivery at full term with normal obstetric monitoring (and therefore normal delivery), via either rate control or, preferably, achievement of sinus rhythm. If the fetus is compromised, there is no evidence that shifting the problem from a fetal one to a neonatal one (via premature delivery) improves outcome. The perfect intrauterine therapy would rapidly cross the placenta, be safe for mother and fetus, and be effective in a wide range of arrhythmias. In practice, of course, no such drug exists, and to date, there have been no randomized trials to assess the efficacy of the many anti-arrhythmic drugs available. Thus, treatment protocols will vary widely from one institution to another, based on clinician familiarity, the availability of the drugs used, and the resources available for maternal monitoring.

Learning point Fetal bradyarrhythmias

Fetal bradyarrhythmias (<110 bpm) can also lead to fetal hydrops, although this group of conditions is generally more difficult to treat than tachyarrhythmias. Careful assessment is required to determine whether the rhythm is sinus bradycardia or associated with AV block (see 'Echocardiographic assessment of arrhythmias in the fetus', p. 8). Whilst intermittent sinus pauses are common in the normal fetus, sustained **sinus bradycardia** can be seen with sinus node disruption associated with left atrial isomerism. It is also seen in congenital long QT syndrome or in the case of significant or end-stage fetal distress from other causes [5, 10]. **Complete heart block** (CHB) is associated with congenital heart defects in around half of all cases, in particular left atrial isomerism (where the combination carries an extremely poor prognosis) or discordant AV connection. In cases of CHB associated with a structurally normal heart, this is most commonly due to transplacental passage of anti-Ro/SSA and anti-La/SSB antibodies from maternal blood, resulting in a passively acquired autoimmune process affecting the fetal conduction tissue, which leads to irreversible fibrosis [11]. Whilst these antibodies are classically associated with systemic lupus erythematosus (SLE), congenital CHB is, in fact, only seen in 2–3% of seropositive women. In patients who have had a previous child with CHB, however, the risk is higher (around 17–20%) [11]. Around half of immune-mediated CHB cases are detected in asymptomatic mothers who were previously unaware of their antibody status. In terms of screening, CHB is unlikely to develop before 18 weeks, or beyond 28 weeks. **Type II second-degree AV block** can progress rapidly to irreversible CHB, although there is stronger evidence that the rhythm may be more responsive to treatment at this stage. **Type I second-degree AV block** can be confused with non-conducted atrial ectopic beats. Both are typically benign and resolve with fetal activity. **First-degree heart block** (prolongation of AV conduction time) can occur in the normal fetus and spontaneously resolve. Whether monitoring the AV conduction time is an effective means of monitoring for higher degrees of AV block remains controversial.

Expert comment

Management of heart block in the fetus is controversial. Once present, CHB is usually irreversible, and there is no clear evidence that earlier treatment can prevent it. In addition, maternal steroids are not without risk, and no prospective randomized studies exist. There is also a confounding 'era' effect, whereby survival appears to have improved in recent cohorts, even with more conservative management [12]; the precise reasons for this are yet to be determined. Fetal hydrops is consistently noted as a reliable predictor of poor outcome, however, and most centres would consider it reasonable to instigate maternal treatment in this scenario.

Treatment

Maternal β-sympathomimetics, such as salbutamol and terbutaline, can be used to increase the fetal heart rate, although there is no evidence of a survival benefit. Maternal treatment with oral steroids (particularly dexamethasone and betamethasone, both of which cross the placenta) may have a role in acute treatment of CHB with hydrops; whilst steroids are less likely to alter the heart rhythm at this stage, the reduction in myocardial inflammation may be of benefit in cases with evidence of poor function or evolving endocardial fibroelastosis. Their use in type II second-degree heart block, which may prevent progression to CHB, is less controversial. The use of prophylactic steroids and/or intravenous immunoglobulin (IVIG) in high-risk patients is not proven [10, 11], and attempts at fetal ventricular pacing, generally as a last resort, have rarely been successful [10].

Learning point Myocardial diseases leading to fetal hydrops

Cardiomyopathy

Cardiomyopathies in the fetus are rare. Dilated cardiomyopathy has been described in genetic, metabolic, and infective diseases, in particular parvovirus B19. It can also rarely be seen with anti-Ro and anti-La antibodies in cases with no evidence of heart block. The appearance of 'non-compaction' cardiomyopathy in the fetus has been associated with Barth syndrome [3]. Hypertrophic cardiomyopathy (HCM) is most commonly seen in fetuses and infants of poorly controlled diabetic mothers and is rarely—if ever—seen with hydrops. Whilst this generally regresses completely after birth, the prognosis for most other fetal cardiomyopathies is poor.

Infection/myocarditis

Primary myocarditis in the fetus is rare, although it has been described in association with parvovirus infection. It is worth noting that certain infections associated with fetal hydrops are also independently associated with cardiac abnormalities (e.g. rubella, parvovirus, and cytomegalovirus).

Myocardial infarction

Due to the nature of the fetal circulation, important coronary malformations, such as anomalous left coronary artery arising from the pulmonary artery (ALCAPA) will have no discernible pathophysiological effects in the fetus. As such, reports of *in utero* myocardial infarction are extremely rare.

Expert comment

Whilst inherited cardiomyopathies presenting in the fetus are rare, it is important that these are not handled any differently than if detected in postnatal life. There may be important implications not just for future pregnancies, but also for the parents and other family members. If inherited disease is suspected, genetic testing should be considered, along with cardiac screening of first-degree relatives. Additionally, should the fetus not survive to term, arrangements need to be made for collection of post-mortem samples.

Clinical tip Echocardiographic assessment of suspected arrhythmia in the fetus

Whilst electrophysiological methods of analysing the fetal heart rhythm have been proposed (see 'Future directions in assessment of fetal arrhythmias', p. 9), in practice, the mainstay of diagnosis is fetal echocardiography, by directly examining the motion of cardiac chambers or flow signals within the heart. **M-mode** involves placing a cursor along a line which transects both atrial and ventricular tissue. The corresponding M-mode trace will then show the relationship between atrial (A) and ventricular (V) contraction (Figure 1.5). The VA time, or the time between the ventricular and atrial contractions, can be helpful in distinguishing between different types of tachyarrhythmia [a mechanical equivalent to the RP interval in the postnatal electrocardiogram (ECG)]. **Doppler** analysis, gated to a region where both an inflow and outflow signal can be detected (e.g. the left ventricular outflow tract/mitral valve, the ascending aorta/superior vena cava, or a branch pulmonary artery/pulmonary vein), allows for calculation of the AV contraction time interval (AVCTI) (Figure 1.6). This uses the onset of the inflow 'A' wave (atrial systole) and the onset of ejection from the outflow tract to provide a mechanical surrogate for the PR interval, and is useful to discriminate between lower degrees of heart block. A full summary of these methods is shown in Table 1.3 [9–11].

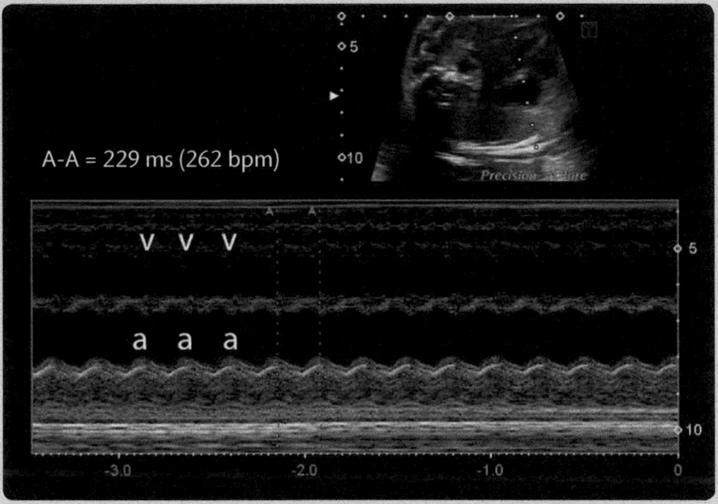

Figure 1.5 M-mode assessment showing 1:1 atrial (a) and ventricular (v) conduction at a fetal heart rate of 262 bpm in a fetus with long VA tachycardia.

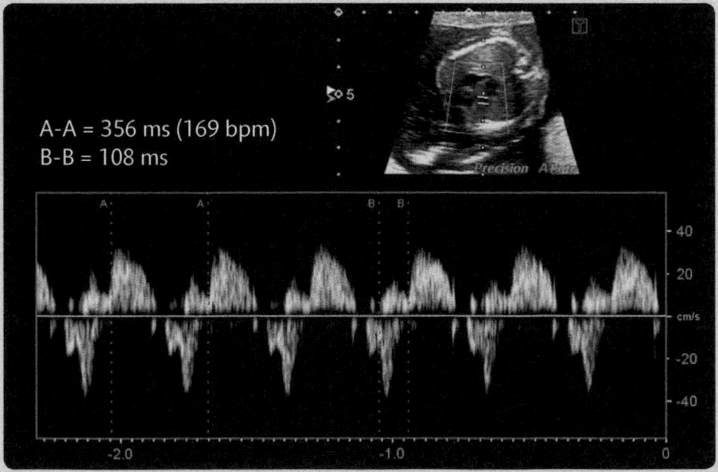

Figure 1.6 PW Doppler placed in the left ventricular outflow tract, showing mitral inflow (negative trace) with aortic outflow (positive trace). The AVCTI is calculated from the start of the mitral A-wave (atrial systole) to the onset of the aortic outflow (ventricle systole, i.e. B-B). The fetal heart rate has also been calculated (A-A).

Table 1.3 Differential diagnosis of fetal arrhythmia from echocardiographic assessment

A rate	A rhythm	V rate	AV relationship	Differential diagnosis
Low (<80 bpm)	Regular	**V = A**	1:1	Sinus bradycardia Junctional rhythm
Normal	Regular	**A > V**	Dissociated	Third-degree AV block
			2:1, 3:1, etc.	Type II second-degree AV block
		A > V	Progressive lengthening of AV interval/AVCTI	Type I second-degree AV block
		A = V	1:1 (prolonged AVCTI)	First-degree AV block
		A = V	1:1 (normal AVCTI)	**Normal sinus rhythm**
		V > A	Dissociated or 1:1	Ventricular tachycardia Junctional tachycardia
	Intermittent ectopics	**V = A**	1:1	Conducted atrial ectopics
		A > V	No V after ectopic A 2:1, 3:1, mixed	Non-conducted atrial ectopics
High (>200 bpm)	Regular	**V = A**	1:1 (short VA)	AV re-entrant SVT AV node re-entrant SVT
	Regular	**V = A**	1:1 (long VA)	Sinus tachycardia PJRT
	Varying	**V = A**	1:1 (long VA)	Ectopic atrial tachycardia
	Chaotic	**A > V**	Variable	AF Multifocal atrial tachycardia
Very high (>300 bpm)	Regular	**A > V**	2:1, 3:1 etc.	Atrial flutter

Learning point Future directions in assessment of fetal arrhythmias

Whilst direct electrocardiographic assessment of the fetal cardiac rhythm (fECG) has shown limited success due to variable recording quality, fetal magnetocardiography (fMCG) has shown greater promise. This relies on a process of signal-averaging to produce electrocardiographic complexes which display the electrical activity of the fetal heart in a manner akin to postnatal ECG. This could allow not only for more accurate diagnosis of fetal arrhythmias, but also for the possibility to detect fetuses with subclinical life-threatening electrophysiologic diseases such as intermittent ischaemia, QT prolongation, QRS conduction delay, or other features of cardiac ion channel dysfunction [8]. It is, however, currently only used in research settings, requiring both a magnetically sealed environment and a period of 1–2 hours to acquire.

Detailed assessment of the cardiac rhythm at 29 weeks showed 1:1 AV conduction between 240 and 260 bpm with a long VA interval. A diagnosis of fetal supraventricular tachycardia (SVT) was made, likely PJRT. Maternal flecainide was commenced at 100 mg three times daily (tds), and follow-up was arranged within a few days.

At 30 weeks, the fetus remained in tachycardia with a heart rate of 240 bpm. Maternal flecainide levels were taken, which were within the therapeutic range. At 31 weeks, the fetus remained in tachycardia and maternal sotalol was added at 80 mg tds. By 32 weeks, the tachycardia still persisted, with an increase in the size of the pleural effusions and ascites. Maternal ECG and liver function tests were requested, both of which were unchanged from their pre-treatment baseline. Both flecainide and sotalol were stopped and maternal amiodarone was started at 600 mg tds, in preparation for direct fetal therapy. The option of preterm delivery was considered; however, the risks of this approach were felt to outweigh ongoing attempts at fetal therapy. The family was counselled that the outcome may be poor.

In the days following maternal loading, the fetus finally achieved cardioversion to sinus rhythm. Direct fetal therapy was not required. Serial follow-up continued with regular maternal ECG and thyroid and liver function tests, and the dose of amiodarone was adjusted according to maternal serum levels. No recurrence of SVT was observed.

The baby was delivered by elective caesarean section at 38 weeks in good condition. All signs of fetal hydrops resolved completely over a period of 2–3 weeks following cardioversion. Postnatal ECG showed normal sinus rhythm. Atenolol was commenced, with a 24-hour tape arranged prior to discharge. Postnatal referrals were arranged for endocrinology (thyroid function) and neurological assessment (in view of the degree of fetal compromise). At a 6-month cardiology review, no postnatal tachycardias had been detected and atenolol was discontinued.

A final word from the expert

Fetal hydrops is a form of cardiovascular decompensation unique to fetal physiology, with a number of important primary cardiac causes. When associated with severe CHD, particularly heterotaxy syndrome, the outcome can be extremely poor, with limited options for treatment. Even in these circumstances, however, the fetal cardiologist can provide important prognostic information to guide both obstetric and parental decision-making. In the structurally normal heart, fetal arrhythmias—particularly SVTs—may be directly amenable to treatment with transplacental therapy. Treatment may not always be straightforward, as in this case. However, if cardioversion is successful, this can lead to restitution of normal cardiac function, resolution of fetal hydrops, and a good long-term prognosis.

References

1. Dempsey E, Homfray T, Simpson JM, et al. Fetal hydrops – a review and a clinical approach to identifying the cause. *Expert Opin. Orphan Drugs* 2020;8:51–66.
2. Bellini C, Hennekam RC. Non-immune hydrops fetalis: a short review of etiology and pathophysiology. *Am J Med Genet A* 2012;158A:597–605.
3. Coady AM, Bower S. *Twining's Textbook of Fetal Abnormalities*, 3rd edition. Philadelphia, PA: Churchill Livingstone, 2014.
4. Hofstaetter C, Hansmann M, Eik-Nes SH, et al. A cardiovascular profile score in the surveillance of fetal hydrops. *J Matern Fetal Neonatal Med* 2006;19:407–13.
5. Knilans TK. Cardiac abnormalities associated with hydrops fetalis. *Semin Perinatol* 1995;19:483–92.
6. Johnson P, Sharland G, Allan LD, et al. Umbilical venous pressure in nonimmune hydrops fetalis: correlation with cardiac size. *Am J Obstet Gynecol* 1992;167:1309–13.
7. McElhinney DB, Tworetzky W, Lock JE. Current status of fetal cardiac intervention. *Circulation* 2010;121:1256–63.
8. Strasburger JF, Cheulkar B, Wakai RT. Magnetocardiography for fetal arrhythmias. *Heart Rhythm* 2008;5:1073–6.
9. Simpson JM. Fetal arrhythmias. *Ultrasound Obstet Gynecol* 2006;27:599–606.

10. Srinivasan S, Strasburger J. Overview of fetal arrhythmias. *Curr Opin Pediatr* 2008;20:522–31.
11. Hunter LE, Simpson JM. Atrioventricular block during fetal life. *J Saudi Heart Assoc* 2015;27:164–78.
12. Ho A, Gordon P, Rosenthal E, et al. Isolated complete heart block in the fetus. *Am J Cardiol* 2015;116:142–7.

CASE

2 A case of severe aortic stenosis: ongoing challenges with management

Sok-Leng Kang

Expert commentary Robin Martin

Case history

A 3-day-old term girl, who was under observation on the postnatal ward due to maternal pyrexia during labour, was found to be mottled and tachypnoeic. The neonate was also lethargic and had lost interest in feeding. Pregnancy had been uneventful, and the baby was born in good condition following induction of labour at 38 weeks due to poor growth. Birthweight was 3.03 kg.

On examination, the vital signs were: heart rate 180 bpm; blood pressure 56/34 mmHg; respiratory rate 80 breaths/min, and oxygen saturation in the right leg 96% on room air. She had poor peripheral perfusion and reduced brachial and femoral pulses. Auscultation revealed a gallop rhythm, no click, and a systolic ejection murmur.

The chest X-ray (CXR) showed a slightly enlarged heart with evidence of upper lobe pulmonary venous diversion (Figure 2.1). The ECG showed sinus tachycardia, left ventricular hypertrophy, and inverted T waves in the left precordial leads. The initial blood gas revealed metabolic acidosis [pH 7.25, base excess (BE) –9, lactate 3.1], but other blood results were unremarkable, including a normal white cell count and C-reactive protein (CRP) level. Given the clinical context, the neonate was started on intravenous antibiotics for presumed sepsis and prostaglandin E2 prior to urgent transfer to a tertiary cardiac centre for further evaluation.

(a) (b)

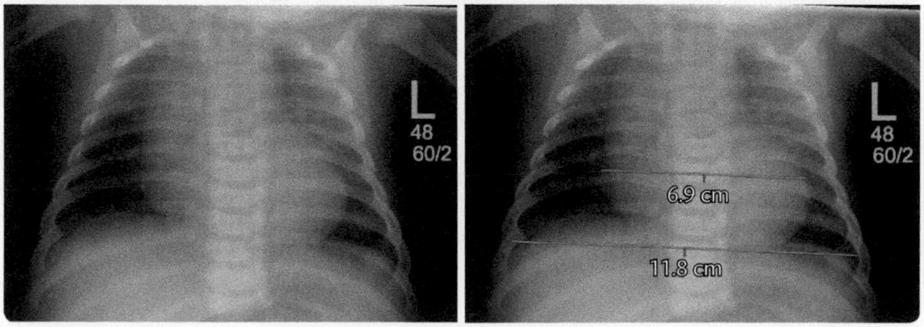

Figure 2.1 Chest X-rays showing mild enlargement of the cardiac silhouette with upper lobe pulmonary venous diversion, reflecting elevation of left atrial pressure.

Learning point Diagnosis of congenital heart disease

CHD encompasses a wide spectrum of lesions, ranging from minor defects that do not need treatment to potentially life-threatening critical defects. Many critical defects are duct-dependent, with consequent acute cardiovascular collapse as the duct constricts; hence, a prostaglandin infusion should be initiated as soon as the diagnosis is suspected. Alprostadil (prostaglandin E1) and dinoprostone (prostaglandin E2) can be given via continuous intravenous infusion at a dose of 5–20 ng/kg/min. The *British National Formulary* (BNF) recommends an initial infusion rate of 5 ng/kg/min, adjusted according to response in steps of 5 ng/kg/min. Higher initial doses are usually no more effective and have increased risks of adverse effects, including apnoea, hypotension, hypoglycaemia, and arrhythmias. The responsiveness of the ductus arteriosus to prostaglandin is primarily dependent on the postnatal age at the start of the infusion. Reduced response is usually suggestive of anatomical closure or that there is irreversible functional closure due to a lack of responsiveness of prostaglandin receptors by this age [1]. Duct-dependent systemic and pulmonary circulations (Table 2.1) are physiologically different from each other, and treatment strategy has to be tailored to the clinical status and underlying cardiac defects.

Table 2.1 Ductus-dependent congenital heart disease

Ductus-dependent systemic circulation/ left-sided obstructive lesions	Ductus-dependent pulmonary circulation/right-sided obstructive lesions
Hypoplastic left heart syndrome (HLHS)	Tetralogy of Fallot with pulmonary atresia (PA)
Critical or severe aortic stenosis (AS)	Pulmonary atresia ± intact ventricular septum (IVS)
Coarctation of the aorta	Critical pulmonary stenosis (PS)
Interrupted aortic arch	Tricuspid atresia with PS/PA
'Shone' complex variants	Severe Ebstein's anomaly Transposition of the great arteries with IVS*

* Duct patency is essential until adequate mixing at atrial level is secured.

The signs and symptoms of CHD in the neonate are variable, depending on the underlying cardiac abnormality. A heart murmur may be helpful in diagnosis, but the more common clinical manifestations are tachypnoea, signs of poor perfusion, and cyanosis. Initial evaluation should include a complete cardiovascular examination, including assessment of all peripheral pulses, pre- and post-ductal pulse oximetry, blood pressure, blood gas, CXR, and ECG.

Echocardiography remains the gold standard for diagnosing CHD; however, access may be limited outside of tertiary cardiology centres. In the UK, recent years have seen the development and expansion of local cardiology services provided by Paediatricians with Expertise in Cardiology (PEC) to meet with this increasing demand. The PEC, working in partnership with tertiary cardiology centres, are an integral part of the proposed 'network' models for the organization and provision of Congenital Heart Disease Services in the United Kingdom (UK), following the CHD Service Review in 2015.

Screening for CHD in the UK relies on a mid-trimester anomaly ultrasound scan in pregnancy and clinical examination of the cardiovascular system at birth and 6 weeks. However, antenatal detection rates vary between centres, ranging from 20% to 55% [2]. Similarly, postnatal examination fails to detect more than half of babies with CHD undiagnosed before birth and more than one-third by 6 weeks [3]. In light of the overall low detection rates with current screening, recent years have seen important developments in the work towards implementation of pulse oximetry as an adjunct to newborn examination screening. The accuracy and cost-effectiveness of pulse oximetry screening have been consistently replicated in many large studies in UK and abroad [4]. In 2015, pulse oximetry screening was piloted in 15 trusts across England to establish its feasibility at a national level and results are due to be published (https://www.gov.uk/government/publications/newborn-and-infant-physical-examination-screening-programme-updates).

On arrival at the tertiary cardiac centre, cross-sectional echocardiography showed usual atrial arrangement with concordant connections and severe aortic stenosis. The aortic valve was dysplastic and bicuspid with fusion of the right and non-coronary cusps (Figure 2.2). There was reduced excursion of the leaflets, with a narrow eccentric jet of flow across the aortic valve and mild dilatation of the ascending aorta. The peak velocity across the aortic valve was 4.3 m/s (estimated peak Doppler gradient 74 mmHg; mean gradient 42 mmHg) from the suprasternal view (Figure 2.3). There was only trivial aortic regurgitation (AR). The aortic valve diameter at the hinge points of the leaflets measured 7 mm (Z-score +0.53) in mid systole and the aortic arch was normal [5]. The left ventricle was well developed with mild hypertrophy. Systolic function was mild to moderately impaired. There was a small patent foramen ovale, with high-velocity left-to-right flow, and estimated left atrial pressure was 15 mmHg. The arterial duct was small with bidirectional flow.

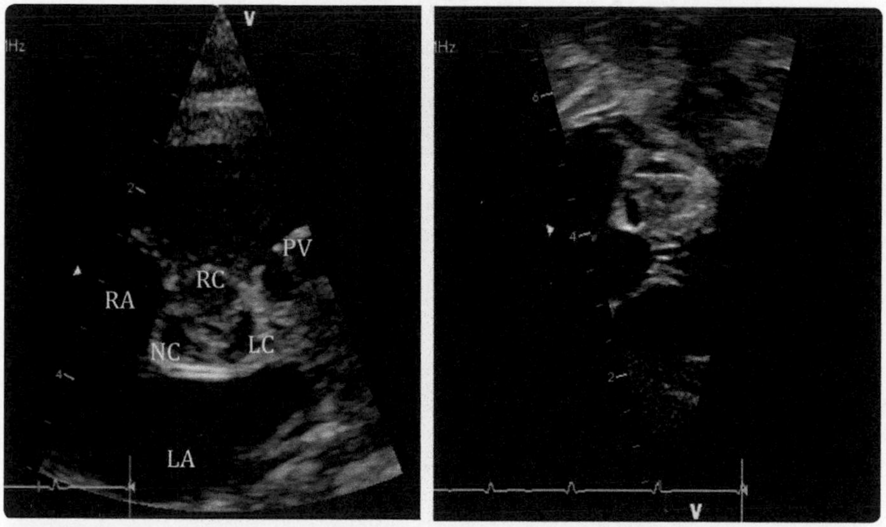

Figure 2.2 Left panel: parasternal short axis view showing severely dysplastic valve, initially thought to be functionally bicuspid with non-separation of right and non-coronary cusps but, at surgery, was found to be trileaflet and densely thickened by fibrous nodules. Right panel: in neonates, the subcostal right anterior oblique view (probe marker towards 2 o'clock) is another useful view to define valve morphology. LA, left atrium; LC, left coronary cusp; NC, non-coronary cusp; PV, pulmonary valve; RA, right atrium; RC, right coronary cusp.

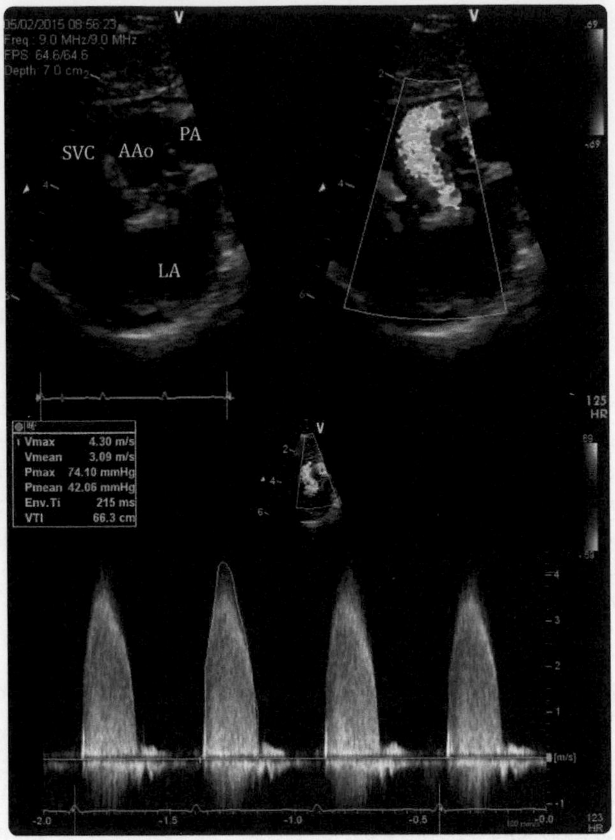

Figure 2.3 Suprasternal view: continuous-wave Doppler through the aortic valve. Taking a trace of the Doppler signal allows for calculation of the peak and mean gradients across the aortic valve. AAo, ascending aorta; PA, pulmonary artery; LA, left atrium; SVC, superior vena cava.

Learning point Management strategies in the neonate with critical left ventricular outflow tract obstruction (LVOTO)

Congenital obstruction of left heart structures represents a diverse spectrum of anatomy, ranging from isolated aortic valve and aortic arch stenosis to hypoplastic left heart complex with aortic and mitral atresia (Table 2.1) The consequent haemodynamic manifestation depends on the level and severity of the obstruction and other associated lesions such as a ventricular septal defect (VSD). These factors influence the treatment strategies, particularly the option of single versus biventricular repair, both of which carry significant risk of mortality and re-intervention. The initial decision is crucial because conversion to a single-ventricle route after a failed attempt of two-ventricle repair is associated with reduced survival [6].

The single-ventricle end of spectrum

This is characterized by a severely underdeveloped left ventricle, mitral valve, and aorta, resulting in obstruction to systemic cardiac output and the inability of the left heart to support the systemic circulation. These patients usually require staged surgical palliation towards univentricular repair or cardiac transplantation, although significantly limited by the supply of donor hearts in this age group [7].

The two-ventricle end of spectrum

Patients in this group have obstruction localized to the aortic valve or supra- or subvalvar area, with two well-developed ventricles, with or without a VSD. The therapeutic options include percutaneous aortic balloon valvuloplasty, surgical aortic valvotomy, neonatal Ross or Ross/Konno procedure, and mechanical aortic valve replacement, which will be discussed later.

The borderline left ventricle

These patients have borderline development of the left ventricle and mitral valve, and decision-making for either one- or two-ventricle repair is perhaps the most complex [6, 8–11]. Several studies have attempted to identify preoperative predictors of suitability for single-ventricle versus biventricular repair in neonates with critical LVOTO and borderline left ventricle. Favourable factors for successful biventricular repair include an angiographically derived 20 ml/m^2 threshold end-diastolic volume and predominant or total antegrade flow in the ascending aorta [10, 11]. Risk factors associated with high mortality following biventricular repair include mitral valve area <4.75 cm^2/m^2, long axis dimension of the left ventricle relative to that of the heart <0.8, diameter of the aortic root <3.5 cm/m^2, and left ventricular mass <35 g/m^2 [6].

Evidence base Single-ventricle pathway

A landmark study by the Congenital Heart Surgeons' Society (CHSS) reported a few independent factors favouring the single-ventricle pathway. This included younger age at entry, higher grade of endocardial fibroelastosis (EFE), lower Z-score of the aortic valve, larger ascending aortic diameter, absence of moderate or severe tricuspid regurgitation, and lower Z-score of the left ventricular length [8]. A few scoring systems have been developed retrospectively from these studies, including the Rhodes [6], CHSS [8], and Discriminant [12] score, to aid selection of the optimum management strategy in this challenging group.

Learning point Echocardiographic evaluation of aortic stenosis/LVOTO

A comprehensive echocardiographic examination is essential to determine the severity of aortic stenosis (AS) and adequacy of the left heart to sustain systemic circulation, including:

- Assessment of the aortic valve:
  - Morphology: tricuspid, bicuspid, or unicuspid and fusion of leaflets
  - Size: aortic valve diameter Z-score
  - Severity of AS: Doppler-derived transvalvular gradient and aortic valve area (AVA)
  - Associated lesions: subvalvar or supravalvar obstruction, AR
- Assessment of other left heart structures:
  - Mitral valve: mitral annulus Z-score and function
  - Left ventricle: left ventricle dimensions and wall thickness; presence of EFE
  - Aortic arch: size, presence of coarctation, retrograde flow in aortic arch or ascending aorta
- Presence of a patent arterial duct and direction of flow.

Clinical tip Differentiating subvalvar, valvar, or supravalvar AS

Use PW Doppler to assess the level of obstruction, whether subvalvar, valvar, or supravalvar. Dilatation of the ascending aorta may be associated with AS. In discreet fibromuscular subaortic stenosis (exceedingly rare in early infancy), fluttering of the aortic valve leaflets can be seen when the M-mode cursor is placed to intersect the aortic valve leaflets in the long axis view, due to the turbulent subaortic jet striking the aortic valve leaflets. AR is also commonly seen. Supravalvar AS is characterized by a discreet hourglass deformity or diffuse hypoplasia originating at the superior margin of the sinus of Valsalva and is often associated with stenosis of peripheral pulmonary arteries in patients with William's syndrome or familial supravalvar stenosis.

Learning point Measuring the severity of AS

Peak pressure gradient

- The aortic peak gradient can be calculated by the simplified Bernoulli equation, provided left ventricular systolic function is normal: **peak gradient (mmHg) = 4 × peak velocity^2**.
- The equation is less accurate if the peak velocity is <3 m/s, and the extended Bernoulli equation should be used: **peak gradient = 4 × (V_2^2 - V_1^2)** where V_2 = peak left ventricular outflow tract (LVOT) velocity and V_1 = velocity proximal to stenosis.

AVA/effective orifice area

- Useful when left ventricular function is impaired or hyperdynamic, but rarely used in the neonate.
- The continuity equation is based on the principle that the volume of blood that flows through the LVOT during 1 s must equal the volume of blood through the aortic valve during 1 s.
- The volume of blood crossing a particular structure = VTI × cross-sectional area (CSA).

The velocity time integral (VTI) is the product of velocity and time and takes into account the pulsatile nature of blood flow in the heart. CSA of the LVOT = π × (LVOT diameter/2)^2

- Hence, the volume of blood flow at the LVOT = LVOT VTI × LVOT CSA, which must equal the volume of blood flow at the aortic valve: AV = AV VTI × AV CSA
- Rearranged continuity equation: AVA = LVOT area × VTI_{LVOT}/VTI_{AV} (Figure 2.4).

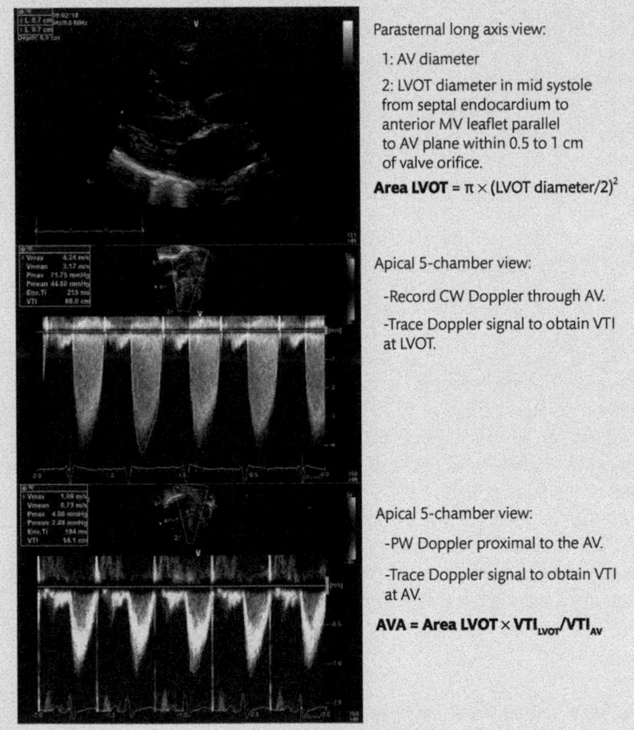
Parasternal long axis view:
1: AV diameter
2: LVOT diameter in mid systole from septal endocardium to anterior MV leaflet parallel to AV plane within 0.5 to 1 cm of valve orifice.
Area LVOT = π × (LVOT diameter/2)^2
Apical 5-chamber view:
-Record CW Doppler through AV.
-Trace Doppler signal to obtain VTI at LVOT.
Apical 5-chamber view:
-PW Doppler proximal to the AV.
-Trace Doppler signal to obtain VTI at AV.
AVA = Area LVOT × VTI_{LVOT}/VTI_{AV}

Figure 2.4 Calculating the aortic valve area (AVA). Two views and three measurements are needed for the continuity equation, as described. In the top panel, the AV diameter* (measurement 1) recorded at the hinge point of the leaflets in systole is important for selection of balloon size during valvuloplasty.

Clinical tip Interpreting the severity of aortic stenosis

- It is paramount to align the continuous-wave (CW) Doppler accurately with aortic outflow. The angle between the ultrasound beam and the blood flow jet of interest should be <20° to avoid underestimation. In neonates, the suprasternal or high right parasternal view usually allows optimal alignment to aortic outflow.
- The transaortic gradient is dependent on flow across the aortic valve. A low pressure gradient can be found in severe AS when transaortic flow is diminished, e.g. in severe left ventricular dysfunction or low cardiac output. Similarly, a high pressure gradient can be found in the absence of severe AS when transaortic flow is increased, e.g. when there is significant concomitant AR. In these situations, the AVA is a useful measurement.
- The direction of flow across the arterial duct provides additional information on the adequacy of the left ventricle to support systemic circulation. Persistent right-to-left flow across the patent ductus arteriosus with a borderline left ventricle suggests a right ventricle-dependent systemic circulation.
- Retrograde flow in the aortic arch is another indicator of inadequate forward flow across the aortic valve.

Learning point Difference between peak instantaneous gradient and peak-to-peak gradient

(See Figure 2.5.)

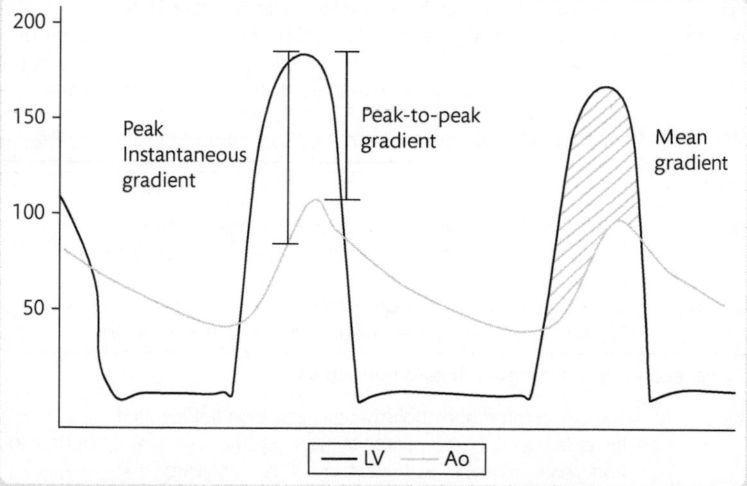

Figure 2.5 Simultaneous left ventricular (LV) and aortic (AO) pressure tracings.

- The peak gradient calculated from maximum Doppler velocity by echocardiography represents the maximum instantaneous pressure difference across the valve and corresponds with the **peak instantaneous gradient** measured at cardiac catheterization.
- The **peak-to-peak gradient** is the difference between the peak left ventricular and peak aortic pressures, which is a non-physiological measurement because the peak pressures occur at different points in time.
- The **mean gradient** is the integrated gradient between the left ventricular and the aortic pressures throughout the entire systolic ejection period. The mean gradient measured at cardiac catheterization correlates well with the mean gradient in children estimated by Doppler echocardiography and should be used to determine the severity of AS.

Clinical tip When to consider intervention or re-intervention in older children

- Evidence of reduced left ventricular function or left ventricular hypertrophy.
- Severe AS measured by Doppler echocardiography or cardiac catheterization, generally a mean gradient of >40 mmHg.
- Symptoms including syncope or evidence of low cardiac output.

Learning point Treatment options for aortic stenosis with otherwise normal left heart structures

There are four main options in the management of AS:

1. Balloon aortic valvuloplasty
2. Surgical aortic valvotomy or valve repair
3. Ross procedure [usually the result of a poor outcome from balloon valvuloplasty (BV)]
4. Aortic valve replacement (rare in infancy).

The choice of valve replacement will depend on patient size and clinical characteristics, taking into account the advantages and disadvantages of different prostheses [13–16] (Box 2.1).

Box 2.1 Advantages and disadvantages of different choices of aortic valve replacement

Mechanical prosthesis	
Advantages	Durability (freedom from reoperation 55–90% at 15 years)
Disadvantages	High risk of thromboembolism Lifelong anticoagulation required Patient–prosthesis mismatch with somatic growth Unavailable in sizes smaller than 16 mm due to inferior flow properties
Tissue prosthesis	
Advantages	Low risk of thromboembolism, anticoagulation not required
Disadvantages	Decreased durability (freedom from reoperation 35% at 10 years and 15% at 15 years) Structural valve degeneration inversely related to patient age and size Patient–prosthesis mismatch with somatic growth Unavailable in sizes smaller than 19 mm
Homografts	
Advantages	Low risk of thromboembolism, anticoagulation not required Suitable for children of all sizes, but availability varies due to limited donor pools
Disadvantages	Decreased durability (freedom for reoperation 15% at 15 years) Rapid structural valve degeneration and calcification in children
Aortic valve reconstruction using autologous pericardium	
Advantages	Low risk of thromboembolism, anticoagulation not required Increased durability, compared to tissue prosthesis or homografts (freedom from reoperation 68% at 10 years and 47% at 16 years)
Disadvantages	Not widely used in paediatric population, therefore evidence on outcome lacking Long-term valve degeneration

Learning point Balloon valvuloplasty versus surgical valvotomy

Since its first description in the 1980s, BV has gradually gained favour as first-line treatment for infants and children with valvar AS of sufficient severity to warrant intervention. The catheter-based technique is minimally invasive but has a higher risk for development of significant AR, as a tear is introduced into the aortic valve at its weakest point, either along the raphe (line of commissural fusion) or into the valve leaflet itself. Surgical valvotomy, on the other hand, allows direct inspection of the valve and precise incision of the fused commissures, but at a cost of a median sternotomy and cardiopulmonary bypass, with its attendant morbidities, in particular neurodevelopmental consequences.

There are no randomized clinical trials comparing BV with surgical valvotomy or alternative therapies. Most retrospective studies centred on the outcomes of either BV or surgical valvotomy, and only a few compared the outcomes of both [17, 18]. In 2001, McCrindle et al. reported equivalent results in terms of survival and rate of reoperation for either approaches, with a greater risk of important AR with BV and of residual stenosis with surgical valvotomy. More recently, Siddique et al. reported superior results with aortic valvotomy, based on a significantly higher rate of freedom from re-intervention, compared to BV. The authors made an important observation that surgical techniques have evolved in the past decade and described additional procedures which may lead to improved outcomes such as resection of nodular dysplasia, thinning of the leaflets, recreation of interleaflet triangles, and even creation of neo-commisures to avoid regurgitation [17].

There is emerging evidence that valve morphology plays an important role in outcomes after both surgical valvotomy and BV. Generally, bicuspid valves with a smaller valve opening area, greater fusion, and decreased leaflet mobility respond more favourably to BV [18]. Less stenotic valves have higher rates of leaflet tears, which, in turn, are associated with significant AR [19]. In unicuspid valves, surgical repair is superior to BV, with lower rates of AR and residual stenosis. Those with tricuspid valves may be better served with surgical valvotomy, as excellent long-term outcomes have been reported in infants in whom surgery results in trileaflet, rather than bileaflet, anatomy [20]. Hence, increased clarity and precision in imaging of the aortic valve may help optimize the therapeutic choice.

Clinical tip Imaging pre-balloon aortic valvuloplasty

Accurate measurement of the aortic valve diameter at the hinge point of the leaflets in the parasternal long axis view (Figure 2.2) in systole is essential for selection of the appropriate-sized balloon for valvuloplasty. Additionally, the degree of AR should be carefully documented. The optimal ratio of the balloon annulus diameter is 0.8–1.0, and larger diameter ratios are associated with a greater risk for AR [21].

The child underwent balloon aortic valvuloplasty via a transaxillary approach on day 4 of life. The aortic valve was dilated with a 6 mm × 2 cm Tyshak balloon, and complete de-waisting of the balloon was seen on inflation to nominal pressure. There was a good initial haemodynamic result with a 30-mmHg reduction in peak-to-peak systolic gradient from 75 mmHg pre-intervention. Post-procedure echocardiogram showed improved excursion of the aortic leaflets with a broader jet of aortic outflow. There was no worsening of AR and left ventricular contractility was better. In spite of good clinical progress in subsequent days, serial echocardiograms on the ward continued to demonstrate parameters indicating moderate to severe AS. As the child was asymptomatic and growing well, she was discharged at 2 weeks of age and the parents were counselled about the likelihood of early re-intervention.

Expert comment Choice of approach for aortic valvuloplasty

The use of the femoral arterial approach for balloon aortic valvuloplasty in neonates is known to be associated with a significant risk for femoral arterial complications, including obstruction. This may be associated with later symptoms of claudication and reduced growth of the affected leg. To reduce the risk for arterial complications, many centres have moved to alternative approaches via the axillary or carotid arteries, whilst others have used a transvenous approach [22–24].

Learning point Aortic regurgitation post-intervention

- Evidence suggests that AR post-balloon or surgical valvotomy is progressive and leads to earlier re-intervention. The severity of AR should be documented, using consistent echocardiographic criteria before and after any intervention (Table 2.2).

Table 2.2 Grading the severity of aortic regurgitation (European Society of Cardiology/American Heart Association guidelines based on adult data) [25, 26]

	Mild	Moderate		Severe
Aortic valve morphology	Normal/abnormal	Normal/abnormal		Abnormal/flail/large coaptation defect
Jet width—CFM	Small in central jets	Intermediate		Large in central jet, variable in eccentric jets
Jet density—CW signal	Incomplete/faint	Dense		Dense
Jet deceleration rate/PHT	>500	Intermediate		<200
Diastolic flow reversal in DAo-PW	Brief, early diastolic reversal	Intermediate		Prominent holodiastolic reversal
Jet width/LVOT width, %	<25	*25–45	46–64	≥65
EROA, mm^2	<10	10–19	20–29	≥30
Regurgitant volume, ml	<30	30–44	45–59	≥60

* Quantitative parameters can subclassify the moderate regurgitation group into mild to moderate and moderate to severe, as above.

CFM, colour flow mapping; CW, continuous-wave; DAo, descending aorta; EROA, effective regurgitant orifice area; LVOT, left ventricular outflow tract; PHT, pressure half-time.

Source data from Lancellotti P, Tribouilloy C, Hagendorff A, et al. European Association of Echocardiography recommendations for the assessment of valvular regurgitation. Part 1: aortic and pulmonary regurgitation (native valve disease). *Eur J Echocardiogr* 2010;11(3):223–44. and Zoghbi WA, Enriquez-Sarano M, Foster E, et al. Recommendations for evaluation of the severity of native valvular regurgitation with two-dimensional and Doppler echocardiography. *J Am Soc Echocardiogr* 2003;16(7):777–802.

- Pressure half-time is more useful as a marker of severity in acute regurgitation, since left ventricular compliance will not have adapted so quickly. With chronic AR, changes in left ventricular function and compliance slow down the equalization of transaortic pressures and lead to misleadingly longer pressure half-time values.
- Normal cardiac function by conventional measures is not necessarily reassuring in the context of AR. In early severe AR, the left ventricle adapts to the volume overload by development of eccentric hypertrophy; however, with time, progressive left ventricular dilatation leads to deterioration of left ventricular function. More advanced techniques, such as strain imaging, have shown abnormal left ventricular function, even in asymptomatic patients.

Expert comment

Assessment of the severity of AR should not be reliant on one measurement or method of assessment. It is important to look at a number of variables, including the clinical signs and symptoms, degree of left ventricular dilatation and function, regurgitant jet size and characteristics, pressure half-time of the regurgitant jet, and amount of retrograde diastolic flow at different points in the aorta.

The child was reviewed regularly in the cardiology clinic, and although she remained generally well, the estimated peak gradient across the aortic valve had risen to 100 mmHg (mean gradient of 50 mmHg). There was mild left ventricular hypertrophy, but preserved function. The ECG demonstrated left ventricular hypertrophy with a strain pattern. On further questioning, her mother reported that she has intermittent episodes of going pale and clammy when she is upset. She was taken back to the catheter laboratory at 7 weeks of age for a repeat balloon aortic valvuloplasty. The AV annulus measured 9 mm on the echocardiogram and 9.6 mm on the left ventricular angiogram. An 8 mm × 2 cm Tyshak II balloon was inflated across the aortic valve, and disappearance of the balloon waist was again noted. Unfortunately, there was no haemodynamic response and the peak-to-peak systolic gradient across the aortic valve remained at 50 mmHg.

The case was subsequently presented at the cardiac and surgical multidisciplinary meeting. The options of aortic valve replacement were discussed, and the consensus was for an attempted repair of the aortic valve or a Ross procedure if the valve was irreparable. The child underwent surgery at 12 weeks of age. The aortic valve was found to be trileaflet with no commissural fusion, but the cusps were densely thickened by fibrous nodules and were not amenable to conventional excision. The surgeon therefore proceeded to a Ross procedure, and the pulmonary outflow was reconstructed with a 14-mm Contegra© conduit. Post-operative echocardiogram demonstrated an excellent surgical result with unobstructed flow through both ventricular outflow tracts. Her immediate post-operative course was complicated by a low cardiac output state and bilateral pneumothoraces requiring drainage, but she made a steady recovery and was discharged home after 10 days.

Learning point The Ross procedure

The Ross procedure utilizes the native pulmonary valve as an autograft to replace the diseased aortic valve, following which the coronary arteries are re-implanted. The continuity of the right ventricular outflow tract (RVOT) is then reconstructed with a pulmonary homograft or conduit. In patients with significant hypoplasia of the aortic annulus or diffuse LVOTO, the Ross–Konno procedure is a modification of the Ross procedure, which involved a complete aortic root replacement with anterior aortoventriculoplasty [27, 28].

The Ross procedure is an attractive option in infants and children, as it can be applied to any age, has the potential for autograft growth with an excellent haemodynamic profile, and avoids the need for anticoagulation. In spite of the surgical complexity, Ross operation has been shown to be safe in experienced centres. The Ross registry and numerous series reported operative mortality of under 2.5%. Nonetheless, infants under 1 year of age continue to have a high mortality risk approaching 15–20%, as compared to a mortality risk approaching 1% in children above 1 year of age [14, 28–32]. Neonates and infants who require intervention at such an early age are represented by a critically ill group of patients with limited surgical options at presentation, and factors associated with poorer outcomes include emergency surgery, left ventricular dysfunction, concomitant arch or mitral valve surgery, and post-operative extracorporeal life support [14].

The autograft has been shown to have a superior haemodynamic profile, and the rate of autograft re-intervention is low. In children with CHD, freedom from autograft reoperation ranges between 75% and 95% at 10 years. The development of neo-aortic root dilatation, with or without subsequent AR, is a concern. Interestingly, older patients at the time of the Ross procedure show a faster increase in neo-aortic root dimensions and AR. It is suggested that the autograft might adapt better to the higher pressure in the systemic circulation at a younger age when smooth muscle cells are more prone to differentiation and hyperplasia, thus allowing for necessary remodelling in its wall to withstand the aortic pressure [14].

The need for repeated RVOT interventions due to somatic growth or conduit failure is a continuous problem post-Ross procedure. Freedom from conduit reoperation was 90–95% at 10 years and 75–85% at 15 years [14]. In experienced hands, RVOT conduit change has been associated with low morbidity and operative mortality. Recent advances in percutaneous pulmonary valve replacement have provided a less invasive solution to address this problem with encouraging results.

At 6 months of age, the child was found to be in significant right heart failure due to severe distal conduit obstruction and right pulmonary artery (RPA) stenosis during routine clinic. Her parents had noticed that she was more breathless in the preceding weeks but attributed this to a respiratory tract infection. She underwent urgent surgery to replace the right ventricle-to-pulmonary artery conduit with patch augmentation of the RPA; however, there was minimal recovery in cardiac function post-operatively. Although the right ventricle-to-pulmonary artery conduit was widely patent, the proximal RPA remained very small, with subtotal ostial occlusion demonstrated on computed tomography (CT). The RPA stenosis appeared to be amenable to balloon angioplasty and stenting, but the procedure was deemed extremely high risk, as rupture of a suture line would be almost certainly irretrievable, even with cardiopulmonary bypass on standby. The general consensus at the multidisciplinary meeting was to allow healing of the surgical repair for at least 6 weeks, provided she was clinically stable on inotropic support. She was also fully anticoagulated due to concerns of potential thrombosis. The child eventually underwent transcatheter RPA stent implantation at 8 months of age, with resultant improvement in right ventricular function, successful weaning of inotropes, and hospital discharge a week later. At her most recent clinic, she was making excellent progress. Echocardiogram showed normal right ventricular function, with mildly increased gradients in the branch pulmonary arteries, but the aortic valve was functioning well with no stenosis or regurgitation.

Expert comment

Pulmonary artery stent implantation or balloon angioplasty early after surgical reconstruction of the pulmonary artery can be associated with vessel or suture line rupture that can be catastrophic. Delayed treatment after 4–6 weeks is generally recommended if the clinical situation allows. Alternatively, early redo surgery can be considered as an alternative.

Stent implantation should be with a stent that has the potential for serial dilatation to adult size, if possible, and the development of bio-absorbable stents may be useful for the future.

Discussion

AS may present throughout life but is generally at the severe end of the spectrum if presenting in the early newborn period. In neonates with critical AS, therapeutic decisions will be focused firstly on the suitability of the left ventricle to sustain the systemic circulation. In those who are suitable for a biventricular repair, the choice between balloon valvuloplasty or surgical valvotomy in the neonatal period is not supported by strong evidence, but there is emerging literature on the role of valve morphology in the outcomes of both approaches [19]. Ultimately, the preferred treatment option is likely to depend on the local expertise and the clinical condition at presentation. For example, the patient with significantly impaired left ventricular function may be better served by initial balloon dilatation.

It is important to emphasize that both BV and surgical valvotomy are palliative interventions. Valve re-stenosis or regurgitation eventually necessitates aortic valve replacement in the majority of children. Selection of the optimal valve replacement requires careful consideration of the specific advantages and drawbacks of each valve type but is often limited by the availability of appropriate sizes for infants and small children. The Ross procedure is a compelling option because it can be performed at any age, with a potential for autograft growth and avoidance of anticoagulation; however, repeated interventions for pulmonary conduit management are commonly required for those having operations in infancy, as in our case. Recent innovative methods such as transcatheter aortic valve implantation (TAVI) have shown promising results in adult patients with prohibitive surgical risk [33, 34]. Rapid developments in valves and delivery systems may well see this become a technical possibility in the paediatric age group in the future.

A final word from the expert

Severe AS is often detected antenatally, but it is an abnormality that can progress during pregnancy and can therefore escape detection at the 20-week anomaly scan. It may not be detected at the postnatal examination when the arterial duct is still open and any murmur may be very quiet or absent. It can also progress rapidly in early infancy and, on rare occasions, may result in death before the heart defect has been diagnosed. It is therefore important that children in the first few months of life have prompt access to cardiological services, and echocardiography is key to an accurate diagnosis. The key clinical features to be aware of are weak arm and femoral pulses and usually an aortic ejection murmur. Referral pathways need to allow prompt assessment to reduce the risk of deterioration or death.

Decision-making in infants and children with severe AS continues to be challenging. An integral part of this process is comprehensive communication of the treatment options to parents and supporting parental involvement in treatment decisions. Parents should understand that congenital aortic valve stenosis is a lifelong disease. The child is committed to regular cardiac follow-up, the potential need for multiple re-interventions, and anticoagulation in those with mechanical valves with its attendant lifestyle modifications to minimize bleeding risks. The impact of aortic valve disease and treatment on the family is huge, and parental counselling and holistic support should not be overlooked.

References

1. Freed MD, Heymann MA, Lewis AB, et al. Prostaglandin E1 infants with ductus arteriosus-dependent congenital heart disease. *Circulation* 1981;64:899–905.
2. Sharland G. Fetal cardiac screening and variation in prenatal detection rates of congenital heart disease: why bother with screening at all? *Future Cardiol* 2012;8:189–202.
3. Knowles R, Griebsch I, Dezateux C, et al. Newborn screening for congenital heart defects: a systematic review and cost-effectiveness analysis. *Health Technol Assess* 2005;9:1–152, iii–iv.
4. Thangaratinam S, Brown K, Zamora J, et al. Pulse oximetry screening for critical congenital heart defects in asymptomatic newborn babies: a systematic review and meta-analysis. *Lancet* 2012;379:2459–64.
5. Pettersen MD, Du W, Skeens ME, et al. Regression equations for calculation of z scores of cardiac structures in a large cohort of healthy infants, children, and adolescents: an echocardiographic study. *J Am Soc Echocardiogr* 2008;21:922–34.
6. Rhodes LA, Colan SD, Perry SB, et al. Predictors of survival in neonates with critical aortic stenosis. *Circulation* 1991;84:2325–35.
7. Alsoufi B, Karamlou T, McCrindle BW, et al. Management options in neonates and infants with critical left ventricular outflow tract obstruction. *Eur J Cardiothorac Surg* 2007;31:1013–21.
8. Lofland GK, McCrindle BW, Williams WG, et al. Critical aortic stenosis in the neonate: a multi-institutional study of management, outcomes, and risk factors. Congenital Heart Surgeons Society. *J Thorac Cardiovasc Surg* 2001;121:10–27.
9. Schwartz ML, Gauvreau K, Geva T. Predictors of outcome of biventricular repair in infants with multiple left heart obstructive lesions. *Circulation* 2001;104:682–7.
10. Kovalchin JP, Brook MM, Rosenthal GL, et al. Echocardiographic hemodynamic and morphometric predictors of survival after two-ventricle repair in infants with critical aortic stenosis. *J Am Coll Cardiol* 1998;32:237–44.
11. Hammon JW, Jr., Lupinetti FM, Maples MD, et al. Predictors of operative mortality in critical valvular aortic stenosis presenting in infancy. *Ann Thorac Surg* 1988;45:537–40.
12. Colan SD, McElhinney DB, Crawford EC, et al. Validation and re-evaluation of a discriminant model predicting anatomic suitability for biventricular repair in neonates with aortic stenosis. *J Am Coll Cardiol* 2006;47:1858–65.
13. d'Udekem Y. Aortic valve surgery in children. *Heart* 2011;97:1182–9.

14. Alsoufi B. Aortic valve replacement in children: options and outcomes. *J Saudi Heart Assoc* 2014;26:33–41.
15. Al Halees Z, Al Shahid M, Al Sanei A, et al. Up to 16 years follow-up of aortic valve reconstruction with pericardium: a stentless readily available cheap valve? *Eur J Cardiothorac Surg* 2005;28:200–5; discussion 05.
16. Ozaki S, Kawase I, Yamashita H, et al. A total of 404 cases of aortic valve reconstruction with glutaraldehyde-treated autologous pericardium. *J Thorac Cardiovasc Surg* 2014;147:301–6.
17. Siddiqui J, Brizard CP, Galati JC, et al. Surgical valvotomy and repair for neonatal and infant congenital aortic stenosis achieves better results than interventional catheterization. *J Am Coll Cardiol* 2013;62:2134–40.
18. McCrindle BW, Blackstone EH, Williams WG, et al. Are outcomes of surgical versus transcatheter balloon valvotomy equivalent in neonatal critical aortic stenosis? *Circulation* 2001;104(Suppl 1):I152–8.
19. Petit CJ, Gao K, Goldstein BH, et al. Relation of aortic valve morphologic characteristics to aortic valve insufficiency and residual stenosis in children with congenital aortic stenosis undergoing balloon valvuloplasty. *Am J Cardiol* 2016;117:972.
20. Bhabra MS, Dhillon R, Bhudia S, et al. Surgical aortic valvotomy in infancy: impact of leaflet morphology on long-term outcomes. *Ann Thorac Surg* 2003;76:1412–16.
21. Feltes TF, Bacha E, Beekman RH, 3rd, et al. Indications for cardiac catheterization and intervention in pediatric cardiac disease: a scientific statement from the American Heart Association. *Circulation* 2011;123:2607–52.
22. Dua JS, Osborne NJ, Tometzki AJ, et al. Axillary artery approach for balloon valvoplasty in young infants with severe aortic valve stenosis: medium-term results. *Catheter Cardiovasc Interv* 2006;68:929–35.
23. Magee AG, Nykanen D, McCrindle BW, et al. Balloon dilation of severe aortic stenosis in the neonate: comparison of anterograde and retrograde catheter approaches. *J Am Coll Cardiol* 1997;30:1061–6.
24. Patel S, Saini AP, Nair A, et al. Transcarotid balloon valvuloplasty in neonates and small infants with critical aortic valve stenosis utilizing continuous transesophageal echocardiographic guidance: a 22 year single center experience from the cath lab to the bedside. *Catheter Cardiovasc Interv* 2015;86:821–7.
25. Lancellotti P, Tribouilloy C, Hagendorff A, et al. European Association of Echocardiography recommendations for the assessment of valvular regurgitation. Part 1: aortic and pulmonary regurgitation (native valve disease). *Eur J Echocardiogr* 2010;11:223–44.
26. Zoghbi WA, Enriquez-Sarano M, Foster E, et al. Recommendations for evaluation of the severity of native valvular regurgitation with two-dimensional and Doppler echocardiography. *J Am Soc Echocardiogr* 2003;16:777–802.
27. Hraska V, Photiadis J, Poruban R, et al. Ross–Konno operation in children. *Multimedia Man Cardiothorac Surg* 2008. doi: 10.1510/mmcts.2008.003160.
28. Hraska V, Krajci M, Haun C, et al. Ross and Ross–Konno procedure in children and adolescents: mid-term results. *Eur J Cardiothorac Surg* 2004;25:742–7.
29. Elder RW, Quaegebeur JM, Bacha EA, et al. Outcomes of the infant Ross procedure for congenital aortic stenosis followed into adolescence. *J Thorac Cardiovasc Surg* 2013;145:1504–11.
30. Abdelbasit MA, Alwi M, Kandavello G, et al. The new Occlutech(R) PDA occluder: initial human experience. *Catheter Cardiovasc Interv* 2015;86:94–9.
31. Piccardo A, Ghez O, Gariboldi V, et al. Ross and Ross–Konno procedures in infants, children and adolescents: a 13-year experience. *J Heart Valve Dis* 2009;18:76–82; discussion 83.

32. Takkenberg JJ, Klieverik LM, Schoof PH, et al. The Ross procedure: a systematic review and meta-analysis. *Circulation* 2009;119:222–8.
33. Leon MB, Smith CR, Mack M, et al. Transcatheter aortic-valve implantation for aortic stenosis in patients who cannot undergo surgery. *N Engl J Med* 2010;363:1597–607.
34. Smith CR, Leon MB, Mack MJ, et al. Transcatheter versus surgical aortic-valve replacement in high-risk patients. *N Engl J Med* 2011;364:2187–98.

CASE

3 Late presentation of the Fontan circulation

Hannah Bellsham-Revell and Aaron Bell

Expert commentary Catherine Head

Case history

A 16-year-old boy was reviewed by the congenital heart disease team after presenting to a routine follow-up clinic with oedema and a cough productive of casts on a background of palliated complex CHD.

He was born abroad with a birthweight of 1.75 kg and was diagnosed with usual atrial arrangement, double-inlet left ventricle, left-sided rudimentary right ventricle, and ventriculoarterial discordance. He proceeded to bidirectional Glenn at the age of 4 years and Fontan completion at the age of 5 (Figure 3.1a–c). Following Fontan completion, he developed protein-losing enteropathy (PLE) that was treated with dietary restriction and diuretics, with some improvement. At the age of 8, he moved to Europe, and unfortunately the following year, he had a further episode of PLE, initially treated by diet and albumin infusions and then with subcutaneous heparin, prednisolone, and intravenous diuretics. Heparin was discontinued the following year, and prednisolone weaned to alternate-day doses at the age of 13. He had a further relapse the following year and was restarted on subcutaneous heparin and prednisolone was increased. Heparin was eventually discontinued due to cutaneous problems and prednisolone weaned to alternate days.

Cardiac catheterization showed mean pulmonary artery pressures of 16–17 mmHg, a pulmonary capillary wedge pressure of 12 mmHg, and a calculated pulmonary vascular resistance (PVR) of 2 $WU.m^2$. Some small venovenous collaterals were noted, but the Fontan circuit appeared unobstructed. A further relapse followed at the age of 15 without major symptoms, but with a fall in albumin to 23. Prednisolone was changed to oral budesonide, and sildenafil was added to his management. Around this time, his family moved to the UK and he was first reviewed by the paediatric cardiology Rapid Access Team.

At this stage, he was asymptomatic, but with signs of long-term steroid use. Echocardiography and cardiac magnetic resonance (CMR) confirmed a normally functioning left ventricle with no significant volume loading, an unobstructed Fontan circuit, and two small venovenous collaterals. The anatomy also suggested the diagnosis of atrioventricular discordance with the aorta from the right ventricle and pulmonary atresia, a large-inlet VSD and a large subaortic outlet VSD. Over the next year, he had remained relatively well until this presentation. He denied alcohol, cigarette and drug use but described low mood with difficulty adapting to life in the UK and the limitation caused by his heart condition.

Clinical examination revealed a relatively short boy with evidence of long-term steroid use and delayed puberty. The jugular venous pressure was elevated, as

Expert comment Red flags when seeing a Fontan patient in clinic

- Significant change in exercise tolerance, compared with last review
- Obstruction to any part of the Fontan circuit [superior vena cava (SVC)/inferior vena cava (IVC)/branch pulmonary arteries)
- Palpitations or syncope
- Cough productive of casts or persistent cough with no clear upper respiratory tract infection (URTI)
- New diarrhoea or abdominal pain
- Oedema
- New cyanosis

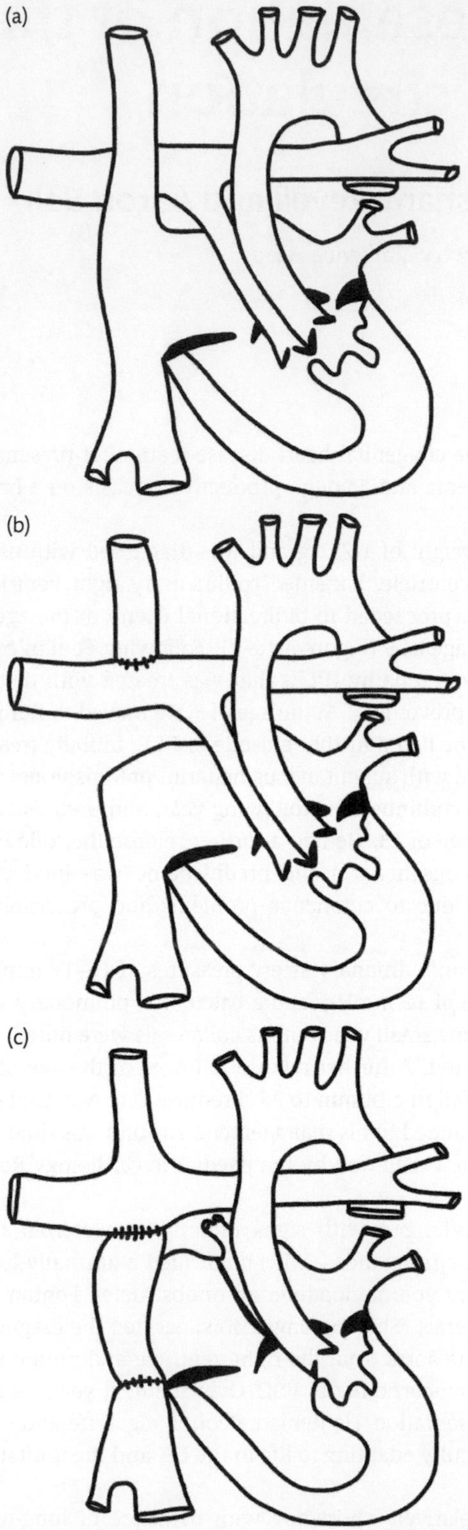

Figure 3.1 Schematic drawing of atrioventricular discordance with the aorta from the right ventricle, a ventricular septal defect, and pulmonary atresia: (a) unoperated; (b) after bidirectional Glenn; and (c) after Fontan completion.

expected, and there was a single second heart sound and no murmurs. There was some oedema of the lower limbs and a cough productive of white casts. The arterial oxygen saturations were in the low 80s, with a heart rate of 83 bpm (the ECG showed sinus rhythm) and a blood pressure of 109/65 mmHg. Echocardiography was challenging with poor transthoracic windows but showed a pulsatile abdominal aorta and a dilated IVC with little change with respiration and spontaneous venous contrast. There was phasic flow in the SVC, with significant spontaneous contrast and no fenestration. Systolic function appeared moderately impaired, with no significant atrioventricular valve regurgitation. There was no aortic obstruction.

Learning point Protein-losing enteropathy

- Definition and diagnosis:
  - Protein loss through the gut wall leading to hypoalbuminaemia with oedema, loose stool, and abdominal pain
  - Loss of coagulation factors (hypercoagulable) and immunoglobulins (immunocompromised)
- Aetiology:
  - Increased permeability to serum proteins?
  - Lymphatic obstruction/high lymphatic pressures caused by the Fontan circulation?
  - Elevated hepatocyte growth factor [1]?
- Investigations:
  - Low serum albumin level
  - Elevated alpha 1-antitrypsin levels in stool (not in normal diet and is not normally secreted; molecular weight is similar to albumin)
  - Nutritional and immune levels
  - Assessment of Fontan circuit and physiology
- Management:
  - Optimization of Fontan circuit and physiology, including use of targeted pulmonary vasodilator agents such as phosphodiesterase (PDE) inhibitors and endothelial receptor antagonists, even in the presence of 'normal' PVR
  - Vitamin supplementation
  - Oral steroids—budesonide has high first-pass metabolism in the liver, with low systemic and good enteric anti-inflammatory effects [2]
  - Heparin thought to stabilize capillary endothelium (NOT as an anticoagulant)
  - Care with coagulation (hypercoagulable) and infection (immunocompromised)
  - Fontan takedown or transplant

Learning point Brain natriuretic peptide (BNP)

- Secreted in response to atrial stretch
- Used widely in adult (and paediatric) heart failure populations
- Shown to be elevated in patients with complex heart disease, with correlation between New York Heart Association class and BNP level [3]
- May vary widely, depending on the lesion, but may be useful sequentially in individual patients

Following hospital admission, biochemical investigations showed a low albumin level of 19 g/l (normal range 40–52 g/l), consistent with a relapse of PLE, and mild elevation in hepatic enzymes, but preserved renal function. Faecal alpha 1-antitrypsin was elevated, and there was hypogammaglobulinaemia with low baseline levels of specific immunoglobulin G (IgG) to *Pneumococcus* and *Haemophilus* and panlymphopenia, consistent with gut loss.

The calcium and vitamin D levels were low, with an appropriately elevated parathyroid hormone level. Haemoglobin was 17.6 g/dl, with mildly low platelets, secondary to chronic hypoxia (urate was also elevated); iron, B12, folate, and selenium levels were low. BNP was not elevated, and thyroid function was normal, with elevated insulin-like growth factor and low testosterone and luteinizing hormone levels. Bone age studies demonstrated significant delay of over 3 years, and bone densitometry showed Z-scores of > −3.5 for the spine, the left hip, and the neck of femur.

Spirometry showed reduced lung function, and bronchoscopy demonstrated casts in the bronchial tree, with histology showing a mild inflammatory infiltrate. These did not dissolve *in vitro* with DNAse or tissue plasminogen activator. Chest CT showed scattered homogenous ground-glass appearances with lower zone predominance. There was moderately extensive smooth interlobular septal thickening at both bases, consistent with pulmonary oedema, but no bronchial thickening was noted. A confluence of venovenous collaterals were seen draining to the coronary sinus. A single-photon emission computed tomography (SPECT) scan showed symmetrical ventilation with normal right lung perfusion. Left lung perfusion was noted to be globally reduced (with no focal deficits), but this was felt to be the result of the contrast injection in the right arm.

A magnetic resonance imaging (MRI) cardiac catheter [4] under general anaesthesia, with cessation of sildenafil 24 hours beforehand, showed the known atrioventricular and ventriculoarterial discordance with an intact atrial septum, but with large-inlet and subaortic VSDs. The left ventricle was dominant with a hypoplastic anterior–superior right ventricle. The aorta arose anteriorly and leftward, and no main pulmonary artery was seen on this scan. The aortic valve was competent and unobstructed, with a single coronary artery origin noted. The arch was left-sided with a normal branching pattern. The Fontan circuit appeared unobstructed, with differential flow from the branch pulmonary arteries of 55% to the right and 45% to the left. No fenestration was seen. Two venovenous collaterals were noted, but no significant aortopulmonary collaterals were seen.

Learning point MRI volumetry

From a short axis (or transverse) cine stack, the end-diastolic and end-systolic endocardial contours are traced (Figure 3.2). Trabeculations can be either included or excluded, but consistency is important. Via summation of discs, the end-diastolic and end-systolic volumes, and therefore ejection fraction, are calculated.

End-diastolic volume: 64 ml/m^2
End-systolic volume: 41 ml/m^2
Stroke volume: 23 ml/m^2

$$\text{Ejection fraction} = (64 - 41)/64 = 0.36 = 36\%$$

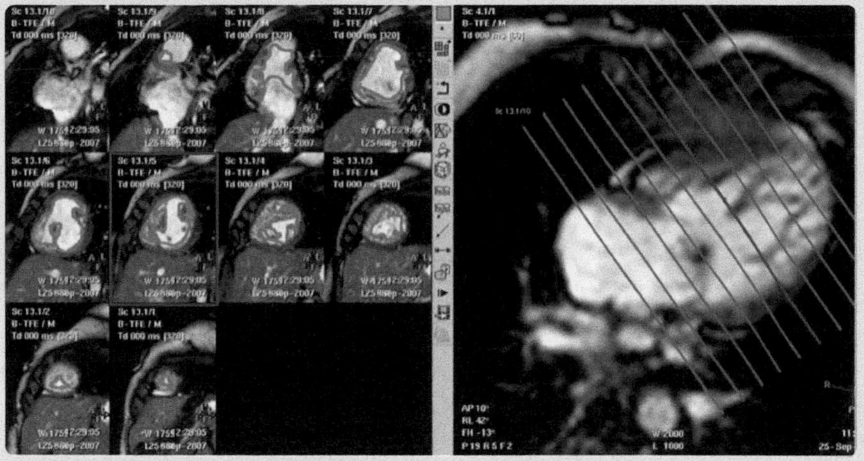

Figure 3.2 MRI volumetry.

Learning point MRI assessment of the Fontan circulation

(See Figure 3.3.)

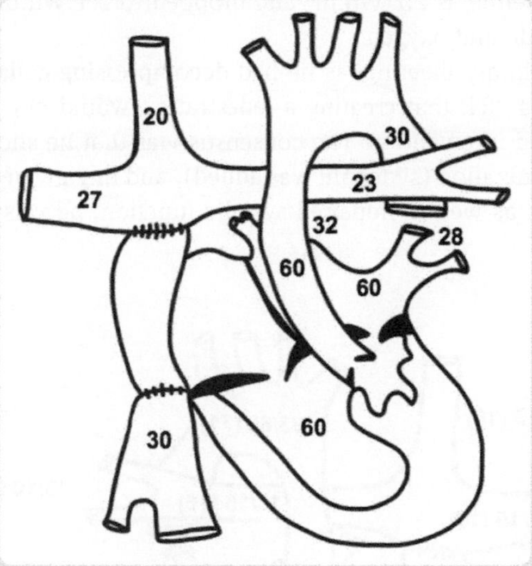

Figure 3.3 MRI assessment of the Fontan circulation.

- Anatomical examination
- Fontan circuit:
  - Obstructions to flow
  - Patent fenestration
  - Any thrombus?
- Functional:
  - Atrioventricular valve function with regurgitant fraction
  - Ventricular volumes and ejection fraction
  - Outflow tracts—obstruction, semi-lunar valve competence
  - Aortic arch—obstruction?

- Flow assessment in SVC, descending aorta (as surrogate for IVC), lateral tunnel above fenestration (if present), left and right pulmonary arteries, aorta, pulmonary artery (if present), atrioventricular valve inflow, left and right pulmonary veins
  - Assessment of differential pulmonary artery flow
  - Assessment of burden of aortopulmonary collaterals

$$\text{Systemic blood flow} = \text{SVC} + \text{IVC flow} = 20 + 30 = 50 \text{ ml}$$

$$\text{Collateral flow} = \text{aortic stroke volume} - \text{systemic blood flow} = 60 - 50 = 10 \text{ ml}$$

$$\text{Collateral flow} = \text{pulmonary venous return} - \text{pulmonary artery flow} = 60 - 50 = 10 \text{ ml}$$

$$\text{Pulmonary blood flow} = \text{SVC} + \text{IVC flow} + \text{collateral flow} = 20 + 30 + 10 = 60 \text{ ml}$$

There was moderately impaired ventricular function with an ejection fraction of 36%. Pressures were measured in the SVC, lateral tunnel, left and right pulmonary arteries, left pulmonary capillary wedge pressure, left atrium, and left ventricle at baseline (Figure 3.4). Baseline end-tidal carbon dioxide (CO_2) was 4.5 kPa, but this could not be maintained during the stress catheter due to increasingly difficult ventilation (from the plastic bronchitis). Dobutamine was infused at 20 mcg/kg/min, and then 100% oxygen with 20 ppm of inhaled nitric oxide added, with repeat measurements (Tables 3.1–3.4). Ejection fraction increased from 36% to 58% with dobutamine. PVR was calculated at baseline as 2.7 Wu.m^2 and dropped to 2.1 Wu.m^2 with addition of the inhaled nitric oxide and oxygen.

At the multidisciplinary meeting, as he had decompressing collaterals and was already cyanosed, it was felt that creating a fenestration would not help and no areas of the Fontan required intervention. The consensus was that he should continue with medical therapy optimization (sildenafil was added), and in view of two complications of Fontan physiology, as well as impaired systolic function, he was referred for transplant assessment.

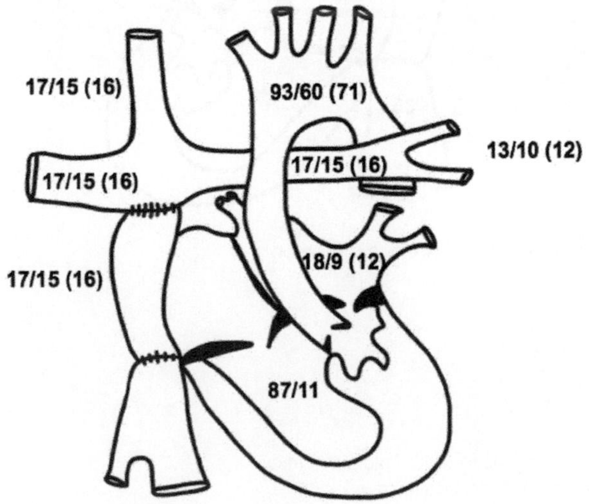

Figure 3.4 Baseline cardiac catheter pressures.

Table 3.1 Stress MRI cath condition 1 (baseline FiO_2 0.3, heart rate 84 bpm, end-tidal CO_2 4.5 kPa)

	Sys/dias/mean (mmHg)	PA wedge (mmHg)	Mean diff (mmHg)	Indexed flow (l/min/m²)	Resistance (Wu.m²)
RPA	17/15/16	12	4	0.79	5.07
LPA	17/15/16	12	4	0.66	6.08
Estimated collateral flow				0.20	
Systemic	93/60/71		71	1.64	43.18

Qp:Qs = 0.88
Total PVR = 2.76 Wu.m²

Table 3.2 Stress MRI cath condition 2 (dobutamine 10 mcg/kg/min, FiO_2 0.3, heart rate 150 bpm, end-tidal CO_2 6.1 kPa)

	Sys/dias/mean (mmHg)	PA wedge (mmHg)	Mean diff (mmHg)	Indexed flow (l/min/m²)	Resistance (Wu.m²)
RPA	19/17/18	11	7	1.32	5.32
LPA	19/17/18	11	7	1.18	5.91
Estimated collateral flow				0.30	
Systemic	133/80/108		108	2.76	39.10

Qp:Qs = 0.90
Total PVR = 2.80 Wu.m²

Table 3.3 Stress MRI cath condition 3 (dobutamine 20 mcg/kg/min, FiO_2 0.3, heart rate 167 bpm, end-tidal CO_2 6.5 kPa)

	Sys/dias/mean (mmHg)	PA wedge (mmHg)	Mean diff (mmHg)	Indexed flow (l/min/m²)	Resistance (Wu.m²)
RPA	20/17/19	12	7	1.32	5.32
LPA	20/17/19	12	7	1.25	5.60
Estimated collateral flow				0.50	
Systemic	112/68/90		90	3.03	29.75

Qp:Qs = 0.85
Total PVR = 2.73 Wu.m²

Table 3.4 Stress MRI cath condition 4 (dobutamine 20 mcg/kg/min, FiO_2 1.0, inhaled nitric oxide 20 ppm, heart rate 171 bpm, end-tidal CO_2 6.5 kPa)

	Sys/dias/mean (mmHg)	PA wedge (mmHg)	Mean diff (mmHg)	Indexed flow (l/min/m²)	Resistance (Wu.m²)
RPA	21/17/19	13	6	1.45	4.15
LPA	21/17/19	13	6	1.38	4.34
Estimated collateral flow				0.30	
Systemic	107/61/84		84	3.16	26.61

Qp:Qs = 0.90
Total PVR = 2.12 Wu.m²

Learning point Other Fontan complications

Arrhythmias after Fontan completion

- Scar-related re-entrant atrial tachycardias, i.e. atypical flutter. Often slower than typical flutter and can be mistaken for sinus rhythm
- Sinus node dysfunction (from repeated surgery in the region of the sinoatrial node)
- Accessory pathways and AV nodal re-entry tachycardias may also exist in Fontan patients [5]

Other non-cardiac issues after Fontan completion

- Constitutional and pubertal delay [6]
- Learning and attention difficulties [7]
- Effects of polycythaemia—thrombosis, gallstones
- Hepatic cirrhosis (with risk of progression to hepatocellular carcinoma) and portal hypertension from high venous pressures
- Psychiatric issues—depression, anxiety
- Reproductive issues—contraception, conception, and pregnancy

Following medical optimization (Box 3.1), he was referred to the immunology team who felt that intravenous immunoglobulins would be lost through the gut, and so he was continued on prophylactic antibiotics and received the Menitorix® and Prevnar 13® vaccines to boost his *Haemophilus* and pneumococcal immunity. He was also commenced on nutritional supplements and bisphosphonates.

His most recent review showed that he had improved, with no further recurrences of plastic bronchitis, and his PLE had remained well controlled (although with some relapses controlled with steroids). Apart from a recent admission with pyomyositis, he has not had any further admissions and has been taken off the active transplant list. Bosentan is currently being held in reserve.

Discussion

Increasing numbers of children are surviving single-ventricle palliation through to Fontan completion and are now entering older childhood and adolescence [8]. The Fontan circulation relies on passive blood flow to the lungs, meaning that low PVR and

Box 3.1 Medication review

- Prednisolone—to control PLE
- Amiloride—to control oedema secondary to PLE (potassium-sparing as also on furosemide)
- Furosemide—to control oedema secondary to PLE (has also previously had bumetanide and spironolactone—latter stopped due to painful gynaecomastia)
- Budesonide—to control PLE
- Sildenafil—to reduce PVR from normal to below normal to improve cardiac output
- Adcal-D3—to treat vitamin D deficiency
- Aspirin or warfarin—for anticoagulation in presence of a low-flow circuit
- Alendronic acid—for steroid-induced osteoporosis
- Fluticasone inhaler—for plastic bronchitis
- Dornase alfa nebulizer—to help reduce casts for plastic bronchitis
- Saline nebulizer—to help reduce casts for plastic bronchitis
- Erythromycin—as an anti-inflammatory
- Fortisip Extra—nutritional supplement

unobstructed pulmonary arteries are required [9]. Distortion of pulmonary arteries can occur through the various stages of palliation [10], and the pulmonary vascular bed is subject to different pressures over these operations. Additionally, the single ventricle or atrioventricular valves may fail over time [11].

Learning point Assessment of Fontan based on Choussat criteria

- Absence of pulmonary artery distortion and good-size pulmonary arteries:
  - Assessed by MRI, CT, or cardiac catheterization
  - Catheter or surgical interventions to augment pulmonary arteries (balloon, stent, plasty)
- Normal systemic and pulmonary venous return:
  - Assessed by MRI, CT, or cardiac catheterization
  - Catheter occlusion or surgical ligation of collateral vessels; ensure unobstructed pulmonary venous return
- Normal ventricular systolic function:
  - Assessed by echocardiography and MRI
  - Medical therapy, e.g. afterload reduction
  - No outflow tract/aorta/arch obstruction
- Competent atrioventricular valve:
  - Assessed by echocardiography
  - Surgical intervention may be possible; if not, then medical therapy with afterload reduction
- Mean pulmonary artery pressure <15 mmHg and pulmonary arteriolar resistance <4 WU.m^2:
  - Assessed by cardiac catheterization, either alone or in combination with MRI
  - Surgical or catheter augmentation of Fontan pathway narrowings
  - Drugs to reduce pulmonary arterial hypertension, e.g. sildenafil, bosentan
- Sinus rhythm:
  - Assessed by ECG, 24-hour tape, event recorders
  - Aggressive management of arrhythmias—medical, ablation
  - Pacemakers for slow nodal rhythm

Patients may present with non-specific symptoms, such as fatigue and reduced exercise tolerance, or with specific syndromes seen in the 'failing Fontan' such as PLE [12] and plastic bronchitis [13]. Assessment of the Fontan circulation [14] is challenging as baseline functional status is often reduced, compared to normal peers. Echocardiographic windows may be challenging in the older child, and many available and validated objective measurements are designed for the normal right or left ventricle and subjective assessment of the single ventricle is poor [15]. Cardiac MRI can be performed in older children without the use of anaesthetic and gives good information on the structure and systolic function [16], but not on diastolic performance. Invasive measurements of pressures, either combined with cardiac MRI or in the cardiac catheter lab (which allows subsequent interventions, if required), provide additional information [17]. Objective assessment of performance during exercise can be obtained using cardiopulmonary exercise testing [18], although a minimum height of around 135 cm is often required for the exercise bike and many of these children also have constitutional delay.

Assessment of other systems is also essential. In patients with PLE, there may be immunocompromise, as seen in this case. Chronic desaturation may coexist with anaemia and can cause gallstones. Progressive hepatic fibrosis resulting from chronic elevation in systemic venous pressure can also be seen in the Fontan patient [19], and routine surveillance for this in the adolescent and adult patient is recommended. Side effects of medication may be seen, particularly with long-term steroid use. There is also increasing evidence of significant pubertal and growth delay in children with palliated congenital heart disease, which is likely multi-factorial. Additionally, many children may have special educational needs (from significant developmental delay to more subtle autistic and attention disorders), as well as the psychological issues that occur with chronic illness, multiple hospitalizations, and reduced life expectancy [7].

Management is often medical with optimization of medication to prevent fluid overload, offload the ventricle, and lower PVR [20]. Inhaled medication may be required for plastic bronchitis, and steroids for PLE. Intervention to optimize the Fontan circuit such as the creation of a fenestration between the venous pathway and the functionally left atrium or occlusion of collaterals and stenting of the venous or pulmonary arterial and aortic pathways can improve patients' status. With severe compromise, takedown of the Fontan circulation or cardiac transplantation may be required, but there is a significant limitation of organ availability in the UK [21]. It is known, however, that patients with congenital heart disease have a poorer outcome than, for example, those with cardiomyopathies; side effects and compliance with anti-rejection drugs remain a significant issue.

Khairy et al. published in 2008 that in patients who had the Fontan procedure, freedom from death or heart transplantation was 93.7%, 89.9%, 87.3%, and 82.6% at 5, 10, 15, and 20 years, respectively [22]. In 2013, in the UK, there were 221 Fontan procedures performed, with four deaths within 30 days. This is an increase from 203 procedures in 2012 and 10 years previously in 2003 (182 procedures). These figures show that the number of patients surviving to Fontan completion is increasing, and survival after Fontan is meaning that there will be an ever increasing number reaching adulthood (http://www.nicor.org.uk).

A Paediatric Heart Network Multicentre study reviewed 546 children (aged 6–18 years) and showed a normal ejection fraction in 73%, with normal diastolic function in only 28%. Twenty percent of patients had a Child Health Questionnaire score lower than control subjects, and the mean percentage predicted peak oxygen consumption was 65% (and decreased with age). The most striking feature was that the ejection fraction Z-score and valvar regurgitation was more prevalent in the group with a single ventricle of right ventricular morphology [23].

Clinical tip Echocardiographic assessment of the Fontan circulation

- Anatomical examination
- Fontan circuit:
  - Obstructions to flow
  - Patent fenestration and mean fenestration gradient
  - Flow in SVC, IVC, and branch pulmonary arteries:
    - Spontaneous contrast?
    - Phasic flow with respiratory variation?
  - Any thrombus?
- Functional:
  - Unobstructed interatrial communication (where appropriate)
  - Atrioventricular valve function (with analysis of structure if regurgitant)
  - Ventricular systolic and diastolic performance
  - Outflow tracts—obstruction, semi-lunar valve competence
  - Aortic arch—obstruction?

Clinical tip Assessment of ventricular performance in the single ventricle

(See Figure 3.5.)

- Caution with assessment of systolic function in the presence of severe atrioventricular valve regurgitation
- Ensure all parameters measured are indexed as appropriate to body surface area, heart rate, and age [24]
- Systole:
  - Subjective—good or mildly, moderately, or severely impaired
  - Fractional area change
  - Tricuspid or mitral annular plane systolic excursion
  - Ventricular change in pressure by change in time
  - Tissue Doppler
  - Speckle tracking
  - Three-dimensional echocardiography
- Diastole:
  - Pulmonary vein Doppler
  - Atrioventricular valve inflow with tissue Doppler

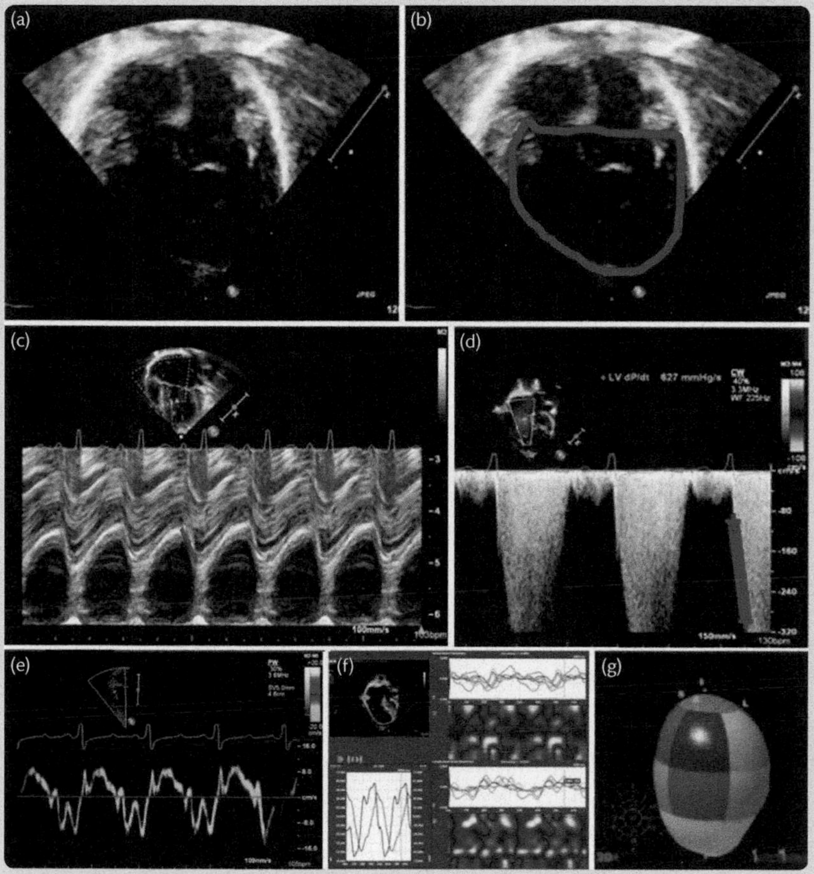

Figure 3.5 Assessment of ventricular performance in the single ventricle.
a) 2D assessment; b) Fractional area change; c) Annular planar excursion; d) dP/dT (change in pressure by time); e) Tissue Doppler; f) Speckle tracking; g) 3D assessment.

A final word from the expert

A true multidisciplinary approach is required in the evaluation and management of older patients after Fontan palliation. There are not only abnormalities of ventricular function and venous and arterial pathways, but also major complications involving the liver, bowel, kidneys, and lungs. Clinical assessment with basic and advanced investigations to assess the aspects of Fontan physiology (based on those described by Choussat) are essential, as well as reviewing all other systems. The management is mainly medical but may include catheter intervention, surgery, or cardiac transplantation in suitable patients.

References

1. Kim GB, Kwon BS, Bae EJ, Noh CI, Choi JY. Significance of circulating hepatocyte growth factor in protein-losing enteropathy after Fontan operation. *Pediatr Cardiol* 2011;32:917–23.
2. Thacker D, Patel A, Dodds K, Goldberg DJ, Semeao E, Rychik J. Use of oral budesonide in the management of protein-losing enteropathy after the Fontan operation. *Ann Thorac Surg* 2010;89:837–42.

3. Eindhoven JA, van den Bosch AE, Jansen PR, Boersma E, Roos-Hesselink JW. The usefulness of brain natriuretic peptide in complex congenital heart disease. *J Am Coll Cardiol* 2012;60:2140–9.
4. Pushparajah K, Wong JK, Bellsham-Revell HR, et al. Magnetic resonance imaging catheter stress haemodynamics post-Fontan in hypoplastic left heart syndrome. *Eur Heart J Cardiovasc Imaging* 2016;17:644–51.
5. Stephenson EA, Lu M, Berul CI, et al. Arrhythmias in a contemporary Fontan cohort. *J Am Coll Cardiol* 2010;56:890–6.
6. Avitabile CM, Leonard MB, Zemel BS, et al. Lean mass deficits, vitamin D status and exercise capacity in children and young adults after Fontan palliation. *Heart* 2014;100:1702–7.
7. Davidson J, Gringras P, Fairhurst C, Simpson J, Witter T. Physical and neurodevelopmental outcomes in children with single-ventricle circulation. *Arch Dis Child* 2015;100:449–53.
8. Coats L, O'Connor S, Wren C, O'Sullivan J. The single-ventricle patient population: a current and future concern a population-based study in the North of England. *Heart* 2014;100:1348–53.
9. Gewillig M. The Fontan circulation. *Heart* 2005;91:839–46.
10. Honjo O, Benson LN, Mewhort HE, et al. Clinical outcomes, program evolution, and pulmonary artery growth in single ventricle palliation using hybrid and Norwood palliative strategies. *Ann Thorac Surg* 2009;87:1885–93.
11. Duncan BW, Mee RBB. Management of the failing systemic right ventricle. *Semin Thorac Cardiovasc Surg* 2005;17:160–9.
12. Rychik J. Protein-losing enteropathy after Fontan operation. *Congenit Heart Dis* 2007;2:288–300.
13. Goldberg DJ, Dodds K, Rychik J. Rare problems associated with the Fontan circulation. *Cardiol Young* 2010;20 Suppl 3:113–19.
14. Kutty S, Rathod RH, Danford DA, Celermajer DS. Role of imaging in the evaluation of single ventricle with the Fontan palliation. *Heart* 2016;102:174–83.
15. Bellsham-Revell HR, Simpson JM, Miller OI, Bell AJ. Subjective evaluation of right ventricular systolic function in hypoplastic left heart syndrome: how accurate is it? *J Am Soc Echocardiogr* 2013;26:52–6.
16. Valsangiacomo Buechel ER, Grosse-Wortmann L, Fratz S, et al. Indications for cardiovascular magnetic resonance in children with congenital and acquired heart disease: an expert consensus paper of the Imaging Working Group of the AEPC and the Cardiovascular Magnetic Resonance Section of the EACVI. *Eur Heart J Cardiovasc Imaging* 2015;16:281–97.
17. Razavi R, Hill DL, Keevil SF, et al. Cardiac catheterisation guided by MRI in children and adults with congenital heart disease. *Lancet* 2003;362:1877–82.
18. Giardini A, Specchia S, Gargiulo G, Sangiorgi D, Picchio FM. Accuracy of oxygen uptake efficiency slope in adults with congenital heart disease. *Int J Cardiol* 2009;133:74–9.
19. Kiesewetter CH, Sheron N, Vettukattill JJ, et al. Hepatic changes in the failing Fontan circulation. *Heart* 2007;93:579–84.
20. Ghanayem NS, Berger S, Tweddell JS. Medical management of the failing Fontan. *Pediatr Cardiol* 2007;28:465–71.
21. Banner NR, Bonser RS, Clark AL, et al. UK guidelines for referral and assessment of adults for heart transplantation. *Heart* 2011;97:1520–7.
22. Khairy P, Fernandes SM, Mayer JE, et al. Long-term survival, modes of death, and predictors of mortality in patients with Fontan surgery. *Circulation* 2008;117:85–92.
23. Anderson PAW, Sleeper LA, Mahony L, et al. Contemporary outcomes after the Fontan procedure. *J Am Coll Cardiol* 2008;52:85–98.
24. Chubb H, Simpson JM. The use of Z-scores in paediatric cardiology. *Ann Pediatr Cardiol* 2012;5:179–84.

CASE

4

Right ventricular outflow tract stenting in the management of tetralogy of Fallot with pulmonary artery hypoplasia and major aortopulmonary collaterals

Gemma Penford

Expert commentary Oliver Stumper

Case history

A 5-day-old male born at 36 weeks' gestation and weighing 2.7 kg presented with episodes of profound cyanosis and a loud systolic murmur. Resting oxygen saturations were 78%, dropping intermittently to 40–50%, with associated inconsolable crying. The 12-lead electrocardiogram (ECG) showed right ventricular hypertrophy and right axis deviation (Figure 4.1). The chest X-ray showed no evidence of a respiratory cause for desaturation; however, the lung fields appeared oligaemic. The cardiac silhouette showed 'lifting' of the apex and a concave appearance in the area of the pulmonary artery (the so-called 'boot-shaped heart') (Figure 4.1).

(a)

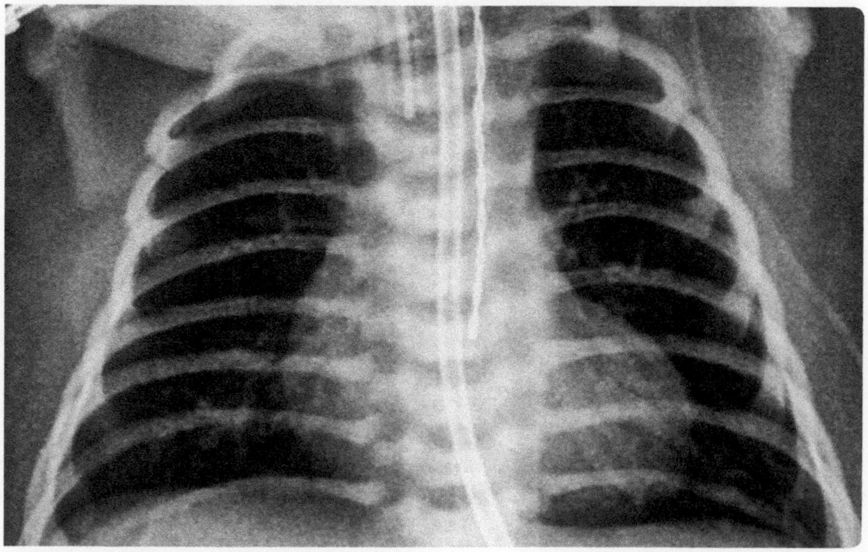

Figure 4.1 (a) Chest X-ray

(b)

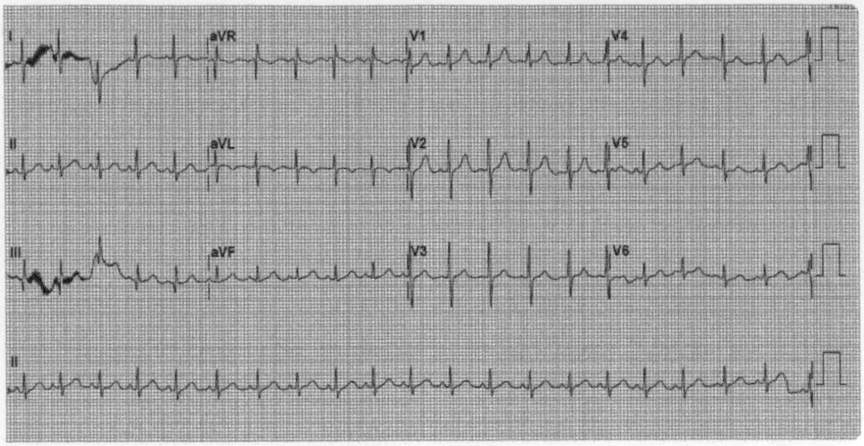

Figure 4.1 (b) electrocardiogram at presentation.

Echocardiogram confirmed the diagnosis of tetralogy of Fallot (Figure 4.2), with severe right ventricular outflow tract obstruction (RVOTO) and hypoplastic pulmonary arteries, plus additional sources of pulmonary blood flow that could not be delineated on echocardiography. Oral morphine and 1 mg/kg of propranolol were administered. A bolus of 10 ml/kg of 0.9% saline was administered after intravenous access was secured. The episodes of desaturation reduced in intensity but did not resolve.

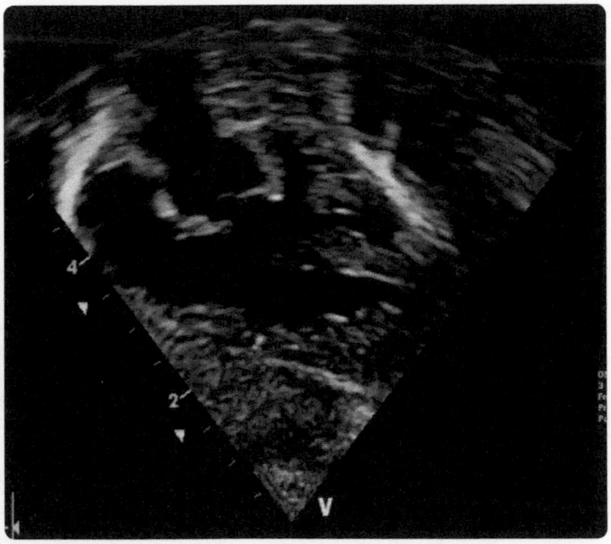

Figure 4.2 Subcostal oblique view of the RVOT in tetralogy of Fallot.

Learning point

The essence of tetralogy of Fallot is antero-cephalad deviation of the outlet septum. This results in RVOTO, a ventricular septal defect (VSD), aortic override, and right ventricular hypertrophy [1] (Figure 4.3).

From this fundamental feature emerges a wide spectrum of disease. The VSD in Fallot's tetralogy is typically large and perimembranous. However, the degree of aortic override can vary. 'Fallot's with double-outlet right ventricle' may be used if there is >50% override of the aorta into the right ventricle (assessed in the long axis view). Aorto-mitral fibrous continuity may or may not be preserved in this setting. Pulmonary atresia (PA) with VSD and major aortopulmonary collateral arteries (MAPCAs) with diminutive, or even absent, central pulmonary arteries are widely considered to be the extreme end of this disease spectrum. (PA with an intact ventricular septum is a morphologically and clinically separate entity and will not be discussed.)

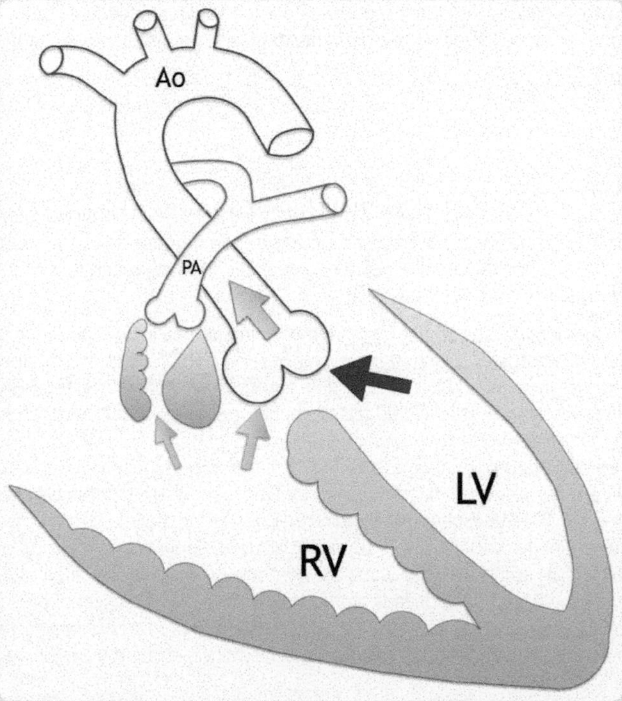

Figure 4.3 The key features of Fallot's tetralogy. Ao, aorta; LV, left ventricle; PA, pulmonary artery; RV, right ventricle.

Interrogation for associated lesions, such as additional VSDs, juxta-ductal branch pulmonary artery coarctation, or aberrant coronary branching, forms part of diagnostic echocardiography [2]. For the majority of Fallot's tetralogy patients, this provides adequate information for repair. Additional cross-sectional imaging may be required if there is concern about coronary artery anatomy, particularly the left anterior descending from the right coronary artery crossing the right ventricular outflow tract (RVOT) at the site of the incision for a transannular patch. Such an anomaly may require insertion of a right ventricular-to-pulmonary artery conduit. MAPCAs may be identified by echocardiography but cannot be reliably delineated, due to tortuosity and intimacy with the airways and lung parenchyma. Computed tomography (CT) or invasive angiography is required to delineate these vessels and the lung segments they supply.

Medical management of cyanotic 'spells' in Fallot's tetralogy is based on efforts to increase left-to-right shunting, primarily by raising systemic vascular resistance, increasing right ventricular diastolic filling, and reducing pulmonary vascular resistance. Maintaining good hydration, treating pyrexia (which can lower systemic vascular resistance), and excluding respiratory causes for desaturation are the mainstays in the initial care of the 'spelling' Fallot's tetralogy patient.

Expert comment

The physiology underlying cyanotic 'spells' remains disputed. Spasm of the muscular infundibulum leading to reduced pulmonary blood flow and worsened right-to-left shunting via the VSD remains a broadly supported theory, though lability in systemic and pulmonary vascular resistance is a likely contributor [3]. Reports of clinically apparent 'spells' in Fallot's tetralogy patients with a doubly committed VSD (where aortic and pulmonary valves are in fibrous continuity) cast doubt on the 'infundibular spasm' theory, as the outlet septum is absent, though a ridge-like fibrous remnant of the outlet septum may be identified between the aortic and pulmonary valves at the time of repair [4].

Clinical tip

An important clinical feature to help discern a true Fallot's tetralogy 'spell' from respiratory causes of cyanosis is the disappearance of the crescendo–decrescendo murmur, as flow across the RVOT diminishes (the VSD of Fallot's tetralogy is typically large and unrestrictive, and thus does not produce an audible murmur) [4].

In the initial management of the spelling Fallot's tetralogy infant, one should place the patient in the 'knee-to-chest' position, with a primary caregiver providing comfort and reassurance. Buccal sucrose may be of use in calming the infant. Folding and compressing limb vessels increases peripheral systemic vascular resistance; this acts to counter resistance to pulmonary flow caused by RVOTO and results in reducing the right-to-left shunting. It also compresses the veins, aiding venous return (pre-load/diastolic filling) to the right ventricle. Morphine may reduce distress, and thus pulmonary vascular resistance, heart rate, and metabolic requirements. Intravenous access should be secured quickly and expertly, to avoid further distressing the infant and worsening the episode. A low threshold for seeking senior support is advised. Cannulation is a good opportunity to obtain venous blood gas and laboratory blood samples, though this may be deferred if the patient is decompensating as the attempt proceeds! Some would argue that the effect of prostaglandin in reducing pulmonary vascular resistance may reduce the intensity of Fallot's tetralogy spells. However, it will also have a corresponding effect on the systemic resistance, so apart from the neonatal period, it is rarely used.

Diastolic right ventricular filling may be augmented by administering saline boluses and inducing a degree of bradycardia with (typically) oral beta-blockade. Supplemental oxygen (largely to reduce pulmonary vascular resistance) or adrenaline (to increase systemic vascular resistance) is often recommended in textbooks but rarely produce impressive improvements. If the child is unstable or shows an increased lactate concentration on peripheral blood gas sampling, the decision may be made to place a nasogastric tube to empty the stomach, in preparation for invasive ventilation or emergency intervention. However, when trying to minimize distress, inducing hunger might not be of assistance!

Cardiac catheterization (Figure 4.4) showed that the branch pulmonary arteries were hypoplastic but distributed to all lung segments. Each branch pulmonary artery measured 2.3 mm [Z score −5]. Additionally, there were multiple MAPCAs. A discussion was held between the cardiac surgeons and interventionists regarding the best course of action to palliate pulmonary blood flow. The decision was to stent the RVOT. A 4 mm × 16 mm coronary stent was deployed via a 4-French hydrophilic long sheath. Systemic oxygen saturations rose from 70% to 96%. The patient was successfully extubated overnight after the procedure, requiring one dose of furosemide due to tachypnoea. Four days after the procedure, the baby was discharged on regular antiplatelet therapy, having established feeding.

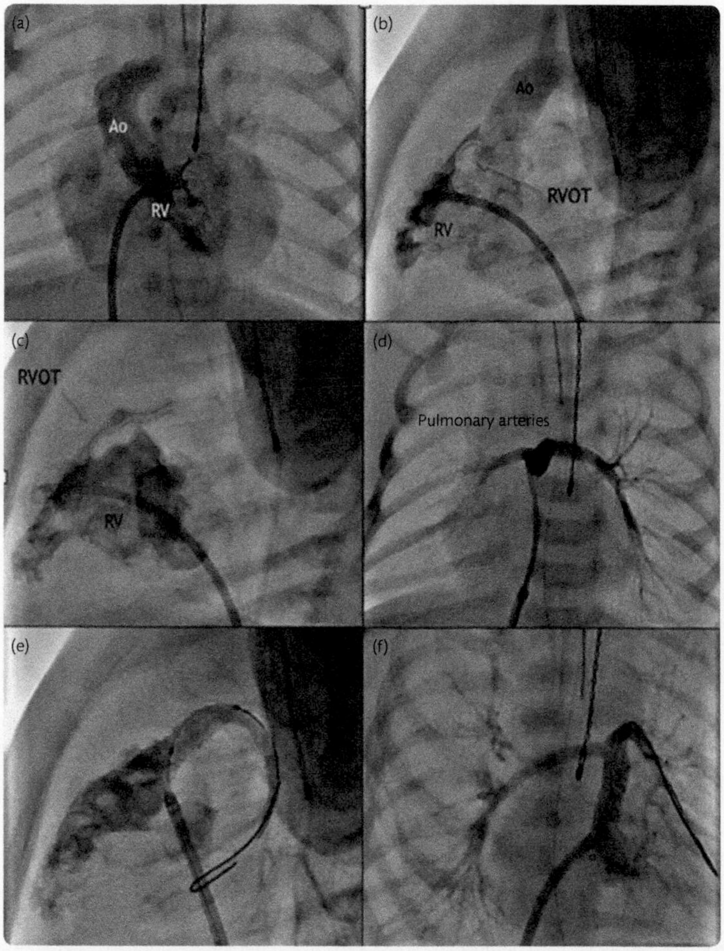

Figure 4.4 (a) Anteroposterior right ventricle angiogram; note filling of the aorta. (b) and (c) RVOT angiograms in lateral projection. (d) Main pulmonary artery angiogram in anteroposterior projection; severely hypoplastic pulmonary arteries. (e) and (f) RVOT angiograms after RVOT stent placement. Ao, aorta; RV, right ventricle.

Learning point

Tetralogy of Fallot was one of the first congenital cardiac lesions to be successfully surgically managed with the classical Blalock–Taussig (BT) shunt in 1945 [5]. This was modified with the use of small Gore-Tex® grafts, to provide shunting between the innominate artery and the corresponding pulmonary artery. It became the mainstay of palliation for decades (Figure 4.5).

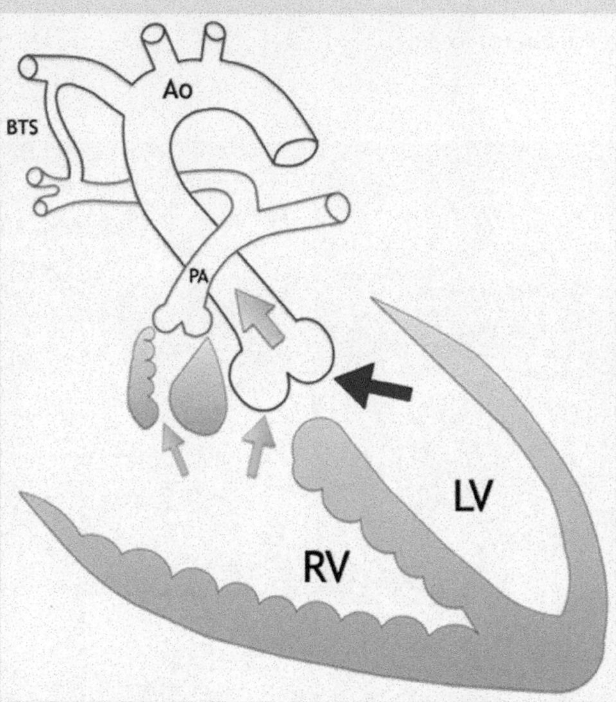

Figure 4.5 Fallot's tetralogy with a Blalock–Taussig shunt between the innominate artery and the right pulmonary artery. Ao, aorta; BTS, Blalock–Taussig shunt; LV, left ventricle; PA, pulmonary artery; RV, right ventricle.

BT shunts, however, come with a set of problems. The position between the great arteries means that left-to-right shunting occurs during both systole **and diastole**. The resultant diastolic 'run-off' into the pulmonary arteries may 'steal' flow from the coronary arteries (which are perfused exclusively during diastole). This may lead to early post-operative haemodynamic instability and left ventricular (LV) dysfunction. Coronary perfusion may be further worsened by raised LV end-diastolic pressures, due to an increase in LV pre-load.

BT shunts are also prone to neo-intimal proliferation. They can also cause stenosis of the anastomosed pulmonary artery in around 21% [6] and may become acutely blocked by a thrombus [6, 7]. Reported rates of thrombosis increase with diminishing shunt size [8]. A multi-centre study of 304 tetralogy of Fallot or PA patients palliated with 3.0- to 3.5-mm BT shunts reported a shunt thrombosis rate of 8.9% over the first year post-implantation [9].

Cardiac catheterization of Fallot's tetralogy patients in the modern era is now reserved for those with complexities, such as MAPCAs, or those requiring palliation for cyanosis. In the recent era, RVOT stenting has emerged as a viable alternative to BT shunt in the palliation of tetralogy of Fallot [10–13]. The primary advantages of RVOT stenting comprise a more physiological circulation, as desaturated blood is directed to the pulmonary arteries, and no diastolic 'run-off' to impact on coronary perfusion. Additionally, the pulsatile nature of the flow plus absence of distortion at the site of implantation, compared to a BT shunt, appear to drive superior pulmonary artery growth prior to repair [14].

Expert comment

In a 10-year retrospective review comparing BT shunt to RVOT stent in the palliation of cyanotic Fallot's tetralogy patients, post-procedural admission rate to the paediatric intensive care unit (PICU) was lower in the RVOT stent group (22% versus 100%; $p < 0.001$). There were six BT shunt thrombotic occlusions (15%) versus no complete occlusion of RVOT stents ($p < 0.001$). Thirty-day mortality in the RVOT stent group was 1.7%, compared to 4.9% in the modified BT shunt group ($p = 0.565$). Length of ward stay was significantly shorter for the RVOT stent group (median 7 days versus 14 days) [13].

Clinical tip

In the immediate period following invasive palliation for low pulmonary blood flow, the pulmonary vasculature is exposed to a sudden increase in pressure and flow. There is potential for pulmonary oedema, reperfusion injury and even pulmonary haemorrhage, so that a chest X-ray is an essential investigation. In those demonstrating high systemic oxygen saturations after invasive palliation, careful observation for tachypnoea and respiratory distress should be paid. Some infants will initially require furosemide therapy and, less commonly, an extended period of invasive ventilation. This is more common for BT shunt-palliated patients due to the physiological features described. Vasopressive inotropes may be used in this scenario but should be considered cautiously. Unwanted pressor effects on pulmonary vascular resistance may worsen left-to-right shunting, precipitating a downward spiral of reduced tissue perfusion, despite the increase in cardiac output.

When evaluating an acutely cyanosed patient after invasive palliation, the absence of a murmur should be of grave concern, raising the suspicion of shunt thrombosis. For both modes of palliation, the administration of single or dual antiplatelet therapy is typical. This has since been supported by a large multi-centre study demonstrating that aspirin administration post-systemic-to-arterial shunt reduces hazard ratios for both late mortality and shunt thrombosis events [15]. There is no evidence regarding platelet use after RVOT stenting, and the practice varies in each centre.

At 6 months of age and weighing 6.2 kg, his oxygen saturations had reduced to 72% and haemoglobin risen to 16 g/dl. The family reported he was feeding normally and seemed well but appeared 'pale' and 'short-tempered' at times. He required frequent naps, compared to his older sibling's habits at the same age.

Repeat cardiac catheterization showed neo-intimal growth into the RVOT stent and muscle bundles, causing obstruction at the proximal portion of the stent. The left and right pulmonary arteries had grown and measured 5.3 mm and 5.7 mm, respectively (Figure 4.6). The MAPCAs had become stenosed but continued to constitute additional sources of pulmonary blood flow. Despite impressive growth of the native pulmonary arteries, it was decided that complete repair at this stage would still carry important risks of post-operative complications. It was decided for further palliation to permit additional pulmonary artery growth, and thus reduce overall operative risk at the time of complete repair.

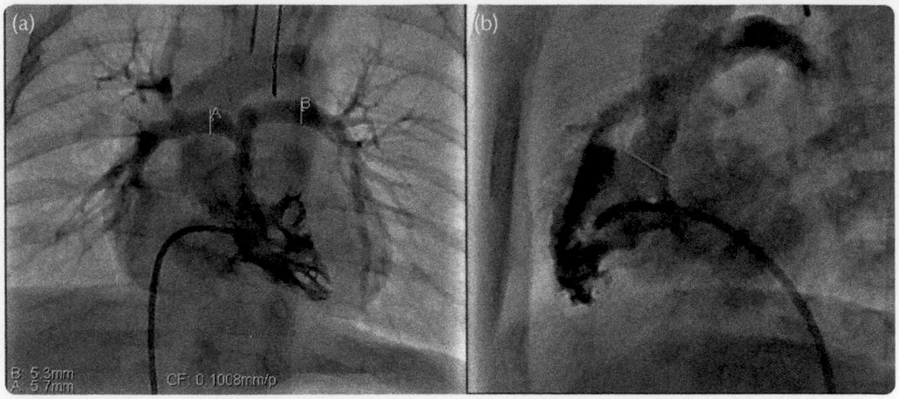

Figure 4.6 (a) Anteroposterior right ventricle angiogram demonstrating good pulmonary artery growth. (b) Right ventricle angiogram in lateral projection demonstrating some neo-intimal growth at the proximal position of the stent (arrow).

Learning point

Historically, complete repair of tetralogy of Fallot was delayed into late childhood. By the 1990s, successful complete repair in early infancy had emerged. In the more recent era, some units have even undertaken early neonatal repair, though this is associated with longer stays on intensive care and remains the exception [16]. Most large centres aim to reserve invasive palliation (RVOT stent/ BT shunt) for symptomatic small or premature infants or those with important comorbidities [17, 18] (such as airway problems associated with di George syndrome). In such patients, a delay to surgery is either essential or desirable. Generally, elective primary repair is performed at 6–18 months of age, depending on the institution, the patient, and their pulmonary artery size [19].

Expert comment

The valve may be spared when implanting an RVOT stent in an attempt to reduce transannular patch or conduit use at the time of repair. In practice, sparing the valve may be technically challenging but is pursued by many in an attempt to preserve valve competence, thus preserving forward flow during diastole to stimulate pulmonary arterial growth. Importantly, the entire length of the right ventricular muscular infundibulum should be covered by the stent. This reduces the recurrence of infundibular muscular obstruction, which most commonly occurs at the proximal portion of the stent [13]. In 60% of patients undergoing a catheter re-intervention after RVOT stenting, some degree of neo-intima could be seen on angiography [13], usually consisting of muscular ingrowth into the struts of the stent.

Clinical tip

Cyanosis drives increased haemoglobin production as a mechanism to meet tissue oxygenation requirements during hypoxaemia. In a patient with tetralogy of Fallot with reassuring saturations at rest, but with raised haemoglobin, cyanotic spells may be occurring without parental recognition. Irritability, poor feeding, pallor, inconsolable crying, or deteriorating neurological state must all be considered as potential manifestations of cyanotic spells. Caregivers of children with strongly pigmented skin may describe the child's lips as appearing 'blackened' at times; this should also be considered a potential sign of episodic cyanosis. Overall, however, recognition of severe cyanosis in non-white infants and children can be very difficult.

To appreciate cyanosis, there must be 3–5 g/dl of desaturated haemoglobin in systemic arterial blood [4]. Therefore, older and physiologically anaemic infants may not demonstrate obvious cyanosis.

The patient underwent re-dilation of the RVOT stent with a 5.5-mm balloon. As expected, the closed cell stent shortened during overdilation, leaving the proximal RVOT uncovered. A 6-mm stainless steel balloon-expandable stent was used to re-stent the outflow tract. The stent was deployed using hand inflation; however, the delivery balloon ruptured, leaving a balloon fragment in the RVOT and precipitating a dramatic drop in systemic oxygen saturations. The balloon fragment was retrieved with a gooseneck snare catheter via the femoral artery.

Systemic oxygen saturations following this were 93%. As such, the remaining significant MAPCAs were occluded with coils (Figure 4.7).

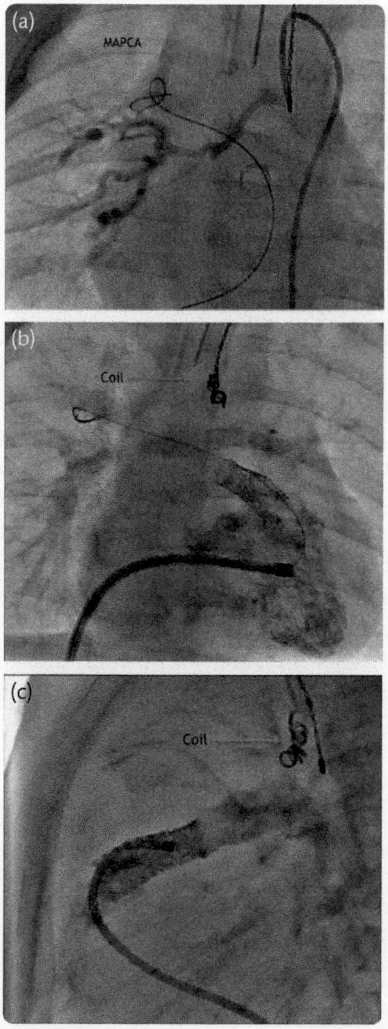

Figure 4.7 (a) Angiogram of MAPCA before coil placement. (b) and (c) Anteroposterior and lateral angiograms showing improved RVOT potency after re-stenting, plus coil (arrow) *in situ* in additional MAPCA.

Expert comment

To account for somatic growth of those likely to require long-term palliation, the use of an overdilatable, non-shortening stent is desirable. However, unlike coronary stents, these stents may not conform well to the anatomic curvature of the RVOT [22].

Learning point

Although difficult to predict, had the patient followed the surgical pathway, he would have likely received a 3-mm Gore-Tex® tube BT shunt as initial palliation. As such, with a low weight-to-shunt size ratio, he would have likely had a 'stormy' initial post-operative course. Additionally, he would have been at risk of shunt thrombosis and likely outgrowing the shunt, potentially requiring an early second palliative procedure. Surgical shunt revision carries significant risks [7], and cumulative thoracotomies and sternotomies increase the chances of restrictive lung disease with each additional procedure [20].

RVOT stenting palliation provided this patient with the option of transcatheter re-intervention. This strategy is particularly useful for those with additional comorbidities known to raise the surgical risk at repair (such as trisomy 21, di George syndrome [21], or tracheobronchomalacia). It may also be useful to provide prolonged palliation to optimize somatic size in patients with complex anatomy such as double-outlet right ventricle or Fallot's tetralogy with complete atrioventricular septal defect. Re-intervention, however, is not without risk, as seen in this case.

When the native pulmonary artery system supplies all segments of the lung, **the priority must be to encourage growth of the native system** and aim for eventual ligation or occlusion of the inherently abnormal MAPCA vessels providing 'dual supply'. In those with pulmonary atresia, VSD, and MAPCAs, certain segments of the lung may exclusively be supplied by MAPCAs. At repair, these vessels are typically mobilized and anastomosed ('unifocalization') to the native vessels, resulting in connection of all segmental lung supply to the implanted RV–PA conduit.

At 15 months of age, the child weighed 11.6 kg, with a systemic oxygen saturation of 85%. The branch pulmonary arteries measured 8 mm on cross-sectional imaging (Z-score −1). A decision was made by the multidisciplinary team for complete repair. At the time of repair, interrogation with Hagar dilators found that the left and right pulmonary arteries were smaller than predicted, measuring 6 mm and 7 mm, respectively. Additionally, the RVOT stent had just crossed the pulmonary valve.

The main and branch pulmonary arteries were incised to allow for patch augmentation. An extensive ventriculotomy and a transannular patch would have been required to excise the RVOT stent in full. As such, the surgeon elected to leave the stent *in situ* and to repair using a 16-mm Contegra® (bovine jugular vein) conduit, creating a 'double-outlet right ventricle'. The VSD was closed with a Dacron patch, and the small atrial communication was closed with a direct suture. Invasive pressure monitoring after weaning from cardiopulmonary bypass showed the right ventricular pressure to be 60% of the systemic arterial pressure. Two pleural drains, one pericardial drain, plus atrial and ventricular pacing wires were sited, and the chest closed. The patient returned to intensive care.

Learning point

Historically, Fallot's tetralogy repair has sometimes involved a large ventriculotomy and transannular incision, through which the VSD would be closed, right ventricular outflow muscle bundles resected, and a transannular patch inserted. The goal was to create a widely patent right ventricular outflow. Since those early years, the technique has evolved, with the realization that both free pulmonary regurgitation and large ventriculotomies were important contributors to impaired right ventricular function and arrhythmias. During the past 3–4 decades, repair of the VSD has been performed via an atriotomy and through the tricuspid valve; transannular patching is minimized, or even avoided, and obstructive outflow muscle bundles may just be divided, rather than completely resected. Mild residual outflow tract obstruction is considered to be acceptable and can even be protective against the long-term impact of free pulmonary regurgitation [23].

In the repair of tetralogy of Fallot or pulmonary atresia with VSD and MAPCAs, in order to septate the heart by closing the VSD, the pulmonary vasculature must be adequate, such that the right ventricle will not fail post-operatively due to high afterload. For some patients with pulmonary atresia and MAPCAs, following unifocalization to a restricted RV–PA conduit, the VSD will be left open for this very reason. In this setting, pulsatile forward flow drives pulmonary artery growth, but the VSD allows for unrestrictive right-to-left shunting, maintaining the right ventricular pressure at or below the systemic pressure.

Expert comment

There is no significant difference in the rate of transannular patch repair between tetralogy of Fallot palliated with RVOT stent or with BT shunt ($p = 0.84$), nor any statistically significant difference in conduit use at the time of repair. The necessity for surgical patch enlargement of the branch pulmonary arteries is higher in the BT shunt group (31%), compared to 15% in the RVOT stent group ($p = 0.08$) [13].

The use of RV–PA conduits at the time of Fallot's tetralogy repair remains, to some extent, a judgement call for the surgeon and cardiologist alike, as practice varies between centres. Conduit use is indicated where an aberrant coronary crosses the RVOT, such that adequate outflow tract incision and patching are impossible. It is otherwise utilized for those with small or borderline-sized branch pulmonary arteries, with the hope of promoting further pulmonary artery growth after repair by providing a competent pulmonary valve. Preservation of forward flow through the pulmonary vasculature simultaneously normalizes pre-load conditions of both left and right ventricles in the early post-operative period, theoretically protecting from early low cardiac output state [24].

Conduit use commits the patient to conduit replacement later in life, and often interim cardiac catheterization procedures for conduit or branch pulmonary artery stenosis. The Contegra® (VenPro) conduit carries a significant risk for infective endocarditis, with reported rates of up to 11% [25]. Its use, particularly in smaller sizes, has been identified as a risk factor for developing distal stenosis at the pulmonary artery bifurcation [26], with such lesions being challenging to address safely with catheter intervention.

Clinical tip

Following tetralogy of Fallot's repair, an epicardial or transoesophageal echo is performed prior to closing the chest. This is to ensure there is no residual septal defect, to estimate the right ventricular pressure if direct measurement was not performed, and to evaluate residual outflow tract obstruction and the extent of tricuspid regurgitation. Once the child arrives to intensive care, a further echo is typically performed to recheck the above plus to evaluate the branch pulmonary arteries and cardiac function and to rule out a pleural or pericardial collection. A 12-lead ECG is required to evaluate atrioventricular conduction, as surgical VSD closure may rarely be complicated by atrioventricular block in the current era.

In most Fallot's tetralogy patients, invasive central venous pressure monitoring will be available after repair and one should expect a reading higher than normal. A central venous pressure of 8–10 mmHg for a post-repair Fallot's tetralogy patient is usually too low to support adequate forward flow into the hypertrophied, stiff right ventricle (where end-diastolic pressures will be high, even if the ventricle is not truly restrictive). Judicious use of crystalloid boluses in the initial hours after repair is a mainstay.

Four hours after return to the intensive care unit, the patient remained invasively ventilated. Sedation had been weaned to minimal settings with a view to early extubation. He was noted to gradually develop tachycardia at 180 bpm. Atrial P-wave activity was not clearly visible on the cardiac monitor. His temperature had risen to 38.5°C. His mean arterial systemic pressure had fallen from 55 mmHg to 35 mmHg, and as such, a low-dose adrenaline infusion was commenced. The central venous saturation was 45%, and the arterial saturation was 100%. The central venous pulse wave was noted to be elevated and erratic.

A 12-lead ECG was suggestive of junctional ectopic tachycardia (JET) (Figure 4.8). It was repeated with the V2 lead connected directly to the atrial pacing wires, and the diagnosis confirmed. Repeat echocardiogram ruled out tamponade and showed mild ventricular systolic dysfunction, with intermittent forward flow across the pulmonary valve during end-ventricular diastole.

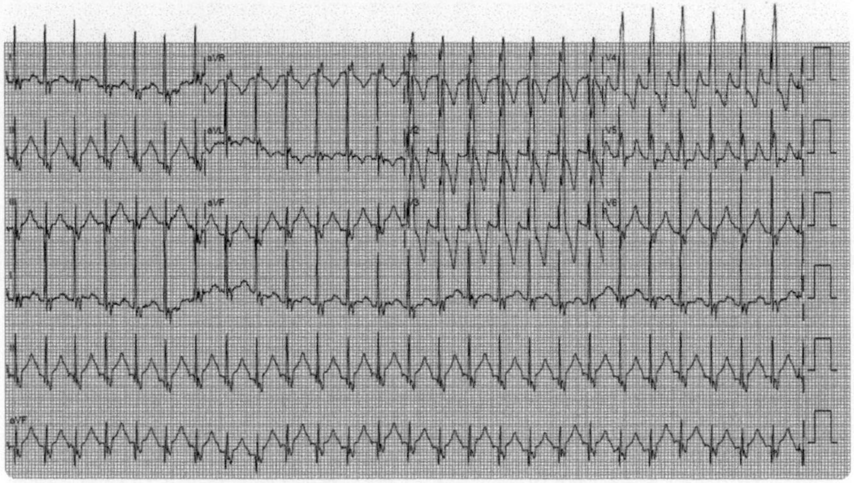

Figure 4.8 Electrocardiogram demonstrating junctional ectopic tachycardia.

An infusion of milrinone was commenced and gradually titrated to a dose of 0.5 mcg/kg/min. Intravenous paracetamol was administered, and intravenous sedation and morphine was uptitrated. He was placed in a cooling jacket, to reduce the core temperature to 36°C. A low-dose infusion of amiodarone was started at 0.3 mg/kg/min. The heart rate reduced to 120 bpm. However, the mean arterial pressure and central venous saturations remained low. He was commenced on dual-chamber pacing at a rate of 130 bpm. Following these measures, his blood pressure and central venous saturations improved. By the following morning, he had been weaned off inotropic support but remained sedated, paced, and cooled.

Learning point

JET is a particularly common arrhythmia noted early after Fallot's tetralogy repair. Though the mechanism remains debated, it is widely thought to arise as a result of myocardial irritation and swelling around VSD patch sutures and regions of muscle bundle resection. As such, it is characteristically self-limiting [27].

JET is a ventricular tachycardia (VT), with a rate exceeding 170 bpm, arising from an ectopic focus distal to the atrioventricular node, but proximal to the bundle branches. The QRS morphology is typically the same as the patient's sinus rhythm QRS morphology, though some rate-related bundle branch block may occur. It may appear on the ECG as a narrow complex tachycardia (as a result of the ectopic focus's proximity to the His bundles), and thus it may be easily mistaken for a supraventricular tachycardia (SVT). However, after Fallot's tetralogy repair, a broad right bundle branch block is typical, making distinguishing JET from other types of slow broad complex VT challenging on baseline ECG alone.

The distinguishing feature of JET is 1:1 retrograde conducted P waves occurring within the QRS complex (if both atria and ventricle are triggered to depolarize by the ectopic focus) or loss of atrioventricular synchrony, with the ventricular rate exceeding the atrial rate. In those with retrograde conducted P waves (where SVT remains a differential), adenosine may be used to disrupt atrioventricular conduction; this will expose the underlying atrial rate as slower than the ventricular rate. As JET arises from an ectopic focus below the atrioventricular node, it may be briefly suppressed, but not terminated, by adenosine.

The cornerstones of JET management are maintaining normal electrolytes (particularly magnesium), haemoglobin, and temperature and providing adequate analgesia and/or sedation to reduce adrenergic tone and metabolic requirements [28]. Rate reduction can be achieved with cooling, sedation, and analgesia. If first-line measures fail and the patient is haemodynamically unstable, amiodarone may be commenced to further suppress the rate [29]. A type III anti-arrhythmic agent with both alpha and beta receptor-blocking properties, amiodarone prolongs the action potential and refractory period of ventricular contraction. It has the highest efficacy for the treatment of JET and is therefore universally accepted as the first-line anti-arrhythmic in this setting. Once the rate has been controlled, 'overdrive' pacing is commonly employed, to restore atrioventricular synchrony and improve cardiac output, if required. In small children and babies, loss of atrioventricular synchrony may result in a fall in cardiac output of up to 30% [27].

LV function may be impaired further by post-cardiac bypass systemic inflammatory response syndrome (CBP SIRS), usually marked by fever of >38°C, ventricular dysfunction, capillary leak, renal dysfunction, and increased inspired oxygen requirements. It is thought to occur as a result of an escalating cascade of inflammatory cytokines. CBP SIRS, along with the positively inotropic drugs used to manage it, typically exacerbate JET [30].

Clinical tip

In diagnosing children with tachycardia, discerning the P wave on the standard ECG can be challenging. To ease identification of P waves, the paper speed on the ECG machine can be slowed, and amplitude settings adjusted, to 'stretch out' and enlarge the complexes. For those with temporary epicardial pacing leads, a more effective measure is to simply attach one of the chest leads (usually V2) directly to the atrial pacing wire. The resulting trace reveals enlarged-amplitude P waves, as a result of the wire's intimacy with the atrial wall. This trace can be compared to the rest of the ordinary trace, helping to identify the relationship between atrial and ventricular activity.

As with those in complete heart block, the absence of atrioventricular synchrony may result in 'cannon waves' of the jugular venous pressure, as the right atrium contracts against a closed tricuspid valve. (In practice, this is difficult to appreciate in small infants, but it may be easily noted on central venous pressure tracings.)

The conduction pattern of JET may persist beyond the immediate post-operative period, but at a slower, more acceptable heart rate. This rhythm takes origin from the same ectopic focus but produces normal or slow rates and is termed 'nodal' or 'junctional' rhythm. If seen at an appropriate rate and with no evidence for pauses, nodal rhythm does not usually require intervention and eventually reverts to sinus rhythm in the great majority.

Some patients may also demonstrate right ventricular diastolic dysfunction or, more correctly, 'restrictive physiology'. This is diagnosed echocardiographically by the presence of anterograde flow in the pulmonary artery during atrial systole, showing the ventricle acting as a non-compliant conduit during end-ventricular diastole, rather than as a compliant chamber being filled effectively prior to ventricular systole [31].

Mixed venous saturation and arterial lactate are valuable substitute markers when assessing the adequacy of cardiac output, reflecting the composite product of the patient's tissue oxygen delivery and extraction.

Expert comment

In selected patients deemed likely to suffer from important restrictive physiology post-operatively, a patent foramen ovale may be left open at the time of repair. Right ventricular diastolic dysfunction can lead to reduced LV filling and low cardiac output, and thus LV dysfunction. An atrial communication provides an opportunity for right-to-left shunting, reducing pre-load on the right ventricle and preserving pre-load to the left ventricle and protecting early post-operative cardiac output (at the expense of normal systemic oxygen saturation).

A note of caution must be made regarding the negatively inotropic effect of amiodarone, particularly in children post-cardiac bypass surgery. Unit practice will vary, but, irrespective of this, there will be patients who suddenly deteriorate once therapeutic levels of amiodarone are achieved (due to bradycardia, the negatively inotropic action of amiodarone, and the vasodilatory effects of the infusion solvent). This can be fatal, and as such, amiodarone should be commenced with caution and with senior supervision, generally at a lower dose than standardized 'textbook' dosing regimens. A maintenance infusion is usually sufficient, and a loading dose is only rarely necessary.

Final word from the expert

Tetralogy of Fallot is the most common cyanotic congenital heart disease in infancy and childhood. Soon after birth, some 20% of children become severely symptomatic due to recurrent episodes of desaturation (spells) and may require initial surgical palliation (systemic-to-pulmonary artery shunt). This carries a mortality of around 9%, even in the current era. Associated significant anatomical associations or comorbidities may dictate the timing of complete surgical repair. Complete surgical repair with the lowest mortality is usually around 6 months.

Transcatheter stenting of the right ventricular outflow tract (RVOT) has been shown to be a lower-risk procedure than surgical systemic-to-pulmonary artery shunting. It has been shown to reduce hospital stay and provides a better foundation for pulmonary arterial growth. As such, it has become a well-established technique in the initial management of Fallot-type lesions. Long-term studies are, however, needed to judge whether initial palliation with RVOT stenting increases the arrhythmia burden in operated Fallot patients. Furthermore, no bespoke stent designs exist. The ideal of a biodegradable stent appears to be a long way away.

The biggest potential benefit of RVOT stenting in Fallot-type lesions could be in emerging countries where there are numerous late-presenting patients with saturations of <70%, resulting in lifelong under-perfusion of their pulmonary vasculature. Single-stage complete surgical repair is often complicated by severe reperfusion injury of their lungs, ensuing a prolonged stay in the intensive care unit with other associated morbidities. In these cases, RVOT stenting could afford a way to improve pulmonary blood flow to acceptable levels (saturations of around 85%) and then proceeding to complete repair 6–8 weeks later when the stent is still easily removable. Despite these being two procedures, the cumulative hospital stay and costs are likely to be significantly less, as would be the morbidity and mortality of these patients.

References

1. Anderson RH, Weinberg PM. The clinical anatomy of tetralogy of Fallot. *Cardiol Young* 2005;15 (Suppl 1):38–47.
2. Flanagan MF, Foran RB, Van Praagh R, et al. Tetralogy of Fallot with obstruction of the ventricular septal defect. Spectrum of echocardiographic findings. *J Am Coll Cardiol* 1988;11:386–95.
3. Kothari SS. Mechanism of cyanotic spells in tetralogy of Fallot—the missing link? *Int J Cardiol* 1992;37:1–5.

4. Reddington A. Tetralogy of Fallot and pulmonary atresia with ventricular septal defect. Moller JH, Hoffman JIE, editors. *Pediatric Cardiovascular Medicine*, 2nd edition. Blackwell Publishing Ltd, 2012; pp. 590–608.
5. Blalock A, Taussig H. The surgical treatment of malformations of the heart in which there is pulmonary atresia. *JAMA* 1945;128:189–202.
6. Gladman G, McCrindle BW, Willimas WG, et al. The modified Blalock–Taussig shunt: clinical impact and morbidity in Fallot's tetralogy in the current era. *J Thorac Cardiovasc Surg* 1997;114:25–30.
7. Petrucci O, O'Brien SM, Jacobs ML, Jacobs JP, Manning PB, Eghtesady P. Risk factors for mortality and morbidity after the neonatal Blalock–Taussig shunt procedure. *Ann Thorac Surg* 2011;92:642–51.
8. McKay R, de Leval MR, Rees PG, et al. Postoperative angiographic assessment of modified Blalock–Taussig shunts using expanded polytetrafluoroethylene (Gore-Tex). *Ann Thorac Surg* 1980;30:137–45.
9. Li JS, Yow E, Berezny KY, et al. Clinical outcomes of palliative surgery including a systemic-to-pulmonary artery shunt in infants with cyanotic congenital heart disease: does aspirin make a difference? *Circulation* 2007;116:293–7.
10. Gibbs JL, Uzun O, Blackburn ME, Parsons JM, Dickinson DF. Right ventricular outflow stent implantation: an alternative to palliative surgical relief of infundibular pulmonary stenosis. *Heart* 1997;77:176–9.
11. Dohlen G, Chatuverdi RR, Benson LN, et al. Stenting of the right ventricular outflow tract in the symptomatic infant with tetralogy of Fallot. *Heart* 2009;95:142–7.
12. Stumper O, Ramchandani B, Noonan P, et al. Stenting of the right ventricular outflow tract. *Heart* 2013;99:1603–8.
13. Quandt D, Ramchandani B, Penford G, et al. Right ventricular outflow tract stent versus BT shunt palliation in Tetralogy of Fallot. *Heart* 2017;103:1985–91.
14. Quandt D, Ramchandani B, Stickley J, et al. Stenting of the right ventricular outflow tract promotes better pulmonary arterial growth compared with modified Blalock–Taussig shunt palliation in tetralogy of Fallot-type lesions. *JACC Cardiovasc Interv* 2017;10:1774–84.
15. Li JS, Yow E, Berezny KY, et al. Clinical outcomes of palliative surgery including a systemic-to-pulmonary artery shunt in infants with cyanotic congenital heart disease: does aspirin make a difference? *Circulation* 2007;116:293–7.
16. Reddy VM, Liddicoat JR, McElhinney DB, et al. Routine primary repair of tetralogy of Fallot in neonates and infants less than three months of age. *Ann Thorac Surg* 1995;60:S592–6.
17. Barron DJ. Tetralogy of Fallot: controversies in early management. 8. *World J Pediatr Congenit Heart Surg* 2013;4:186–91.
18. Sousa Uva M, Chardigny C, Galetti L, et al. Surgery for tetralogy of Fallot at less than six months of age. Is palliation 'old-fashioned'? *Eur J Cardiothorac Surg* 1995;9:453–9.
19. Van Arsdell GS, Maharaj GS, Tom J, et al. What is the optimal age for repair of tetralogy of Fallot? *Circulation* 2000;102(19 Suppl 3): II123–9.
20. Hawkins SM, Taylor AL, Sillau SH, Mitchell MB, Rausch CM. Restrictive lung function in paediatric patients with structural congenital heart disease. *J Thorac Cardiovasc Surg* 2014;148:207–11.
21. Khositseth A, Tocharoentanaphol C, Khowsathit P, Ruangdaraganon N. Chromosome 22q11 deletions in patients with conotruncal heart defects. *Pediatr Cardiol* 2005;26:570–3.
22. Quandt D, Ramchandani B, Bhole V, et al. Initial experience with the Cook Formula balloon expandable stent in congenital heart disease. *Catheter Cardiovasc Interv* 2015;85:259–66.
23. Latus H, Gummel K, Rupp S, et al. Beneficial effects of residual right ventricular outflow tract obstruction on right ventricular volume and function in patients after repair of tetralogy of Fallot. *Paediatric Cardiol* 2013;34:424–30.
24. Gatzoulis MA, Elliott JT, Guru V, et al. Right and left ventricular systolic function late after repair of tetralogy of Fallot. *Am J Cardiol* 2000;86:1352–7.

25. Albanesia F, Sekarskib N, Lambrouc D, Von Segessera LK, Berdajs DA. Incidence and risk factors for Contegra graft infection following right ventricular outflow tract reconstruction: long-term results. *Eur J Cardiothorac Surg* 2014;45:1070–4.
26. Yong MS, Yim D, d'Udekem Y, et al. Medium-term outcomes of bovine jugular vein graft and homograft conduits in children. *ANZ J Surg* 2015;85:381–5.
27. Dodge-Khatami A, Miller OI, Anderson RH, et al. Surgical substrates of postoperative junctional ectopic tachycardia in congenital heart defects. *J Thorac Cardiovasc Surg* 2002;123:624–30.
28. Cools E, Misact C. Junctional ectopic tachycardia after congenital heart surgery. *Acta Anaesthesiol Belg* 2014;65:1–8.
29. Pfammatter JP, Paul T, Ziemer G, Kallfelz HC. Successful management of junctional tachycardia by hypothermia after cardiac operations in infants. *Ann Thorac Surg* 1995;60:556–60.
30. Bruins P, te Velthuis H, Yazdanbakhsn AP, et al. Activation of the complement system during and after cardiopulmonary bypass surgery: postsurgery activation involves C-reactive protein and is associated with postoperative arrhythmia. *Circulation* 1997;96:3542–8.
31. Carminati M, Pluchinotta FR, Piazza L, et al. Echocardiographic assessment after surgical repair of tetralogy of Fallot. *Frontiers in Pediatrics* 2015;3:3.

CASE

5 Neonatal enteroviral myocarditis: a potentially devastating disease

Grazia Delle Donne

Expert commentary Piers Daubeney

Case history

A neonate born at term and weighing 2.7 kg, following an uneventful pregnancy, presented with fever and grunting at 1 hour of age. In view of maternal fever 12 hours prior to delivery, the mother was treated with antibiotics at the time of delivery. The baby on arrival to the neonatal intensive care unit (NICU) was started on antibiotics, following a full septic screen, the results of which were unremarkable. On day 7, he was commenced on continuous positive airway pressure (CPAP) after being noted to be persistently tachycardic with ongoing respiratory distress.

The ECG was suspicious of supraventricular tachycardia (SVT), with a heart rate of 237 bpm (Figure 5.1). The chest X-ray demonstrated cardiomegaly with pulmonary oedema (Figure 5.2). Echocardiography showed severely impaired left ventricular function with an ejection fraction of 20%. The respiratory distress worsened, and he was referred to the network paediatric cardiac intensive care unit for management of the SVT and ongoing symptoms of heart failure.

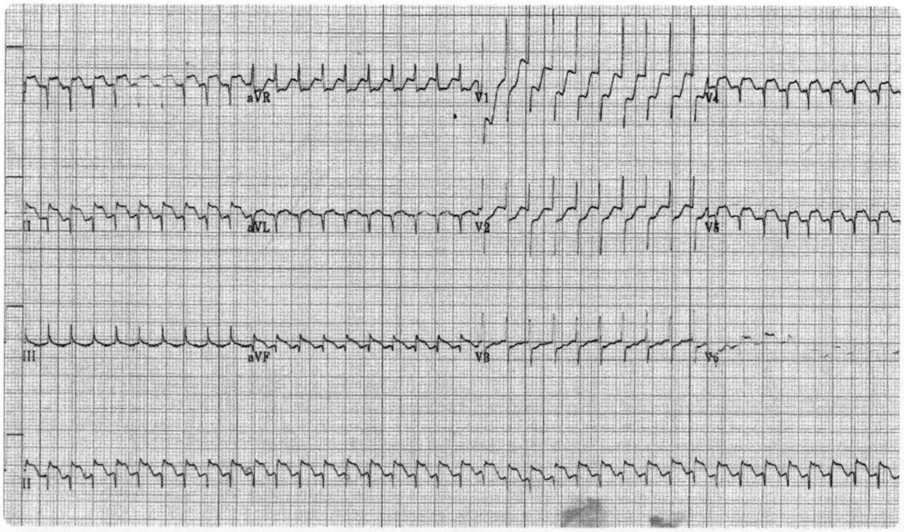

Figure 5.1 ECG showing supraventricular tachycardia with repolarization changes in all leads, consistent with myocardial ischaemia or infarction.

Learning point Differential diagnosis

- Myocarditis with sinus tachycardia or SVT
- Atrial ectopic tachycardia with heart failure
- Dilated cardiomyopathy (DCM) with incidental infection and tachycardia
- Neonatal sepsis
- Respiratory distress syndrome

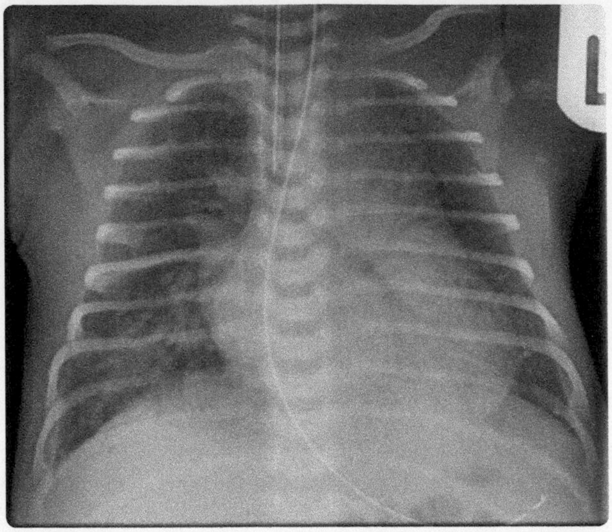

Figure 5.2 Chest X-ray showing cardiomegaly, pulmonary oedema, and a small right pleural effusion.

Progress

In PICU, the baby was intubated due to worsening respiratory distress, tachycardia, and metabolic acidosis. He was started on milrinone, adrenaline, noradrenaline, heparin, and a furosemide infusion (see Learning point: Treatment of myocarditis, p. 64). Despite the use of adenosine, the SVT persisted and as such, he was started on an amiodarone infusion—successfully reverting him to sinus rhythm 12 hours later. His ECG (Figure 5.3) showed sinus tachycardia and generalized small voltages with ST changes inferolaterally.

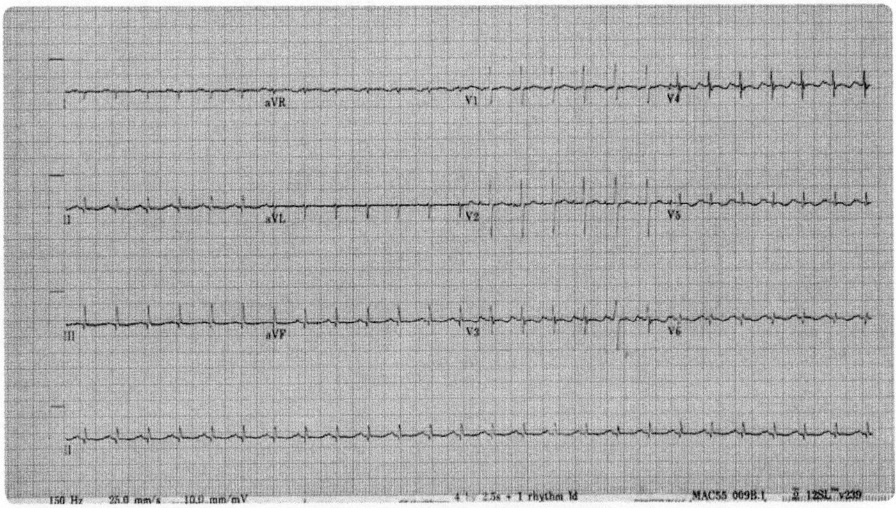

Figure 5.3 ECG showing sinus tachycardia and generalized small voltages with ST changes inferolaterally, with resolution of earlier severe ST segment changes.

Clinical tip Arrhythmia in myocarditis

Cardiac arrhythmias are a common complication of myocarditis, ranging from 29% to 100% [1]. Although our patient presented with SVT, the most common arrhythmias in myocarditis are ventricular tachycardia, ventricular fibrillation, and atrioventricular block. Clinically significant arrhythmia occurred in nearly half of the patients, most commonly ventricular in origin. Although ventricular tachycardia is a rare initial manifestation of myocarditis, it may often develop in chronic patients and may occasionally result in sudden cardiac death [2].

Investigations

Blood tests are shown in Table 5.1. A cardiomyopathy screen was performed, which was normal, other than the parameters listed below.

Table 5.1 Initial blood panel results

Full blood count	Normal
Renal function	Normal
Liver function	Normal
Troponin I peak	13,000 ng/l
CK-MB peak	106.2 mg/l
BNP	>5907 ng/l
CRP	20 mg/l
Vitamin D level	<5 nmol/l (deficient)
Viral PCR	Enterovirus
Blood cultures	Negative

An echocardiogram showed a dilated left atrium with severe mitral regurgitation. The left ventricle was dilated, with a bright appearance of the myocardium and papillary muscles (Figure 5.4). The left ventricular function was poor, with an ejection fraction of 10% (Simpson's biplane) and no left ventricular outflow tract obstruction. The right ventricular function was preserved, with mild tricuspid regurgitation and a gradient of 30 mmHg (systemic blood pressure 50 mmHg). There were no intracavity thrombi. The duct was closed. There were small pleural effusions bilaterally. His initial progress was poor, and mechanical support [extracorporeal membrane oxygenation (ECMO)] was considered as the next step if there were further deterioration. However,

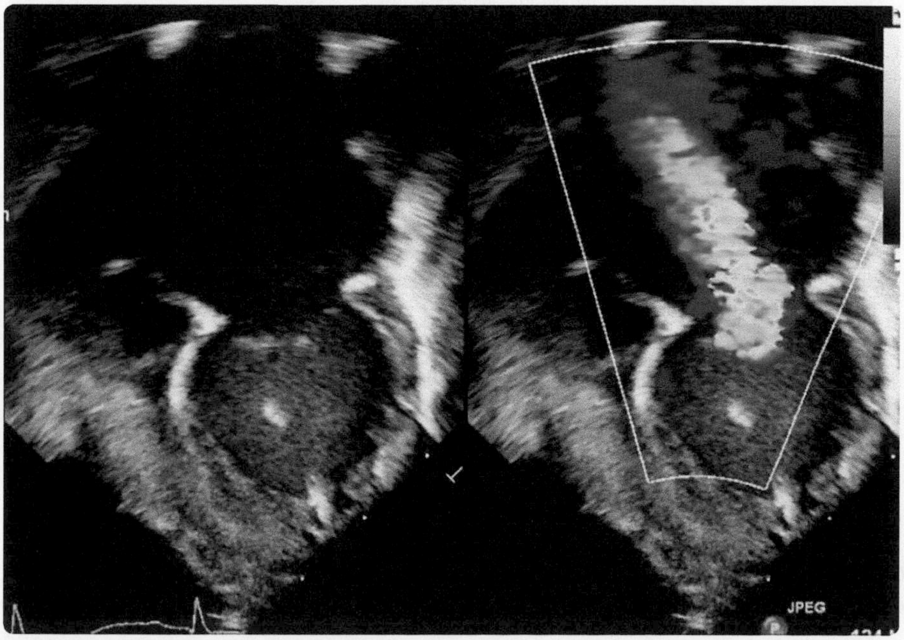

Figure 5.4 Echocardiogram showing dilated left ventricle and left atrium, bright myocardium, and papillary muscle. Severe mitral regurgitation on colour Doppler.

over the following days, he showed signs of improvement, albeit with an episode of non-sustained ventricular tachycardia.

Learning point Investigations

Laboratory findings

The general markers of inflammation—erythrocyte sedimentation rate (ESR) and C-reactive protein (CRP)— are usually elevated. Normal values, however, do not exclude myocarditis. Cardiac troponin T is used as a diagnostic marker of myocarditis. It is released in the bloodstream within hours following myocardial injury and is persistent for more than a week. Troponin T has been documented to have a specificity of 83% and a sensitivity of 71% for myocarditis in children. In patients with myocarditis, serum concentrations of troponin T and I are elevated more frequently than creatine kinase myocardial binding fraction [3].

The utility of viral serology remains unproven. Mahfoud et al. demonstrated that viral serology should not be commonly used for the diagnosis of myocarditis, as in only five of 124 patients (4%) was there serological evidence of infection similar to that detected on endomyocardial biopsy (EMB) [4]. Moreover, the diagnostic value of serology is also limited in that most viruses involved in the pathogenesis of myocarditis are highly prevalent in the population.

Electrocardiogram

ECG is widely used as a screening tool for myocarditis despite its low sensitivity (47%) [5]. The most common findings are sinus tachycardia and non-specific ST–T wave changes [6]. The QRS amplitude is reduced [7]. The presence of new Q waves or a new left bundle branch block is associated with a higher risk for heart transplantation [8]. A QT prolongation of >440 ms, an abnormal QRS axis, and ventricular ectopics are associated with poor clinical outcome. A prolonged QRS duration of >120 ms was found to be an independent predictor for cardiac death or heart transplantation. Some patients can also present with ST elevation mimicking myocardial infarction [9]. Several mechanisms may account for the ischaemic changes in myocarditis. Myocardial inflammation may lead to left ventricular mural thrombus and coronary artery embolization. Vasoactive kinins or catecholamine released during the acute phase of a viral infection can lead to coronary spasm, and finally arteritis caused by parvovirus B19 and platelet activation may cause thrombi formation in coronary arteries.

Echocardiography

Children suspected of having myocarditis warrant a comprehensive echocardiogram, detailing the structure and function in all available echo modalities. There are no specific echocardiographic features of myocarditis. Echocardiography should exclude other causes of heart failure. It should document the wall thickness, chamber size, systolic and diastolic function, and the presence of thrombi within the left ventricle. Left ventricular diastolic dysfunction with a restrictive pattern is observed in most cases of myocarditis. Left ventricular wall thickness was found to be highest on days 1–3 after the onset of acute myocarditis and is more marked in fulminant myocarditis. Pericardial effusion is commonly seen. Patients with fulminant myocarditis often have normal cardiac chamber sizes, but with increased septal thickness due to oedema. By contrast, patients with acute myocarditis have marked left ventricular dilatation and normal wall thickness [10]. In addition, right ventricular systolic dysfunction is a powerful independent predictor of death or the need for heart transplantation in patients with myocarditis [11].

Further progress

On balance, it was considered that the diagnosis was most likely to represent an enteroviral myocarditis [history, echo appearances, and polymerase chain reaction

(PCR) finding of enterovirus]. He was treated, in addition, with immunoglobulin, consistent with our departmental policy, and thereafter made a slow, but steady, progress before being extubated and weaned off inotropic support.

At discharge 2 weeks later, his cardiac function had improved with a fractional shortening of 18% and an ejection fraction of 36%. The appearances of his left ventricular myocardium and papillary muscles remained bright and speckled, and the left ventricle and atrium continued to be dilated, with moderate mitral regurgitation. His liver function had completely recovered. Troponin was 10 ng/l, and brain natriuretic peptide (BNP) 50 ng/l. He was discharged home on furosemide, spironolactone, captopril, aspirin and low does carvedilol. The ECG still showed widespread repolarization changes (Figure 5.5).

The patient was reviewed regularly, and at 3 years following his initial presentation, he remains clinically asymptomatic. The echocardiogram continues to show moderate to severe impairment of left ventricular systolic function with an ejection fraction of 40%, mild mitral regurgitation and enlargement of the left atrium. There is persistence of akinetic regions and scarring, particularly on the basal and mid-posterior walls. On his most recent review, his blood test results showed BNP at 115 ng/l, with normal troponin I (< 20 ng/l) and creatine kinase (123 U/l; normal value 25–171 U/l). His 12-lead ECG showed sinus rhythm, with repolarization changes inferolaterally (Figure 5.6). He remains on an angiotensin-converting enzyme (ACE) inhibitor, a beta-blocker, furosemide, spironolactone, ivabradine, vitamins, and iron supplement (see Learning point: Treatment of myocarditis, p. 64).

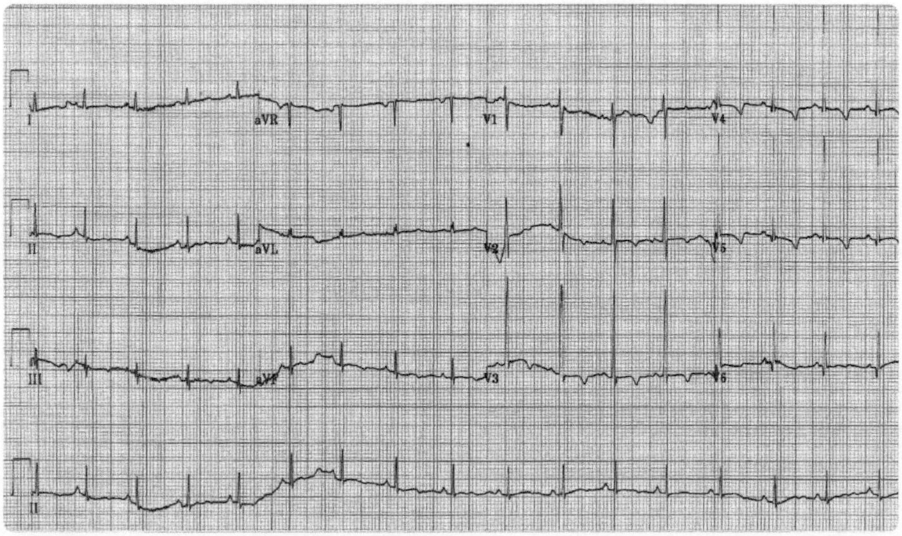

Figure 5.5 ECG at follow-up showing persisting and widespread repolarization changes.

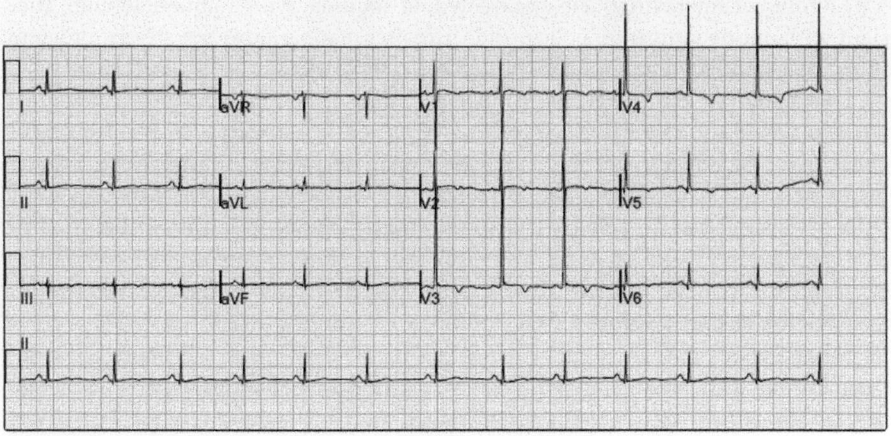

Figure 5.6 12-lead ECG showing sinus rhythm, heart rate of 60 bpm, and repolarization changes inferolaterally.

Learning point Myocarditis

Myocarditis is defined as inflammation of the myocardium in association with myocellular necrosis and degeneration [12]. The aetiology of myocarditis comprises a number of infectious and non-infectious agents—viruses, bacteria, protozoa, and toxins—as well as myocardial involvement in systemic disease (Table 5.2) [13]. Lipshultz et al. found that viral myocarditis was the cause of 27% of cases of DCM [14].

Table 5.2 Aetiology of myocarditis

Infectious causes	Non-infectious causes
Virus: adenovirus, human herpesvirus, Epstein-Barr virus, parvovirus B19, Coxsackie virus, respiratory syncytial virus	Autoimmune disease: Wegener's granulomatosis, inflammatory bowel disease, giant cell myocarditis, systemic lupus erythematosus
Bacteria: *Brucella, Clostridium, Neisseria* meningitis, *Mycobacterium* tuberculosis, *Haemophilus influenzae, Borrelia burgdorferi*	Drugs: anthracycline, catecholamines, chloramphenicol, doxorubicin, phenytoin
Fungi: *Aspergillus, Candida, Cryptococcus, Histoplasma*	Hypersensitivity reaction (drugs): cephalosporins, lithium, diuretics, tetracycline
Protozoa: *Leishmania, Toxoplasma gondii, Trypanosoma brucei*	Systemic disease: collagen disease, sarcoidosis, Kawasaki disease
Helminthic: *Schistosoma, Echinococcus granulosus*	Others: transplant rejection, radiation injury

Enteroviruses and adenoviruses are recognized as the major causes of viral myocarditis. Recently, parvovirus B19 and human herpesvirus have been described as new pathogens detected in adults [15, 16]. Parvovirus B19 can cause devastating myocarditis in children. In some parts of the world, human immunodeficiency virus (HIV) is the most frequent association of myocarditis. Children with fulminant myocarditis, ST segment changes, or a short prodrome have the worst outcome.

Bacterial infection may cause myocarditis. Fulminant septicaemia may result in myocarditis with a fatal course. The most common cause is in association with *Meningococcus, Streptococcus,* and *Borrelia* bacteraemia [17].

Many drugs and toxins can cause myocarditis, including anthracycline, cyclophosphamide, antibiotics (penicillin, ampicillin, sulfonamides, tetracyclines), lithium, catecholamines, phenytoin, and clozapine [18, 19]. Myocarditis may occur as a direct toxic effect or as a result of hypersensitivity reactions. The latter can occur days or weeks after administration. It is thought to be a reaction to their metabolites. The inflammatory infiltrate consists mainly of eosinophils and can be focal or diffuse within the myocardium. Eosinophilic necrotizing myocarditis is an extreme form of hypersensitivity myocarditis that can cause cardiovascular collapse [20].

Systemic diseases can be related to myocarditis. These include connective tissue disorders (systemic lupus erythematosus, systemic sclerosis, coeliac disease, and Whipple disease).

Learning point Role of endomyocardial biopsy

EMB is the gold standard for the diagnosis of myocarditis. According to the Dallas criteria, acute myocarditis is defined by lymphocytic infiltrates in association with myocyte necrosis. The Dallas criteria for the diagnosis of myocarditis were introduced in 1987. They have since been found to be limited due to sampling error and intraobserver variability in interpreting biopsy specimens. Thus, the Dallas criteria are no longer considered adequate for state-of-the-art diagnosis and risk stratification of acute myocarditis [21]. A scientific statement from the American Heart Association, the American College of Cardiology, and the European Society of Cardiology, published in 2007, has evaluated the role of EMB in myocarditis [22]. Despite the above concerns about the Dallas criteria, biopsy is still recommended in scenarios that are compatible with fulminant and giant cell myocarditis and in acute heart failure unresponsive to treatment [22].

Compared to adults, there is an increased risk in children [23] in performing EMB. Brighenti et al. have retrospectively evaluated 41 patients (mean age at EMB 5.2 ± 4.9 years; range 16 days to 17 years). The overall incidence of EMB-related complications was 15.5% (31.2% in infants). The authors concluded that in a paediatric population with suspected myocarditis/idiopathic cardiomyopathy, EMB was useful in confirming the diagnosis only in 41% of cases but showed an overall diagnostic power of 63%. They also concluded that as complications of EBM are not negligible, particularly in infants, the risk/benefit ratio should be taken into account in each patient [24].

Expert comment Making the diagnosis: myocarditis versus dilated cardiomyopathy

It has been a long-standing problem in distinguishing childhood myocarditis from a new presentation of DCM. The aetiology of myocarditis in this age group is often viral, whereas patients with DCM often have a viral cause of their cardiac decompensation as a consequence of an intercurrent infection. Initial investigations are often non-discriminatory. In myocarditis, the ECG **may** show low precordial voltages. The cardiothoracic ratio on chest X-ray **may** initially be normal, but once the child with myocarditis has decompensated, this may enlarge to be indistinguishable from DCM. Echocardiogram **may** show right ventricular dysfunction, with a normal left ventricular end-diastolic diameter and an increased left ventricular wall thickness due to oedema. However, as myocarditis progresses, the appearances tend to be those of DCM. Overall, these investigations are insufficiently discriminatory to be relied upon.

The gold standard for distinguishing these two diseases is still EMB, utilizing both viral PCR and histopathological appearance. The reader should consult the excellent American College of Cardiology and European Society of Cardiology consensus documents for further guidance. The former recommends EMB in children with Class of recommendation 2a and Level of evidence C [22]. However, there is significant morbidity and mortality from cardiac biopsy, particularly in infants—so much so that certainly in the United Kingdom and the United States, it is not performed generally to distinguish between these two diseases in this age group [23]. Cardiac MRI has recently been proposed as being able to distinguish between the two, and this is an exciting non-invasive alternative, albeit logistically difficult in the acute setting. In our institution, this is now the preferred option.

This discussion is, of course, only pertinent if different treatment strategies are to be adopted. With the advent of mechanical support, this may now be the case.

Learning point Role of magnetic resonance imaging in myocarditis

Cardiac MRI may be particularly useful in paediatric patients, considering the risk of EMB in children. Its tissue characterization with utilization of T1 and T2 sequences is able to assess the tissue injury (hyperaemia, capillary leakage, fibrosis, necrosis, and intracellular and interstitial oedema) [25]. Gadolinium is used as the contrast agent due to its ability to penetrate cells whose membranes are ruptured, thus allowing the contrast to diffuse into the cells. Necrosis and fibrosis, which are the result of irreversible tissue damage, are demonstrated by late gadolinium enhancement. The distribution of myocarditic lesions is predominantly in the lateral free wall and localized to the subepicardial (patchy distribution) or intramyocardial regions of the septal wall [26]. By contrast, the pattern in myocardial infarction is typically subendocardial. The International Consensus Group on Cardiovascular Magnetic Resonance proposed the diagnostic criteria for myocarditis (the Lake Louise Consensus Criteria) and that cardiac magnetic resonance (CMR) should be performed in patients with suspected myocarditis who have persistent symptoms and evidence of significant myocardial injury. CMR may also be useful to guide tissue sampling of an EMB [25]. In a retrospective study published in 2009, researchers have found that myocarditis in children is characterized mainly by subepicardial and transmural enhancement. Global hypokinesia, left ventricular dilatation, ejection fraction of <30%, and transmural myocardial involvement were associated with poor outcome [27].

Expert comment Myocarditis: what is the optimal treatment strategy?

In childhood, distinguishing myocarditis from DCM is important for two reasons—if differing treatment strategies are being considered and for prognostication. Initial treatment for both diseases is essentially the same: cardiorespiratory support, fluid management, end-organ support, and treatment of intercurrent complications. Treatment may then differ with regard to use of immunoglobulins and ongoing strategy, particularly with regard to mechanical support such as ECMO, the Berlin Heart, or similar.

The efficacy of immunoglobulin therapy is controversial, and supporting evidence limited. Nevertheless, proponents would treat biopsy-proven myocarditis with immunoglobulin, sometimes even without performing a biopsy.

Short-term mortality and morbidity in myocarditis may be significant, but if the child survives the initial illness, then the long-term outlook is good—in contrast to DCM. This difference is important for decision-making; if myocarditis is confirmed from biopsy or cardiac MRI, then mechanical support should be considered as a bridge to **recovery**, rather than **transplantation**. In other words, knowledge of the presence of myocarditis does change the strategy. At the current time, definitive confirmation of myocarditis is commonly not the case—it should be our longer-term goal.

Learning point Treatment of myocarditis

The mainstay of treatment of myocarditis presenting with DCM is supportive with use of inotropes and phosphodiesterase inhibitors and respiratory support, as required. Once stable, the management of heart failure is standard with ACE inhibitors, beta-blockers, diuretics, and anticoagulation.

ACE inhibitors and angiotensin II receptor blockers (ARBs)

ACE inhibitors, by early initiation of renin–angiotensin blockade, may limit chronic cardiac remodelling, and hence progression to DCM. In mice models, captopril, as well as losartan and olmesartan, significantly reduced inflammation, necrosis, and fibrosis in experimental autoimmune or viral-induced myocarditis [28, 29].

In the adult population, the combination sacubitril (neprilysin inhibitor) and valsartan was proven to be superior to enalapril in reducing the risk of death and hospitalization for heart failure [30]. Its use in the paediatric population has not been determined yet (PANORAMA study in progress) [31].

Diuretics

Diuretics are used to prevent or treat fluid overload.

Beta-blockers

Beta-blocker treatment should be avoided in the acute phase of decompensated heart failure and in very early treatment of fulminant myocarditis. Beta-blockade improves ventricular function, reduces hospital admission for worsening heart failure, and increases survival. Carvedilol was shown to be cardioprotective in rats with immune myocarditis by suppression of inflammatory cytokines and its antioxidant properties. Administration of carvedilol has been reported to improve left ventricular function and clinical symptoms [32]. However, a randomized, double-blind, placebo-controlled trial on 161 patients with paediatric heart failure by Shaddy et al. concluded that carvedilol does not significantly improve clinical heart failure outcomes in children and adolescents with symptomatic systolic heart failure [33]. Propranolol and metoprolol were not shown to have the same beneficial effect [34]. Metoprolol administration in rats with Coxsackie virus B3 myocarditis resulted in increased inflammation, necrosis, and death, compared to the placebo group [35]. In practice, it is usually bisoprolol or carvedilol that are administered in chronic heart failure in children.

Ivabradine

Ivabradine is a selective inhibitor of the I(f) channels in the atrioventricular node. It decreases the heart rate and myocardial oxygen consumption at rest and during exercise. Bonnet et al. have investigated its use in heart rate reduction in patients between 6 months and 18 years with DCM, in New York Heart Association (NYHA) classes II–IV, and left ventricular ejection fraction of ≤45% [36]. This was a randomized, double-blind, placebo-controlled phase II/III study. A total of 116 patients were enrolled (22% post-viral myocarditis). The authors demonstrated that ivabradine safely reduces the heart rate in children with DCM, with improved left ventricular ejection fraction and a favourable trend in clinical status and quality of life [36].

Aldosterone antagonists

Aldosterone antagonists reduce hospital admission for worsening heart failure and increases survival [37]. The anti-inflammatory effect of eplerenone on murine viral myocarditis resulted in an improvement of myocardial remodelling by suppressing fibrosis [38].

Cardiac glycosides

Cardiac glycosides reduced morbidity in patients with symptomatic heart failure. High doses of digoxin increased myocardial production of pro-inflammatory cytokines and worsened myocardial injury in viral-infected mice [39]. Therefore, digoxin should be used in low dose and with caution in patients with viral myocarditis.

Phosphodiesterase inhibitors

Milrinone can be helpful, if tolerated. Oral enoximone is used off-label. Furck et al. have reviewed retrospectively 48 patients receiving oral enoximone treatment for acute or chronic myocardial dysfunction (29% patients had myocarditis). No adverse haemodynamic effects were noted. Myocardial functional recovery allowed for weaning of enoximone treatment in 15 patients (31%) [40].

Calcium sensitizer

Levosimendan, being a calcium sensitizer and an adenosine triphosphate (ATP) agonist, has inotropic and vasodilating effects. Its maximal haemodynamic effects have been shown to occur 1–3 days after starting the infusion and are sustained for at least a week. Séguéla et al. showed that levosimendan seems to improve haemodynamics in children with decompensated DCM and repeated infusions may delay the need for mechanical circulatory support while awaiting heart transplantation. They suggested that levosimendan should be systematically considered in children with DCM in advanced heart failure, in addition to conventional inotropic drugs [41].

Anticoagulation and antiplatelet therapy

Where there is poor ventricular function, heparin is usually commenced to avoid complications of thromboembolism. If ventricular function remains poor, then warfarin therapy is instituted. As the clinical condition and ventricular function improve, warfarin may be changed to low-dose aspirin therapy.

Non-steroidal anti-inflammatory drugs and colchicine

They are used for treatment of pericarditis as non-specific anti-inflammatory therapy, whereas there is no indication for patients with myocarditis. Non-steroidal anti-inflammatory drugs (NSAIDs) can be used at the lowest dose for patients with perimyocarditis in whom the left ventricular function is normal and who have chest pain from pericarditis.

Pacemaker and implantable cardioverter-defibrillator

Temporary pacemaker insertion is indicated for patients with acute myocarditis who present with symptomatic atrioventricular block (e.g. Lyme and Chagas' disease). Persistent third-degree heart block is rare. An implantable cardioverter-defibrillator (ICD) is indicated after a cardiac arrest due to ventricular fibrillation or after symptomatic sustained ventricular tachycardia. Cardiac resynchronization therapy with defibrillator function is indicated for adult patients with impaired left ventricular function (left ventricular ejection fraction ≤35%) and left bundle branch block in NYHA classes II–IV [42]. There are no formal guidelines in childhood.

Heart transplantation and mechanical circulatory support

In patients with cardiogenic shock due to acute fulminant myocarditis who deteriorate despite optimal medical therapy, ECMO may be required as a bridge to transplantation or to recovery [43]. Despite the severe initial presentation, these patients have a good prognosis, with between 60% and 80% surviving with a high rate of recovery of native function [44, 45]. Cardiac transplantation is reserved for patients who are intractable despite maximal medical management and mechanical circulatory support. Half of the heart transplants performed at 1 year of age are due to DCM, at least 10% of which represent myocarditis [18].

Other treatments

Immunosuppressive therapy has been evaluated in trials. One of the largest randomized controlled treatment trials in adults, the Myocarditis Treatment Trial failed to show benefit from immunosuppressive therapy additional to heart failure therapy. There was neither a difference in mortality nor an improvement of left ventricular ejection fraction after 1 year of treatment with prednisolone with either azathioprine or ciclosporin versus placebo [46]. Immunosuppression is a well-established treatment for giant cell myocarditis. Ciclosporin and prednisolone have significantly prolonged transplant-free survival in those patients [47]. Immunosuppression is also used in hypersensitivity myocarditis and myocarditis associated with systemic diseases (systemic lupus erythematosus and sarcoidosis). Immunoglobulins can be used in viral myocarditis due to their antiviral and immunomodulating effects. Children with acute myocarditis treated with immunoglobulin showed an improvement of left ventricular function and survival in the first year after treatment [48].

Immunoadsorption, the removal of circulating antibodies from plasma, has been reported to improve cardiac function and humoral markers of heart failure severity (N-terminal pro-BNP) [49, 50].

Expert comment Myocarditis: what is the long-term outcome?

Childhood myocarditis is a severe and life-threatening disease, but outcome is considerably better than for DCM, in terms of both survival and left ventricular function. As distinguishing between the two conditions remains problematic, outcome studies usually examine a composite of both. The two largest registries of paediatric cardiomyopathy patients—the population-based National Australian Childhood Cardiomyopathy Study (NACCS) and the North American Pediatric Cardiomyopathy Registry (PCMR)—have shown very similar outcomes from childhood DCM [13, 51].

Survival free from cardiac transplantation for DCM (including myocarditis) in the NACCS study was 74% at 1 year, 65% at 5 years, 62% at 10 years, and 56% at 20 years. The highest-risk period was the first year after diagnosis, with just over one-quarter dying or needing transplant, compared with an average of about 1% per year subsequently. Risk factors for poor outcome were age at diagnosis, family history of cardiomyopathy, and baseline left ventricular function. There was a complex interaction between age at diagnosis and transplantation-free survival, with patients such as ours diagnosed at <4 weeks and those diagnosed older than 5 years having a higher risk of death or transplantation.

Of the 175 patients in the NACCS study, only 40 underwent EMB. Thirteen had diagnostic features of lymphocytic myocarditis, and the remaining 27 non-specific histological findings, implying that they had DCM, rather than myocarditis. Those with biopsy-confirmed lymphocytic myocarditis had better survival than those with non-specific findings. This is consistent with results of multiple single-centre case series and the PCMR registry. The latter demonstrated that in children with biopsy-confirmed or clinically diagnosed lymphocytic myocarditis, freedom from death or transplantation was about 75% 3 years after diagnosis and better than in those with idiopathic DCM [52]. In a single-centre series, 97% of patients with active lymphocytic myocarditis on myocardial biopsy survived to a median follow-up of 13 years, compared with only 32% of those without features of lymphocytic myocarditis on biopsy [53].

In the NACCS study, echocardiographic normalization of left ventricular function for those with biopsy-confirmed lymphocytic myocarditis occurred more commonly (92%) than in those with non-specific histologic findings (36%).

Children presenting with myocarditis, such as the infant described, are often highly unstable and can deteriorate precipitously. Surviving the presenting episode, however, usually leads to good long-term outcomes with mostly resolved left ventricular function. Bridging to recovery with mechanical support, not prevalent at the time of the NACCS and PCMR studies, is therefore an important addition in the clinician's armamentarium.

Discussion

Myocarditis—the disease

Myocarditis accounts for 30–35% of children with DCM phenotypes in the Australian and North American paediatric cardiomyopathy registries, and for 22% of new-onset left ventricular dysfunction in the United Kingdom [13, 54, 55]. It is a significant cause of morbidity and mortality in the paediatric population, and it accounts for 12% of sudden cardiac deaths among adolescent and young adults [56]. It is the most common cause of cardiac failure in a healthy child [57]. The diagnosis can be challenging, and it is often missed as it can be masqueraded as more common paediatric illnesses. Symptoms can vary from asymptomatic cases to cardiovascular collapse.

Learning point Clinical manifestations of myocarditis

The clinical manifestation can vary with a broad spectrum of symptoms ranging from asymptomatic to cardiogenic shock or sudden death. A viral prodrome, including fever and respiratory or gastrointestinal symptoms, often precedes the onset of the disease. Chest pain, cardiac arrhythmias, and acute or chronic heart failure can occur during the course of the disease. A recent study of paediatric patients presenting with myocarditis and a chest pain/myocardial infarction pattern found that all had elevations of cardiac troponin I (peak range 6.54–64.59 ng/ml) in the presence of normal values of ESR and CRP. Echocardiography demonstrated a mild reduction in left ventricular function in 57% of the patients, and cardiac MRI findings were consistent with myocarditis. The prognosis was good, with resolution of cardiac abnormalities within a few weeks, similar to the adult experience [58]. Non-specific gastrointestinal or respiratory symptoms are more frequent than chest pain [27]. Durani et al. have observed that the diagnosis of myocarditis was missed on the first presentation to a physician in 83% of cases. In the most severe cases of myocarditis, a patient can develop heart failure with a normal-sized left ventricle or a dilated left ventricle and haemodynamic compromise. This is the case in active lymphocytic myocarditis, necrotizing eosinophilic myocarditis, or giant cell myocarditis.

A rare type of childhood myocarditis is giant cell myocarditis. It is characterized by heart failure, a dilated left ventricle and arrhythmias, heart block, and a lack of response to therapy within 1–2 weeks [47].

Typical findings on examination comprise tachycardia, tachypnoea, hepatomegaly, a laterally displaced apex, gallop, pallor, and hypersensitivity rash. Neonates and infants present with poor feeding and irritability.

The main causative agents are viral but can also be due to bacterial infection and toxic/hypersensitive reactions or autoimmune-mediated [57]. Long-term follow-up studies of patients who present with myocarditis show that approximately 21% of these patients develop DCM, which is the most frequent cause of heart transplantation.

Little data is available on the natural history of myocarditis in children. The outcome in paediatric patients presenting with acute heart failure secondary to acute myocarditis is better than that due to DCM [51]. Prognosis depends on the clinical presentation, clinical parameters, and EMB findings positive for myocarditis. It is noteworthy, however, that many paediatric cardiac units do not perform routine myocardial biopsies.

Overall prognosis is good, with survival rates of up to 80% in the first year, but 25–50% of cases may develop DCM and chronic heart failure [57].

The long-term survival rate is usually good in fulminant myocarditis if the patient survives the initial phase, with a complete recovery in 40% of patients [58]. In contrast, long-term outcome is worse in acute myocarditis in which the symptoms are more protracted and the clinical picture is less dramatic [59].

Heart transplantation was required in 1–8% of patients with acute myocarditis [18]. The 1- and 3-year survival rates after transplantation of children with myocarditis were 83% and 65%, respectively, whereas those without myocarditis had 93% and 88% 1- and 3-year survival rates, respectively [14].

A final word from the expert

This case history describes a typical case of fulminant neonatal enteroviral myocarditis. Such children can be extremely sick and deteriorate very quickly. Surviving the initial episode enables excellent long-term outcomes, in terms of both survival and recovery of left ventricular function. The advent of mechanical support, such as ECMO, the Berlin Heart, or similar, is a great addition to the cardiologist's and intensivist's armamentarium, allowing for longer time for spontaneous recovery of the affected heart. This would be expected to improve future outcomes from this sudden and devastating disease.

References

1. Miyake CY et al. In-hospital arrhythmia development and outcomes in pediatric patients with acute myocarditis. *Am J Cardiol* 2014;113:535–40.
2. Drory Y et al. Sudden unexpected death in persons less than 40 years of age. *Am J Cardiol* 1991;68:1388–92.
3. Lauer B. Cardiac troponin T in patients with clinically suspected myocarditis. *J Am Coll Cardiol* 1997;30:1354–9.
4. Mahfoud F. Virus serology in patients with suspected myocarditis: utility or futility? *Eur Heart J* 2011;32:897–903.
5. Shauer A et al. Acute viral myocarditis: current concepts in diagnosis and treatment. *Isr Med Assoc J* 2013;15:180–5.
6. Punja M et al. Electrocardiographic manifestations of cardiac infectious-inflammatory disorders. *Am J Emerg Med* 2010;28:364–77.
7. Nugent AW et al. Clinical, electrocardiographic, and histologic correlations in children with dilated cardiomyopathy. *J Heart Lung Transplant* 2001;20:1152–7.

8. Nakashima H et al. Q wave and non-Q wave myocarditis with special reference to clinical significance. *Jpn Heart J* 1998;39:763–7.
9. Kindermann I et al. Update on myocarditis. *J Am Coll Cardiol* 2012;59:779–92.
10. Felker GM et al. Echocardiographic findings in fulminant and acute myocarditis. *J Am Coll Cardiol* 2000;36:227–32.
11. Mendes LA et al. Right ventricular dysfunction: an independent predictor of adverse outcome in patients with myocarditis. *Am Heart J* 1994;128:301–7.
12. Batra AS et al. Acute myocarditis. *Curr Opin Pediatr* 2001;13:234–9.
13. Towbin JA et al. Incidence, causes, and outcomes of dilated cardiomyopathy in children. *JAMA* 2006;296:1867–76.
14. Lipshultz SE et al. Pediatric cardiomyopathies: causes, epidemiology, clinical course, preventive strategies and therapies. *Future Cardiol* 2013;9:817–48.
15. Kindermann I et al. Predictors of outcome in patients with suspected myocarditis. *Circulation* 2008;118:639–48.
16. Magnani JD et al. Myocarditis: current trends in diagnosis and treatment. *Circulation* 2006;113:876–90.
17. Brodison A, Swann JW. Myocarditis: a review. *J Infect* 1998;37:99–103.
18. Ellis CR et al. Myocarditis basic and clinical aspects. *Cardiol Rev* 2007;15:170–7.
19. Kindermann I et al. Update on myocarditis. *J Am Coll Cardiol* 2012;59:779–92.
20. Al Ali AM, Straatman LP, Allard MF, Ignaszewski AP. Eosinophilic myocarditis:case series and review of literature. *Can J Cardiol* 2006;22:1233–7.
21. Kindermann I et al. Predictors of outcome in patients with suspected myocarditis. *Circulation* 2008;118:639–48.
22. Cooper LT et al. The role of endomyocardial biopsy in the management of cardiovascular disease. *Circulation* 2007;116:2216–33.
23. Pophal SG et al. Complications of endomyocardial biopsy in children. *J Am Coll Cardiol* 1999;34:2105–10.
24. Brighenti M et al. Endomyocardial biopsy safety and clinical yield in pediatric myocarditis: an Italian perspective. *Catheter Cardiovasc Interv* 2016;87:762–7.
25. Friedrich MG. Cardiovascular magnetic resonance in myocarditis: a JACC White Paper. *J Am Coll Cardiol* 2009;53:1475–87.
26. Mahrholdt H et al. Cardiovascular magnetic resonance assessment of human myocarditis. A comparison to histology and molecular pathology. *Circulation* 2004;109:1250–8.
27. Vashist S. Acute myocarditis in children: current concepts and management. *Curr Treat Option Cardiovasc Med* 2009;11:383–91.
28. Godsel LM. Captopril prevents experimental autoimmune myocarditis. *J Immunol* 2003;171:346–52.
29. Bahk TJ et al. Comparison of angiotensin converting enzyme inhibition and angiotensin II receptor blockade for the prevention of experimental autoimmune myocarditis. *Int J Cardiol* 2008;125:85–93.
30. McMurray JJV et al. Angiotensin–neprilysin inhibition versus enalapril in heart failure. *N Engl J Med* 2014;371:993–1047.
31. Saddy R et al. Design for the sacubitril/valsartan (LCZ696) compared with enalapril study of pediatric patients with heart failure due to systemic left ventricle systolic dysfunction (PANORAMA-HF study). *Am Heart J* 2017;193:23–34.
32. Bajcetic M et al. Effects of carvedilol on left ventricular function and oxidative stress in infants and children with idiopathic dilated cardiomyopathy: a 12-month, two-center, open-label study. *Clin Ther* 2008;30:702–14.
33. Shaddy RE et al.; Pediatric Carvedilol Study Group. Carvedilol for children and adolescents with heart failure. A randomized controlled trial. *JAMA* 2007;298:1171–9.
34. Yuan Z et al. Cardioprotective effects of carvedilol on acute autoimmune myocarditis: anti-inflammatory effects associated with antioxidant property. *Am J Physiol Heart Circ Physiol* 2004;286:H83–90.

35. Rezkalla S et al. Effect of metoprolol in acute coxsackievirus B3 murine myocarditis. *J Am Coll Cardiol* 1988;12:412–14.
36. Bonnet D et al. Ivabradine in children with dilated cardiomyopathy and symptomatic chronic feart failure. *J Am Coll Cardiol* 2017;70:1262–72.
37. Dickstein K et al. ESC Guidelines for the diagnosis and treatment of acute and chronic heart failure 2008: the Task Force for the Diagnosis and Treatment of Acute and Chronic Heart Failure 2008 of the European Society of Cardiology. Developed in collaboration with the Heart Failure Association of the ESC (HFA) and endorsed by the European Society of Intensive Care Medicine (ESICM). *Eur Heart J* 2008;29:2388–442.
38. Xiao J et al. Anti-inflammatory effects of eplerenone on viral myocarditis. *Eur J Heart Fail* 2009;11:349–53.
39. Matsumori A et al. High doses of digitalis increase the myocardial production of proinflammatory cytokines and worsen myocardial injury in viral myocarditis: a possible mechanism of digitalis toxicity. *Jpn Circ J* 1999;63:934–40.
40. Furck A et al. Oral enoximone as an alternative to protracted intravenous medication in severe pediatric myocardial failure. *Pediatr Cardiol* 2016;37:1297–301.
41. Séguéla PE et al. Single-centred experience with levosimendan in paediatric decompensated dilated cardiomyopathy. *Arch Cardiovasc Dis* 2015;108:347–55.
42. Dickstein K et al. 2010 focused update of ESC Guidelines on device therapy in heart failure: an update of the 2008 ESC Guidelines for the diagnosis and treatment of acute and chronic heart failure and the 2007 ESC Guidelines for cardiac and resynchronization therapy. Developed with the special contribution of the Heart Failure Association and the European Heart Rhythm Association. *Eur J Heart Fail* 2010;12:1143–53.
43. Cooper LT et al. Myocarditis. *N Engl J Med* 2009;360:1526–38.
44. Mirabel M et al. Outcomes, long-term quality of life, and psychologic assessment of fulminant myocarditis patients rescued by mechanical circulatory support. *Crit Care Med* 2011;39:1029–35.
45. Rajagopal SK et al. Extracorporeal membrane oxygenation for the support of infants, children, and young adults with acute myocarditis: a review of the Extracorporeal Life Support Organization registry. *Crit Care Med* 2010;38:382–7.
46. Mason JW et al. A clinical trial of immunosuppressive therapy for myocarditis. The Myocarditis Treatment Trial Investigators. *N Engl J Med* 1995;333:269–75.
47. Cooper LT. Idiopathic giant-cell myocarditis—natural history and treatment. Multicenter Giant Cell Myocarditis Study Group Investigators. *N Engl J Med* 1997;336:1860–6.
48. Drucker NA et al. Gamma-globulin treatment of acute myocarditis in the pediatric population. *Circulation* 1994;89:252–7.
49. Felix SB et al. Removal of cardiodepressant antibodies in dilated cardiomyopathy by immunoadsorption. *J Am Coll Cardiol* 2002;39:646–52.
50. Doesch AO et al. Effects of protein A immunoadsorption in patients with advanced chronic dilated cardiomyopathy. *J Clin Apher* 2009;24:141–9.
51. Alexander PM et al. Long-term outcomes of dilated cardiomyopathy diagnosed during childhood. *Circulation* 2013;128:2039–46.
52. Foerster SR et al. Ventricular remodeling and survival are more favorable for myocarditis than For idiopathic dilated cardiomyopathy in childhood. *Circ Heart Fail* 2010;3:689–97.
53. Gagliardi MG et al. Long term follow up of children with myocarditis treated by immunosuppression and of children with dilated cardiomyopathy. *Heart* 2004;90:1167–71.
54. Daubeney PE et al.; National Australian Childhood Cardiomyopathy Study. Clinical features and outcomes of childhood dilated cardiomyopathy: results from a national population-based study. *Circulation* 2006;114:2671–78.
55. Andrews RE, Fenton MJ, Ridout DA, Burch M; British Congenital Cardiac Association. New-onset heart failure due to heart muscle disease in childhood: a prospective study in the United Kingdom and Ireland. *Circulation* 2008;117:79–84.
56. Marla C Levine et al. Update on myocarditis in children. *Curr Opin Pediatr* 2010;22:278–3.

57. Dancea AB. Myocarditis in infant in children: a review for the paediatrician. *Paediatr Child Health* 2001;6:543–5.
58. Vigneswaran TV et al. Parvovirus B19 myocarditis in children: an observational study. *Arch Dis Child* 2016;101:177–80.
59. McCarthy RE et al. Long-term outcome of fulminant myocarditis as compared with acute (nonfulminant) myocarditis. *N Engl J Med* 2000;342:690–5.

CASE

6 The spectrum of disease in double outlet right ventricle

Andrew Ho

Expert commentary Tara Bharucha

Case history

A male infant was born at 39 weeks' gestation by spontaneous vaginal delivery with a birthweight of 3.4 kg, following the antenatal diagnosis of double outlet right ventricle (DORV) with a non-committed ventricular septal defect (VSD). No resuscitation was required, and he was transferred to the neonatal unit with oxygen saturations in the 80s (pre- and post-ductally measured in the right hand and right foot, respectively) in room air. Both the mother's previous two children had variants of DORV (see Learning point: Familial recurrence risk of congenital heart disease, p. 73). Neither parent was known to have structural cardiac disease.

Learning point Familial recurrence risk of congenital heart disease

The development of congenital heart disease is a multi-factorial phenomenon. Incidence in the general population is generally placed at around 8–10 per thousand live births, and familial recurrence is well established. The largest population-based study to date [1] found a risk ratio for recurrence in first-degree relatives of 3.2, with the same lesion more likely to occur (RR 8.6) than a different lesion. However, the overall contribution is small, with a population attributable risk of 2.2%.

The risk in siblings has been estimated across several studies to be in the region of 2.7% [2], which is slightly less than that with an affected mother and slightly more than with an affected father.

Recurrence risk in different lesions has also been shown to vary markedly, with heterotaxy and atrioventricular septal defects (AVSDs) showing a higher risk. The risk in DORV is, however, difficult to quantify, primarily due to differences in diagnostic criteria between units (see Learning point: Diagnosis of DORV, p. 74), making the true incidence difficult to ascertain. Despite this, a number of putative causative genes have been identified [3].

Although consanguinity at first-cousin level is associated with an increased incidence of congenital heart disease, its effect size is unclear [4].

A postnatal echocardiogram demonstrated the usual atrial arrangement with atrioventricular concordance and DORV (see Learning point: Diagnosis of DORV, p. 74; Expert comment: The diagnosis of DORV, p. 75), with a non-committed VSD (see Learning point: The VSD in double outlet right ventricle, p. 76; Clinical tip: Echocardiographic localization of the VSD, p. 79; Learning point: Classification schemes in DORV, p. 79), and side-by-side great vessels (the aorta rightward to the pulmonary artery). There was both subpulmonary and pulmonary stenosis (see Clinical tip: Anatomical variants in DORV, p. 79), with a peak velocity of 2.7 m/s across the pulmonary outflow tract. Bilateral infundibulums were present, supporting both the aortic and pulmonary

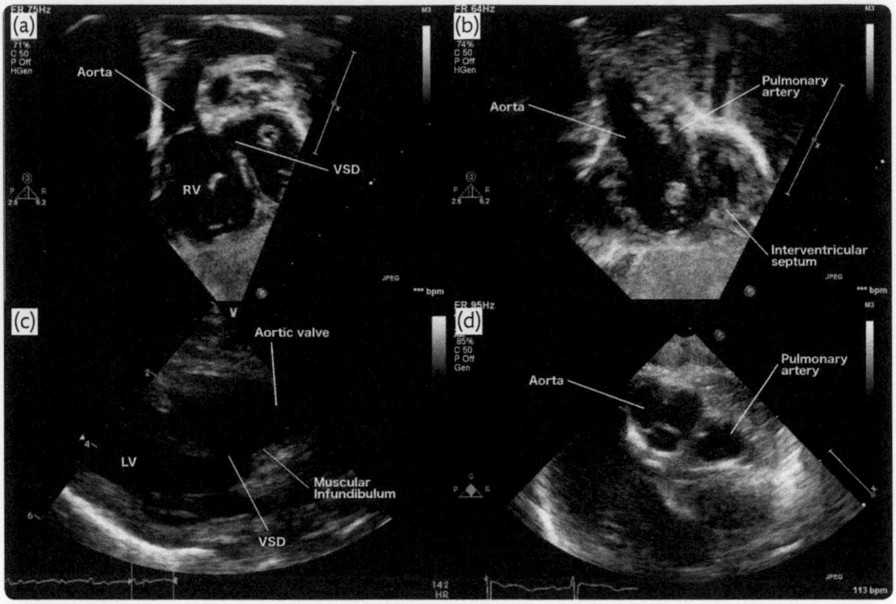

Figure 6.1 (a) An oblique subcostal view demonstrating the VSD distant from the aortic valve, sitting in the anterior septum. (b) When the pulmonary artery is brought into view, the VSD is no longer visible. (c) A parasternal long axis view, again demonstrating the VSD distant from the aorta, with a clear muscular infundibulum. (d) The parasternal short axis demonstrates the side-by-side arrangement of the great vessels with marked disproportion in size.

valves. The arterial duct was widely patent. Figure 6.1 summarizes the echocardiographic findings.

Learning point Diagnosis of DORV

The subject of DORV is frequently confusing, particularly in regard to its definition and diagnosis. The Congenital Heart Surgery Nomenclature and Database Project has defined DORV as 'a type of ventriculo-arterial connection in which both great vessels arise either entirely or predominantly from the right ventricle' and that in 'true' DORV, the VSD should 'form an integral part of the left ventricular outflow tract' (i.e. it functions as the outlet of the left ventricle) [5]. Two important points follow from this—firstly that DORV is merely the description of the ventriculo-arterial connection, not a diagnosis in its own right, and secondly that DORV can be found in both single- and two-ventricle circulations.

Although several diagnostic criteria have been used for DORV in the past, the '50% rule' is the most widely used [6]. To apply this criterion, the clinician must decide what proportion of the outflow tracts are committed to the right ventricle. As shown in Figure 6.2, the plane of the ventricular septum is taken through the overriding outflow valve, and should >50% of the orifice of the outflow valve lie beneath the right ventricle, the ventriculo-arterial connection is described as DORV. On the echocardiogram, this is usually best assessed from the parasternal long axis views.

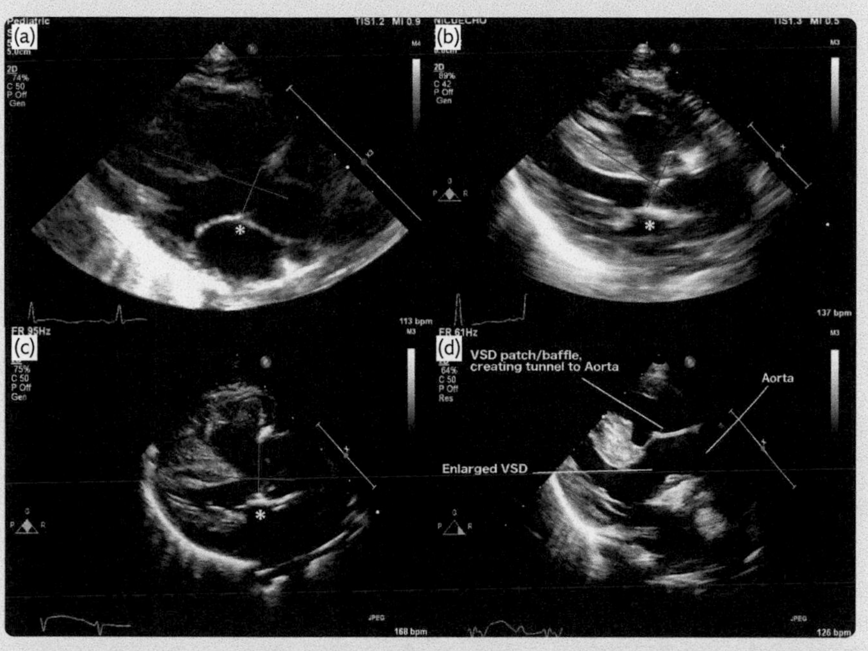

Figure 6.2 The diagnosis of DORV. (a) Patient with tetralogy of Fallot. Markings in red demonstrating the basic process for the diagnosis of DORV. A line is taken through the plane of the ventricular septum and continued through the overriding outflow valve. Less than 50% of the outflow valve is committed to the right ventricle. Note the mitral–aortic continuity at the point marked with an asterisk. (b) An example of a patient with DORV with a subaortic VSD and mitral–aortic continuity, again marked with an asterisk. The image is marked up in the same way as (a), this time demonstrating >50% origin from the right ventricle. (c) A patient with DORV and a subpulmonary VSD. There is >50% override, and in this example, mitral–pulmonary discontinuity is demonstrated, marked with an asterisk. (d) Our example patient following surgical repair, with this parasternal long axis view demonstrating the enlarged VSD and long tunnel through to the aorta. Note the difference between the plane of the 'VSD' and the location of the patch.

Expert comment The diagnosis of DORV

Given that DORV is not a diagnosis per se, but merely a description of the ventriculo-arterial connection, it is important to describe the anatomy completely when describing a patient with DORV to a colleague.

How to appropriately label the ventriculo-arterial connection as DORV has been extensively debated. In many examples, one of the great arteries retains some commitment to the left ventricle, but if at least 50% of this outlet artery is committed to the right ventricle, then this is considered a double outlet ventriculo-arterial connection.

DORV can be found in congenitally malformed hearts that are capable of supporting either single- or two-ventricle circulations. Completing the 'diagnosis' requires further description using sequential segmental analysis for colleagues to have a complete picture of the anatomy and a proper understanding of the physiology or potential management strategies for the patient.

Historically, there was a suggestion that a diagnosis of DORV requires mitral–arterial discontinuity, with muscle interposed between the mitral valve and the aortic outflow valve (as shown in Figure 6.2c), producing bilateral infundibulums or bilateral 'conuses'. The authors of this work do not feel that bilateral infundibulums are a necessary part of the diagnosis, as, to reiterate the vital concept again, DORV is simply a description of the ventriculo-arterial connection [6–8].

Definitions have varied in the published literature over time, and so care must be taken when evaluating published, particularly historical, data and making comparisons with your own patient population.

Learning point The VSD in double outlet right ventricle

Understanding the position of the VSD relative to the great arteries in DORV is vital to know the expected clinical behaviour of the patient and is one of the major determinants of medical management and surgical strategy. The VSD has been typically classified into four groups: subaortic, subpulmonary, doubly committed, and non-committed (or remote) [6].

Although, in much of congenital cardiology, we describe the VSD by its position in the ventricular septum, in DORV with subaortic, subpulmonary, and doubly committed VSDs, the location of the VSD within the septum is actually remarkably consistent, usually lying between the two limbs of the septomarginal trabeculation. In these three groups, it is instead the arrangement of the overlying muscular infundibulum(s) and great vessels which defines the location of the VSD.

DORV with subaortic VSD

In DORV with subaortic VSD, the VSD sits between the limbs of the septomarginal trabeculation, with normally related and spiralling great vessels. Most commonly, there is anterocephalad deviation of the outlet septum, as seen in tetralogy of Fallot (Figure 6.3), and the clinical picture is very much like that of tetralogy of Fallot. In the absence of anterocephalad deviation of the outlet septum (or significant pulmonary stenosis), the patient is likely to progress as with a large VSD, becoming symptomatic with pulmonary over-circulation and congestive heart failure (Figure 6.4).

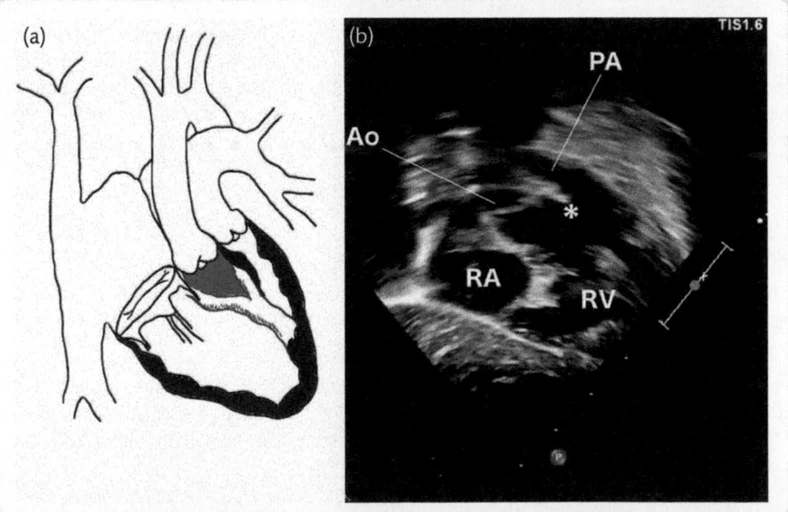

Figure 6.3 DORV with subaortic VSD and anterocephalad deviation of the outlet septum (tetralogy-type'). (a) A cartoon demonstrating the anatomy. The septomarginal trabeculation is shown in blue. The VSD, coloured in red, is cradled in the limbs of the septomarginal trabeculation. The arrangement is of tetralogy of Fallot, with anterocephalad deviation of the outlet septum, but with >50% of the aorta arising from the right ventricle. (b) An oblique subcostal echocardiographic view of the right ventricle, demonstrating the anterocephalad deviation of the outlet septum (marked with an asterisk).

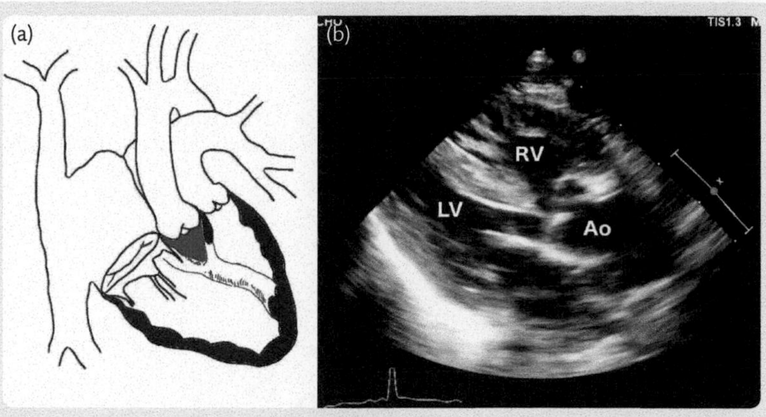

Figure 6.4 DORV with subaortic VSD without pulmonary obstruction ('VSD-type'). The cartoon in (a) demonstrates the anatomy, with the septomarginal trabeculation in blue. The VSD is coloured in red and sits in the limbs of the septomarginal trabeculation. The echocardiographic still frame in (b) is a parasternal long axis view of the heart, demonstrating the large VSD with >50% override.

DORV with subpulmonary VSD

In DORV with subpulmonary VSD (Figure 6.5), a number of arrangements are possible, but the most common variant has a VSD positioned between the two limbs of the septomarginal trabeculation and side-by-side parallel great vessels, such that the pulmonary artery arises centrally and overrides the VSD. This will usually exhibit 'transposition' physiology, with pulmonary arterial saturations higher than aortic saturations, although the clinical behaviour can vary markedly with the relative effects of systemic or pulmonary outflow obstruction, atrial mixing, and 'streaming' of blood through the heart.

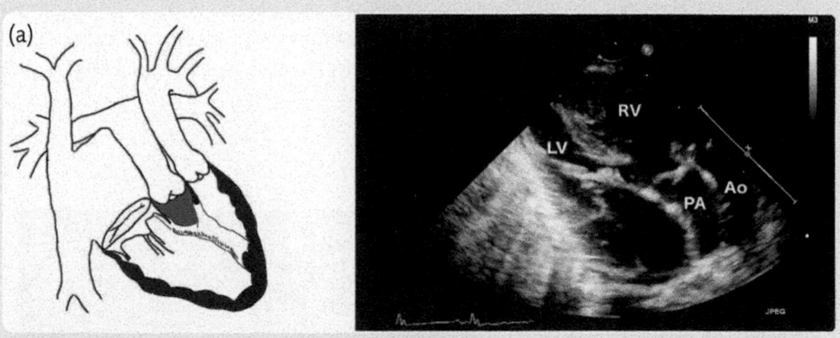

Figure 6.5 DORV with subpulmonary VSD ('TGA-type'). The cartoon in (a) demonstrates the anatomy, with the margins of the VSD and the septomarginal trabeculation in blue and areas in continuity with the left ventricle in bright red. The VSD again lies between the limbs of the septomarginal trabeculation, although the overriding vessel is now the pulmonary artery, with malposition of the great vessels. (b) shows a parasternal long axis view of the heart, with the aorta seen to lie anteriorly and the pulmonary artery coming from the centre of the heart.

Although some would term this the 'Taussig–Bing' variant, there has at times been much debate regarding appropriate use of the term and the specific implied anatomy. The original description comprised a patient with a subpulmonary VSD, side-by-side parallel great vessels, and bilateral subarterial infundibulums [9]. Once again, to avoid confusion, it is important to describe the anatomy in full, using consistent terminology.

DORV with doubly committed subarterial VSD

In this less common variant, the VSD again usually sits in between the limbs of the septomarginal trabeculation. The core difference between the above two variants is not the relative position of the outflow tracts, but the absence of muscular outlet septum such that the upper margin of the VSD is formed by both outflow tracts. This variant can be found both with and without pulmonary outflow obstruction (Figure 6.6).

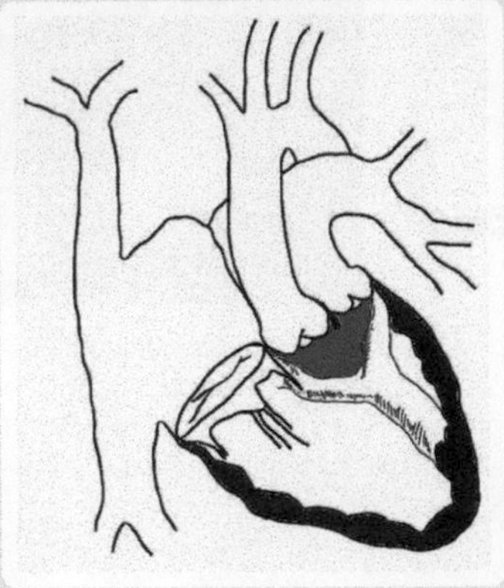

Figure 6.6 DORV with a doubly committed subarterial VSD. This cartoon demonstrates the location of the VSD, again between the limbs of the septomarginal trabeculation, but in this case, both great vessels are committed to the defect.

Within this subset, clinical presentation can vary markedly, dependent on relative obstruction through the outflow tracts. Mixing of blood is often less of a problem, as the VSD outlets to both great vessels.

DORV with non-committed (remote) VSD

This group is notable in that the VSD does not lie between the limbs of the septomarginal trabeculation and therefore does not have either great vessel as its superior border. The accompanying anatomy is extremely variable. Of the possibilities, the most common comprises malposition of the great vessels, with the aorta lying to the right of the pulmonary trunk, with either spiralling or parallel great vessels (Figure 6.7).

Clinical behaviour is dependent on a number of factors, including VSD location, possible streaming, relative outflow stenosis, and other associated lesions.

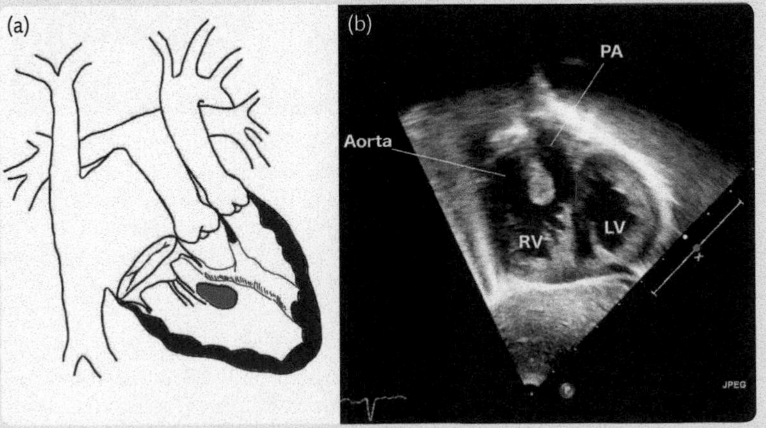

Figure 6.7 An example of DORV with a non-committed VSD. In the cartoon in (a), the septomarginal trabeculation is drawn in blue. The VSD is shown in bright red, outside of the margins of the septomarginal trabeculation. Each great vessel sits astride a separate conus, with significant distance of both great vessels from the VSD. (b) is an oblique subcostal echocardiographic view, demonstrating both great vessels arising from the right ventricle.

Clinical tip Echocardiographic localization of the VSD

This can be challenging, and a well-organized and logical scan is crucial.

The subcostal views can demonstrate the anatomy extremely clearly in the newborn and should be laboured in attempts to show the VSD in the same image as either one or both great vessels.

In cases of subaortic and subpulmonary VSDs, the interventricular communication is usually best demonstrated in the parasternal long axis view, showing overriding of one of the great vessels (i.e. forming the superior margin of the VSD, shown in Figure 6.4c and Figure 6.5c). Prior identification of the great vessels from the subcostal windows is often extremely helpful before the parasternal windows are reached.

After locating the VSD in the standard planes, the operator should try to understand and demonstrate the relationship of the outlet vessels, in simple terms (left/right, anterior/posterior) to one another. Again, although the parasternal short axis views usually offer the clearest description (Figure 6.1d), the operator will have to be clear which vessel is which, particularly if the aorta and pulmonary valves are of similar size. Discrepancy in the sizes of the great vessels can often be extremely helpful.

One final suggestion is that slow sweeps from the subcostal, apical, and parasternal windows in two dimensions and colour are valuable to help later reviewers understand the anatomy, as they demonstrate the relationship of the intracardiac structures to each other, in particular the relationship of the great arteries to each other and to the VSD.

Learning point Classification schemes in DORV

The description of the VSD location is commonly used as a classification scheme in its own right. It should, however, be noted that several other classifications have been used, quite variably through the literature and between practitioners.

One notable, relatively recently defined scheme is from the Society of Thoracic Surgeons and European Association of Cardiothoracic Surgery and uses four subtypes:

1. Fallot type (pulmonary stenosis with DORV with either subaortic or doubly committed VSD Figure 6.3). This is the most common group and can be associated with a complete AVSD.
2. Transposition type (DORV with a subpulmonary VSD Figure 6.5). This is the second most common group.
3. VSD type (DORV with subaortic or doubly committed subarterial VSD without pulmonary stenosis Figures 6.4 and 6.6).
4. DORV with non-committed VSD (Figure 6.7).

A potential advantage of this approach is that the name allied to each group better subdivides into clinical behaviour and possible surgical interventions.

Others have suggested that such classification schemes are unhelpful and fail to capture the enormous spectrum of anatomical and physiological states associated with DORV [8]. Proponents of this would argue that patients with DORV are all unique and avoidance of subdivision into groups highlights this variety.

Clinical tip Anatomical variants in DORV

Patients with the ventriculo-arterial arrangement of DORV are an excellent example of the importance of sequential segmental analysis in congenital heart disease, as variants exist at all levels.

Particular attention should be paid to:

- Anatomy of the subpulmonary and subaortic areas—subvalvar stenosis may be caused by the muscular infundibulum
- Straddling of the atrioventricular valves, which can preclude biventricular repair
- Restriction across the VSD, which can lead to significant loading of the left ventricle
- Restriction across the atrial communication which can lead to significant cyanosis in those with transposition physiology, requiring urgent septostomy
- The coexistence of coarctation which may also require urgent intervention.

Expert comment

It is important to be aware of the association of DORV with criss-cross atrioventricular connection, either concordant or discordant.

Expert comment The initial assessment

Initial assessment of the patient with DORV should involve a careful assessment of the clinical state, as well as a thorough echocardiogram. Although it is common for the echocardiogram to be comparatively long, this is vital to the understanding of the patient and may allow more expedient management decisions to be made by reducing repeated visits to the patient. A comprehensive and detailed echocardiogram should aim to describe both the anatomy and the physiology.

The immediate questions to be asked should be around potential duct dependency and the adequacy of the mixing of blood. Difficult-to-palpate femoral pulses should initiate a search for coarctation or subaortic obstruction, and marked desaturation is a pointer towards either severe pulmonary outflow obstruction or inadequate mixing. Patients exhibiting desaturation with transposition physiology and a restrictive atrial septum may benefit from balloon atrial septostomy, due to the effects of streaming and the requirement for adequate mixing at atrial level.

On day 2 of life, his oxygen saturations fell to the 50s. A repeat echocardiogram demonstrated ductal constriction and a marked increase in the peak velocity across the pulmonary outflow tract to 4 m/s. A prostaglandin infusion was commenced to maintain ductal patency, with recovery of his oxygen saturations. Following discussion at a multidisciplinary team meeting, the decision was made for him to proceed to placement of a modified Blalock–Taussig (BT) shunt, which was performed on day 9 of life, with a right-sided 3.5-mm Gore-Tex® shunt placed from the brachiocephalic artery to the right pulmonary artery via a median sternotomy incision.

Excellent post-operative progress was made, and he was extubated into air the next morning. Inotropic support was weaned and discontinued. He was discharged home 7 days later, with frequent paediatric cardiologist review as an outpatient and monitoring of feeding, weight gain, and oxygen saturations by the community nursing team (see Expert comment: Short- and medium-term risk in patients with systemic-to-pulmonary shunts, p. 80–81).

Expert comment Short- and medium-term risk in patients with systemic-to-pulmonary shunts

Patients with systemic-to-pulmonary shunts are recognized to be at particularly high risk of death, with 30-day mortality rates of between 10% and 15% from contemporary UK data, with one recent study finding improvements in 30-day mortality rates for all operations, other than systemic-to-pulmonary shunts, which have shown a statistically significant increase in mortality over the decade from 2000 to 2010 [10]. The mechanisms for this increase in mortality is likely to be multi-factorial and may, in part, relate to increasing case complexity.

From retrospective analyses, risk factors for mortality following systemic-to-pulmonary shunt in the UK population include younger age at operation, central shunts and a diagnosis of pulmonary atresia with an intact ventricular septum, Ebstein's anomaly, pulmonary atresia with single-ventricle physiology, or transposition with an intact ventricular septum [11].

Evidence of thrombus in the shunt is often found at post-mortem, and so shunt obstruction is felt to be the most common mechanism of death in these patients. Most practitioners prescribe an antiplatelet agent such as aspirin, with observational evidence of efficacy [12]. Few practitioners formally anticoagulate outside the immediate post-operative period. Careful parental counselling should take place prior to discharge, with advice to report acute desaturation, irritability, or intercurrent illness (particularly diarrhoea or vomiting), and an urgent medical review should be initiated. Waiting until the next day may not be appropriate for review of even minor reported issues.

Concerns regarding a possible obstructed shunt should be managed urgently with appropriate resuscitation and a bolus of intravenous heparin administered. Support with extracorporeal membrane oxygenation may be urgently required prior to catheter or surgical intervention.

Home monitoring programmes have been used in patients with hypoplastic left heart syndrome (HLHS) since the turn of the century [13], with wide-scale adoption over the last decade. Given the high observed mortality in patients with systemic-to-pulmonary shunts, some have also added patients with systemic-to-pulmonary shunts to their home monitoring programmes [14]. Although the finer details of these programmes vary between units, the general themes include parental training and daily saturations and weight monitoring, with the parents given certain calling criteria to report to the medical team. Our institutional feeling is that both patients with HLHS and those with systemic-to-pulmonary shunts carry similar high rates of mortality and should be monitored in the same way.

An MRI scan performed at 5 months of age confirmed the echocardiographic findings and also demonstrated mild stenosis at the insertion of the BT shunt into the right pulmonary artery (see Expert comment: Multimodality imaging in DORV, p. 81).

Expert comment Multimodality imaging in DORV

The standard two-dimensional echocardiogram is by far the most important study in patients with DORV. A number of other modalities can, however, be used in addition, to better understand the anatomy and plan surgical intervention.

One extremely valuable technique is three-dimensional echocardiography, with an approach described by Pushparajah et al. [15] for cropping the volumes in such a way as to help visualize the VSD and also to plan potential patch placement. MRI also allows cross-sectional imaging and reformatting, although it is likely to require general anaesthesia using current technologies in young patients.

Transoesophageal imaging can also be extremely helpful to delineate the anatomy in the context of atrioventricular valves straddling the ventricular septum.

One other method currently available is three-dimensional printing, which allows the surgeon to plan his intervention in detail prior to the operation [16].

He remained well and gained weight steadily before elective admission at 15 months of age and weighing 9.6 kg for surgical repair (see Learning point: Surgical repair and outcomes in DORV, p. 81). Via a median sternotomy, his VSD was enlarged and a tunnelled closure performed to commit the left ventricle to the aorta. The pulmonary outflow tract was enlarged, with a porcine pericardial patch and a pericardial monocusp valve placed, along with augmentation of the right pulmonary artery and takedown of the BT shunt.

Learning point Surgical repair and outcomes in DORV

The wide spectrum of anatomy represented by patients with DORV, as well as the array of lesions associated with DORV, inevitably leads to the employment of a wide array of surgical strategies.

The first decision to be made is the feasibility of a biventricular repair. Barriers to this will usually comprise either ventricular hypoplasia or significant surgically irrevocable straddling of the atrioventricular valves. One large single-unit cohort of 393 patients has suggested that higher re-intervention rates associated with biventricular repair in borderline candidates encourage their leaning towards Fontan-style palliation [17].

Upon a decision to proceed to biventricular repair, the first aim (and in the case of a VSD-type DORV, the sole aim) is to close the VSD such as to commit the left ventricle to the nearest outflow tract. A comparatively large patch is often required, forming a 'tunnel' through to the outflow tract (Figure 6.2d). At times (such as in our example patient), enlargement of the VSD at the septum is required prior to closure to avoid left ventricular outflow tract obstruction. One should also note that the patch will also occupy a portion of the right ventricle.

Potential methods to complete the repair are numerous and can include:

- **Augmentation of the pulmonary outflow tract** (analogous to tetralogy of Fallot repair)—the most common intervention for tetralogy-type DORV
- **Arterial switch procedure**—to make the left ventricle the subaortic ventricle in DORV with subpulmonary VSD
- **Rastelli procedure** (tunnelled closure of the VSD committing the left ventricle to the aorta, alongside placement of a right ventricle-to-pulmonary artery conduit)—performed on any variant where the intended pulmonary outflow is severely atretic and not amenable to repair.

A number of other approaches have been described for specific situations, including the double root translocation (Nikaidoh procedure), the Yasui procedure (Rastelli procedure with a Damus–Kaye–Stansel anastomosis), or the *réparation à l'étage ventriculaire* (REV) procedure.

The age and weight at which complete repair is performed can vary markedly between patients, depending on the planned procedure, clinical status (including growth trajectory), and previous palliative procedures undertaken. The parents should be carefully counselled that there may be changes to both planned procedure and timing of the procedure, depending on clinical progress.

Surgical planning is therefore of vital importance. Detailed description of the anatomy is required, as well as careful review of available data with the surgeon in a multidisciplinary team prior to intervention.

At the time of surgery, the bypass time was 225 minutes with cross-clamp of 177 minutes. Intra- and post-operative imaging demonstrated satisfactory post-operative repair, with normal function of both ventricles, unobstructed outflow tracts, and no residual VSD. On day 2, he developed a junctional ectopic tachycardia, without haemodynamic compromise, and was successfully managed with an amiodarone infusion. His 7-day intensive care stay was further complicated by the development of a metapneumovirus respiratory tract infection.

He was extubated 7 days after his surgery and went on to make good progress, with discharge home 11 days after his operation.

Clinical tip Long-term follow-up in patients following surgical repair of DORV

Patients following DORV repair will require lifelong follow-up by a paediatric cardiologist. For mixed populations undergoing both single- and two-ventricle repairs, long-term survival in large, single-centre cohort studies have varied hugely from 56% at 15 years [17] to over 90% [18].

All those undergoing biventricular repair will require specific attention to the subaortic region, as the VSD patch (Figure 6.2d) becomes an integral part of the left ventricular outflow tract, with late left ventricular outflow tract obstruction a well-recognized complication [19].

A good understanding of the repair performed is vital to understand potential areas of concern at follow-up. Specific examples include the branch pulmonary arteries and evidence of regional wall motion abnormality following the arterial switch procedure, and assessment of the right ventricle-to-pulmonary artery conduit following a Rastelli procedure.

Although a clinical history, examination, and an echocardiogram form the core of long-term evaluation, MRI is becoming a frequently utilized adjunct, particularly once children are old enough to tolerate this investigation without a general anaesthetic. A specific example is for the assessment of the branch pulmonary and coronary arteries late following the arterial switch procedure, imaging of which can be difficult in patients of adult size using echocardiography.

Discussion

Patients with DORV comprise only approximately 1% of congenital heart disease but, as described, comprise a wide spectrum of both anatomical and management options. DORV is merely a description of the ventriculo-arterial connection.

Careful, detailed, and comprehensive preoperative imaging is vital to demonstrate the anatomy to the surgeon prior to intervention, so that appropriate planning can take place. A number of modalities can be utilized and are often complementary, with two-dimensional echocardiography remaining the primary modality for understanding of both anatomy and haemodynamics.

A large variety of surgical interventions can be performed, depending on the specific anatomy and associated lesions, and associated long-term outcomes are consequently variable.

A final word from the expert

The huge spectrum of disease and the number of management options often make patients with DORV both an extremely enjoyable intellectual challenge and a source of difficulty for trainees.

Nomenclature in the field can feel opaque to the beginner, and we have endeavoured to clarify some of the frequently encountered areas of confusion. Use of the language and system of sequential segmental analysis provides a framework for simplification of understanding of DORV and is a significant improvement since the use of the term 'partial transposition' in the early literature.

The two-dimensional echocardiogram continues to be the most important investigation, and a careful, logical study is vital. Echocardiography in DORV is often a good test of the ability of a trainee to perform a complete anatomical study, describe the physiology, and demonstrate an understanding of the concepts behind the sequential segmental analysis.

Acknowledgement

Our thanks to Mr Nicola Viola for his advice and drafting of the cartoons in Figures 6.3 to 6.7.

References

1. Øyen N, Poulsen G, Boyd HA, Wohlfahrt J, Jensen PKA, Melbye M. Recurrence of congenital heart defects in families. *Circulation* 2009;120:295–301.
2. Gill HK, Splitt M, Sharland GK, Simpson JM. Patterns of recurrence of congenital heart disease. *J Am Coll Cardiol* 2003;42:923–9.
3. Obler D, Juraszek AL, Smoot LB, Natowicz MR. Double outlet right ventricle: aetiologies and associations. *J Med Genet* 2008;45:481–97.
4. Shieh JTC, Bittles AH, Hudgins L. Consanguinity and the risk of congenital heart disease. *Am J Med Genet A* 2012;158A:1236–41.
5. Walters HL, Mavroudis C, Tchervenkov CI, Jacobs JP, Lacour-Gayet F, Jacobs ML. Congenital Heart Surgery Nomenclature and Database Project: double outlet right ventricle. *Ann Thorac Surg* 2000;69(4 Suppl):S249–63.

6. Anderson RH, McCarthy K, Cook AC. Continuing medical education. Double outlet right ventricle. *Cardiol Young* 2001;11:329–44.
7. Mahle WT, Martinez R, Silverman N, Cohen MS, Anderson RH. Anatomy, echocardiography, and surgical approach to double outlet right ventricle. *Cardiol Young* 2008;18:39–13.
8. Wilkinson JL, Eastaugh LJ, Anderson RH. Double outlet right ventricle. In: Anderson RH, Baker EJ, Penny DJ, Redington AN, Rigby ML, Wernovsky G, editors. *Paediatric Cardiology*, 3rd edition. Philadelphia, PA: Churchill Livingstone, 2010; pp. 837–57.
9. Van Praagh R. What is the Taussig–Bing malformation? *Circulation* 1968;38:445–9.
10. Brown KL, Crowe S, Franklin R, et al. Trends in 30-day mortality rate and case mix for paediatric cardiac surgery in the UK between 2000 and 2010. *Open Heart* 2015;2:e000157–7.
11. Dorobantu DM, Pandey R, Sharabiani MT, et al. Indications and results of systemic to pulmonary shunts: results from a national database. *Eur J Cardiothorac Surg* 2016;49:1553–63.
12. Li JS, Yow E, Berezny KY, et al. Clinical outcomes of palliative surgery including a systemic-to-pulmonary artery shunt in infants with cyanotic congenital heart disease: does aspirin make a difference? *Circulation* 2007;116:293–7.
13. Ghanayem NS, Hoffman GM, Mussatto KA, et al. Home surveillance program prevents interstage mortality after the Norwood procedure. *J Thorac Cardiovasc Surg* 2003;126:1367–75.
14. Dobrolet NC, Nieves JA, Welch EM, et al. New approach to interstage care for palliated high-risk patients with congenital heart disease. *J Thorac Cardiovasc Surg* 2011;142:855–60.
15. Pushparajah K, Barlow A, Tran V-H, et al. A systematic three-dimensional echocardiographic approach to assist surgical planning in double outlet right ventricle. *Echocardiography* 2012;30:234–8.
16. Farooqi KM, Uppu SC, Nguyen K, et al. Application of virtual three-dimensional models for simultaneous visualization of intracardiac anatomic relationships in double outlet right ventricle. *Pediatr Cardiol* 2016;37:90–8.
17. Bradley TJ, Karamlou T, Kulik A, et al. Determinants of repair type, reintervention, and mortality in 393 children with double-outlet right ventricle. *J Thorac Cardiovasc Surg* 2007;134:967–73.e6.
18. Brown JW, Ruzmetov M, Okada Y, Vijay P, Turrentine MW. Surgical results in patients with double outlet right ventricle: a 20-year experience. *Ann Thorac Surg* 2001;72:1630–5.
19. Li S, Ma K, Hu S, et al. Surgical outcomes of 380 patients with double outlet right ventricle who underwent biventricular repair. *J Thorac Cardiovasc Surg* 2014;148:817–24.

CASE

7 Cardiac transplantation

Filip Kucera

Expert commentary Michael Burch

Case history

A 4-year-old girl presented to her local emergency department with a 2-week history of cough, increasing shortness of breath, and low-grade fever. She had been previously investigated for failure to thrive and anorexia. There was no other significant medical history of note, and her antenatal course was unremarkable. On examination, she was well perfused and, although pale, was fully saturated. She had normal heart sounds, with a 2/6 systolic murmur over the apex and good-volume peripheral pulses. Her work of breathing was mildly increased, and there were a few sparse crackles on the left side of her chest. The abdomen was soft, with a significantly enlarged liver.

Blood results were unremarkable, showing only mild anaemia and a slightly raised C-reactive protein (CRP). Chest X-ray (Figure 7.1) showed a severely enlarged heart and increased vascular markings bilaterally. Echocardiography showed a markedly dilated left ventricle with severe mitral regurgitation, suggestive of dilated cardiomyopathy. Based on these findings, she was transferred to a paediatric cardiology centre.

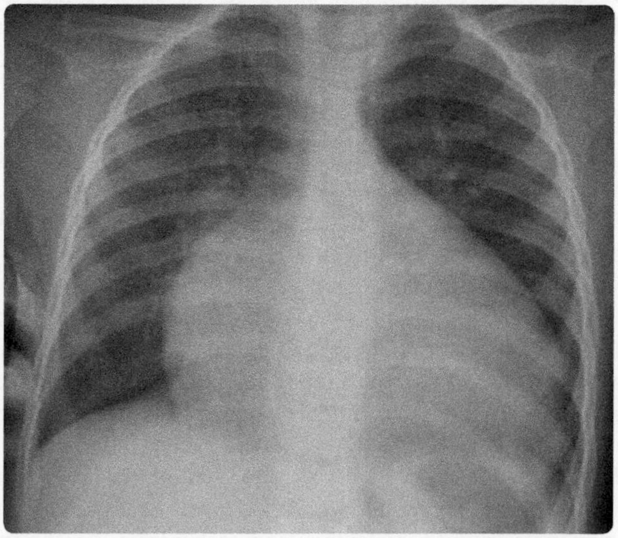

Figure 7.1 Chest X-ray showing prominent cardiomegaly with pulmonary plethora.

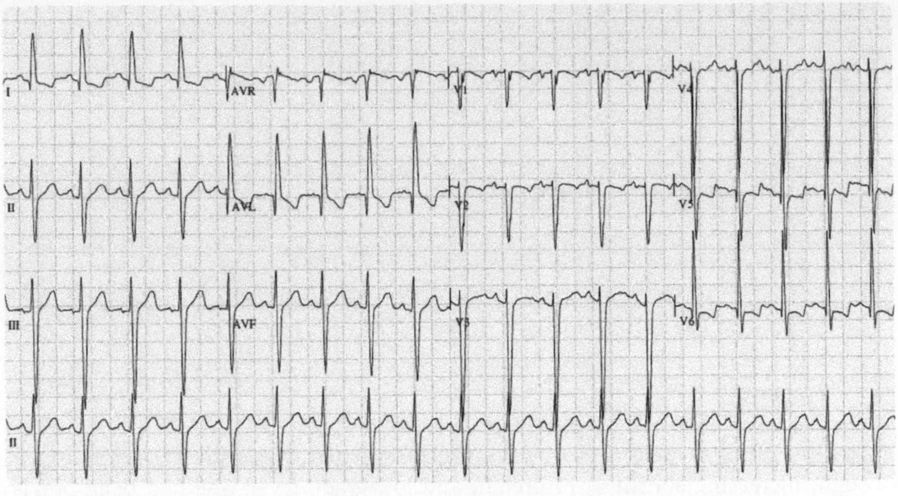

Figure 7.2 A 12-lead ECG showing abnormal T wave inversions in leads I, aVL, and V5–V6.

On admission, a repeat echocardiogram demonstrated a markedly reduced left ventricular systolic function with an ejection fraction of 25%, with preserved right ventricular systolic function. Her coronary artery origins were normal, and there was no evidence of aortic stenosis or coarctation of the aorta. She was in sinus tachycardia and was noted to have widespread ischaemic changes on the ECG (Figure 7.2).

She was clinically well perfused and alert, with a normal blood pressure and a low lactate on arterial blood gas. As such, inotropic support was not required. She was started on oral digoxin, captopril, and intravenous furosemide and was fluid-restricted, aiming for a negative balance. As spontaneous contrast was noted on echocardiography, aspirin was added to prevent clot formation in the dilated left ventricle. Over the next few days, her respiratory rate came down and her liver reduced in size. After 2 weeks, she was successfully discharged home on oral drug therapy.

Clinical tip

Patients with an anomalous origin of the left coronary artery from the pulmonary artery usually present with unexplained left ventricular dysfunction in early infancy at about 2–3 months of age. Therefore, it is extremely important to demonstrate normal left coronary artery origin, especially in this age group. The left coronary artery origin can be well visualized from the parasternal short axis, but also from the apical five-chamber view. Antegrade diastolic flow should also be demonstrated.

An extensive dilated cardiomyopathy blood screen showed high pro-BNP and normal troponin I and CK-MB. Viral serologies and metabolic screen were both negative. In the meantime, both parents and her older sister were seen by a cardiologist and had a normal examination.

Despite an initial amelioration at the time of discharge from hospital, there was no further decrease in pro-BNP when reviewed in outpatients. Clinically, she remained similar as she was when discharged. Low-dose carvedilol was introduced, in addition to other heart failure drugs. No arrhythmias were recorded on a 24-hour ECG tape.

Expert comment

B-type natriuretic peptide (BNP) is a hormone secreted by the ventricles in response to high left ventricular filling pressures and excessive wall tension. The levels are used in the diagnosis of heart failure, including diastolic dysfunction. The N-terminal fragment of BNP (NT-pro-BNP) is also used in clinical practice to monitor heart failure. Both can also predict the risk of death and cardiovascular events.

Three months later, she was readmitted to her local hospital because of increased breathlessness and a lack of appetite. This was accompanied by an increase in pro-BNP. She was again stabilized on intravenous furosemide and was successfully discharged a week later on an increased dose of diuretics. The carvedilol was suspended in view of this acute decompensation. Despite maximal drug therapy, she made no clinical progress. Echocardiography continued to show impaired ventricular systolic function.

Although she was stable for a while, she was readmitted from clinic just over a month after her previous admission with a 2-day history of abdominal pain and vomiting. She was pale, sweaty, breathless, and tachycardic. As she was also cool peripherally and hypotensive, she was stabilized on a milrinone infusion, resulting in improved haemodynamics and lactate levels. She had a mildly deranged renal and hepatic function, with a markedly raised pro-BNP.

She became less symptomatic over the next few days, although she did not tolerate weaning of milrinone. In view of her worsening symptoms, static clinical progress despite maximal medical therapy, and milrinone dependence, she was discussed at the multidisciplinary meeting and was urgently listed for transplant. The decision was made to 'bridge' her to transplantation using a Berlin Heart™ ventricular assist device (VAD) supporting the left ventricle only, as there was no right ventricular dysfunction. The procedure was planned for the following day.

Expert comment Transplant listing

In the UK, priority is given to patients on the urgent list in whom survival without transplantation is likely to be very short. To qualify, they need to be bridged to transplantation with a mechanical circulatory support, such as extracorporeal membrane oxygenation (ECMO), Berlin Heart™ VAD, or high-dose inotropes, and ventilated. The non-urgent waiting list is for more stable patients and has longer waiting times. Sadly, as many as a third of children are never transplanted and die whilst waiting for a new heart. The waiting times depend on several factors that determine the suitability of a donor organ for the child such as weight, blood group, human leucocyte antigen (HLA) antibody testing, and tissue typing results. Most nations have priority listing schemes, but the criteria vary [1].

The pre-transplant serology was negative; her blood group was O Rh (D)-positive, and she had high anti-A and anti-B blood group antibody titres, making ABO-incompatible transplant not possible. Panel-reactive antibodies (PRAs) were negative (0%), demonstrating that she had no antibodies against common HLAs. Historically, she had never received any blood transfusions or cardiac surgery using 'foreign' material like homografts that would lead to anti-HLA antibody production. As such, she was considered **not** to be 'sensitized' and was unlikely to have an immunological reaction against potential donor hearts. No other contraindications to transplant were found.

Learning point Pre-transplant investigations

Blood tests:

1. Routine blood tests: full blood count, coagulation profile, extended biochemistry
2. Serology: herpes simplex virus (HSV), varicella-zoster virus (VZV), Ebstein–Barr virus (EBV), cytomegalovirus (CMV), rubella, measles, *Toxoplasma*, hepatitis B, hepatitis C, HIV
3. Immunology:
   a. HLA typing
   b. PRA testing—measures the amount of pre-existing antibodies targeting HLA antigens present in the general population. It is a marker of sensitization of the recipient. High titre of anti-HLA antibodies against a potential donor contraindicates the transplant going ahead
   c. Anti-A or anti-B blood group antibodies (isohaemagglutinin titres) in ABO-incompatible transplant candidates

Other investigations:

- Chest X-ray
- Echo
- ECG, 24-hour Holter
- Abdominal ultrasound
- Exercise test, 6-minute walk test
- Cardiac catheter (not routinely in dilated cardiomyopathy)
- Bacterial swabs, sputum, and urine sample.

Expert comment

Although the majority of transplants are ABO-compatible, an ABO mismatch transplant can be performed in very young children. Their immune system is immature and does not reject organs from a different blood group, unless high titres of preformed anti-A and anti-B antibodies (isohaemagglutinins) are present. Therefore, anti-A and anti-B antibodies are closely monitored in ABO mismatch transplant candidates.

The exact level at which an ABO-incompatible cross-match is acceptable is also dependent on recipient circumstances and institutional policies.

She rapidly deteriorated and decompensated after multiple runs of ventricular tachycardia. With diminishing cardiac output unresponsive to conventional therapy, it was decided to initiate emergent veno-arterial (VA) ECMO. She stabilized over the next few days and was transferred to theatre for Berlin Heart™ left ventricular assist device (LVAD) insertion.

An apical inflow cannula and an ascending aortic outflow cannula were inserted. Biventricular support was not required, as there was reasonable right ventricular function on transoesophageal echocardiography and the central venous pressure remained low throughout. On return from theatre, she required low-dose inotropic support. Histopathology revealed no signs of myocarditis, but non-specific changes with a moderate degree of myocardial fibrosis.

She was extubated soon after LVAD implantation. As per protocol, she was started on heparin 24 hours later. Over the following days, aspirin and dypiridamole were introduced as dual antiplatelet therapy. The Berlin Heart™ VAD was working well and no clots were seen in the circuit. Clinically, she had a normal cardiac output. Two weeks later, she progressed to the cardiac ward and heparin was switched to warfarin.

Learning point Mechanical circulatory support in children

Despite recent advances in medical therapy, treatment options are very limited in patients with end-stage heart failure. In those cases refractory to maximal medical treatment, mechanical circulatory support is used as a bridge to heart transplantation or to recovery. The mechanical pump receives blood from the heart and pumps it back out into the circulation (Table 7.1).

The device usually does not fully replace the weakened heart but significantly assists in maintaining the circulation. Three types of support are used by most centres in children: ECMO, Berlin Heart™, and HeartWare™.

ECMO

ECMO stands for extracorporeal membrane oxygenation. The machine oxygenates blood from the patient, clears carbon dioxide, and rewarms it before returning it back to the circulation. The ECMO circuit consists of a pump, an oxygenator, a heater, and an inflow (venous) and outflow (arterial cannula) (Figure 7.3).

The venous cannula is positioned in the right internal jugular vein (Figure 7.4) and continuously sucks blood from the right atrium. In older children, an additional cannula in the femoral vein is usually required as blood flow across the neck cannula alone is not sufficient. The arterial cannula is inserted into the right common carotid artery and the right side of the brain is perfused, thanks to the presence of the circle of Willis. This type of ECMO is also called veno-arterial (VA) ECMO and bypasses the heart, allowing it to 'rest'. The veno-venous ECMO acts like a ventilator and replaces the lungs only.

ECMO is the most frequent type of circulatory support used in children requiring constant use of heparin. It provides immediate biventricular and respiratory assistance and may be lifesaving in cardiac arrest unresponsive to conventional resuscitation (ECMO-CPR) [2]. It can be used in small children (including newborns), as well as in adults. There is, however, a significant risk for uncontrolled bleeding and clot formation in the circuit, leading to neurological sequelae, as well as sepsis.

The use of ECMO support provides only short-term treatment to a maximum of 3–4 weeks often, but not exclusively, following major cardiac surgery.

Table 7.1 Mechanical circulatory support in children: summary

	ECMO	Berlin Heart™	Heart Ware™
Weight at implantation	Usually >2.5 kg	Usually >4 kg	Usually >15–20 kg
Duration of support	Short term	Long term	Long term
Discharge home	Not possible	Not possible	Possible

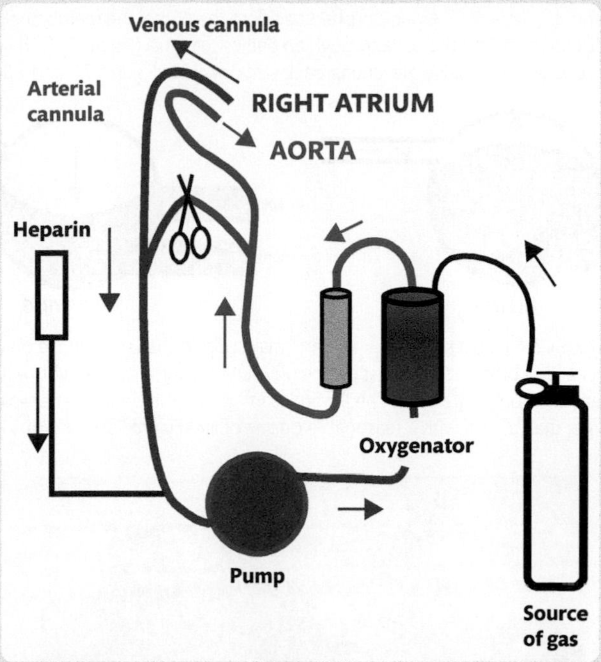

Figure 7.3 VA-ECMO circuit.

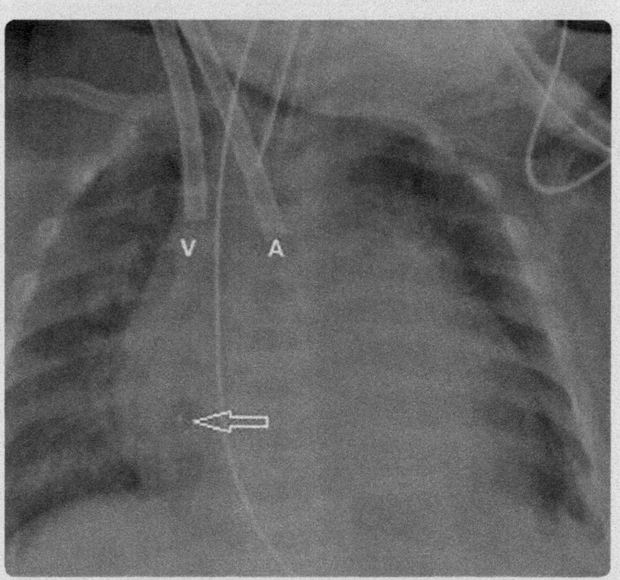

Figure 7.4 Patient with neck ECMO cannulation. A, arterial cannula; V, venous cannula. Arrow shows the tip of the venous cannula.

Berlin Heart™

The paucity of donor organs and long waiting times led to the development of long-term VADs. The Berlin Heart™ consists of a simple air-driven pulsatile flow device that is outside the body. It has a blood- and an air-filled side, separated by a flexible membrane. As air is pulled out of the pump, the membrane separating the two sides is drawn back and blood is sucked into the pump from the left ventricle through an apical inflow cannula (Figure 7.5). As air is pushed back into the pump, the membrane is pushed forward, pumping blood back into the aorta through an outflow cannula (Figure 7.6). The pump and both cannulae are separated by a valve preventing backward flow. (See Figures 7.7 and 7.8.)

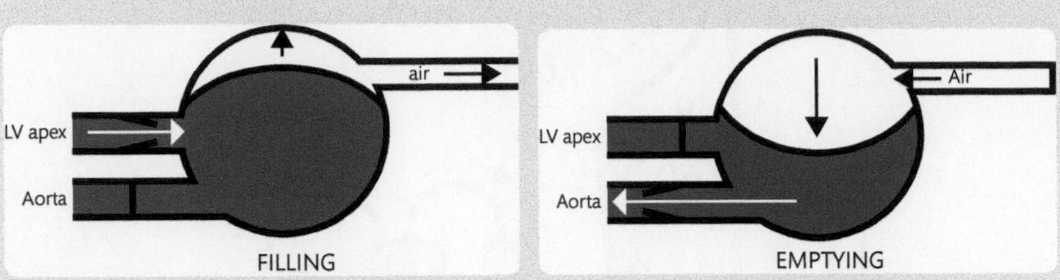

Figures 7.5 (left) and 7.6 (right) The Berlin Heart™ may support the left ventricle only (LVAD) (Figure 7.7) or can act as a biventricular assist device (BiVAD) assisting also the right ventricle, in which case two separate pumps are used. The Berlin Heart™ allows the bridge to transplantation to sometimes be longer than a year, with a reasonable quality of life (Figure 7.8).

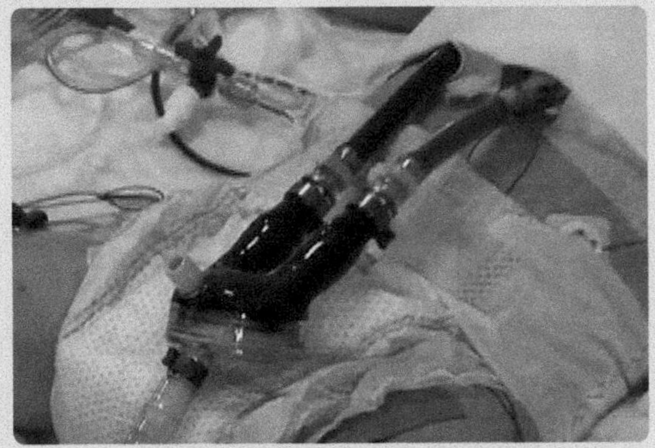

Figure 7.7 Berlin Heart™ chamber and cannulae after implantation.

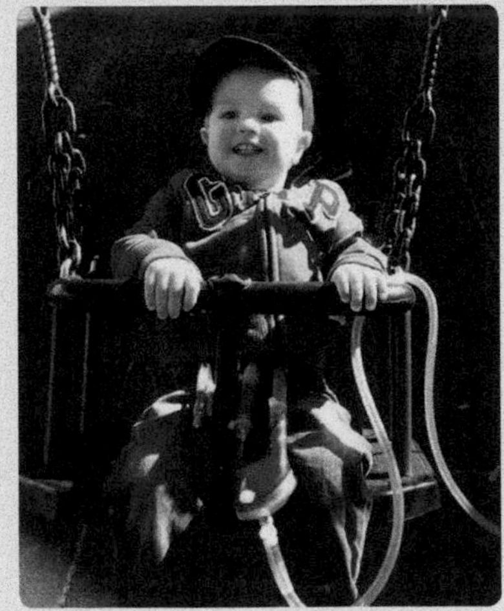

Figure 7.8 Patient with Berlin Heart™ on a swing (with parents' permission).

The device allows stable children to go out from the ward under supervision. Unfortunately, the risk of stroke is approximately 30%; that is why the whole circuit needs to be checked for the presence of clots on a regular basis several times a day and patients need to be anticoagulated (warfarin or heparin) with dual antiplatelet therapy. Children on Berlin Heart™ are on the urgent transplant list in the UK [3].

Heart Ware™

Heart Ware™ is an internal long-term support, and unlike the Berlin Heart™, patients can be discharged from hospital. In children, it is used to support the left ventricle only. It is a continuous-flow device, and the pulse is clinically present only if there is spontaneous ejection. It uses a centrifugal blood pump that is implanted in the pericardial space. Therefore, the system is limited to patients with a weight of more than approximately 15–20 kg.

An inflow apical cannula is integrated with the pump and sucks blood from the left ventricle (Figures 7.9–7.11). Blood is pumped back into the aorta through an outflow cannula. The pump is connected via a percutaneous driveline to an external controller unit.

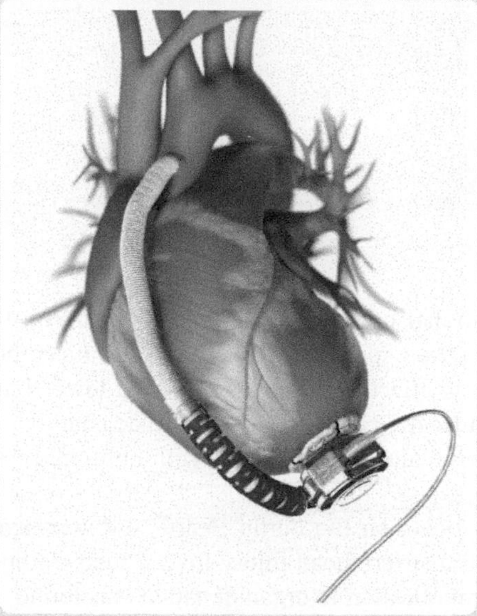

Figure 7.9 Heart Ware™ (with Heart Ware™).
© Heartware (https://www.heartware.com/resources)

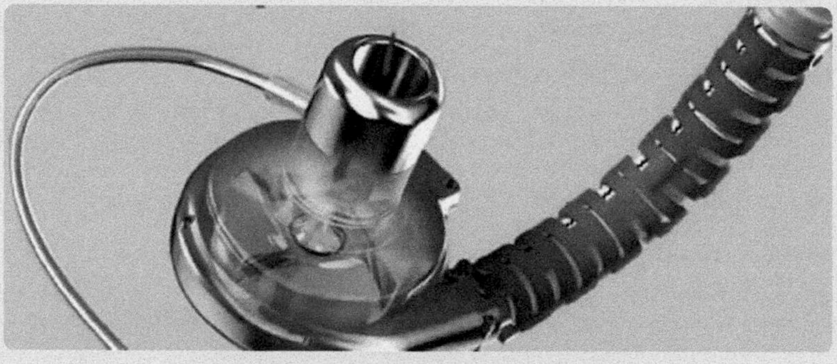

Figure 7.10 Detail of Heart Ware™ pump with inflow (apical) cannula.
With permission from Heart Ware™.

Patients on Heart Ware™ have a good quality of life and can stay at home. For this reason, Heart Ware™ is the first-choice device in older children with reasonable right ventricular function and good social background. Heart Ware™ patients are non-urgently listed in the UK, unless some device-related problems occur (like frequent driveline infections, etc.). Patients need to be anticoagulated and require daily driveline dressing change.

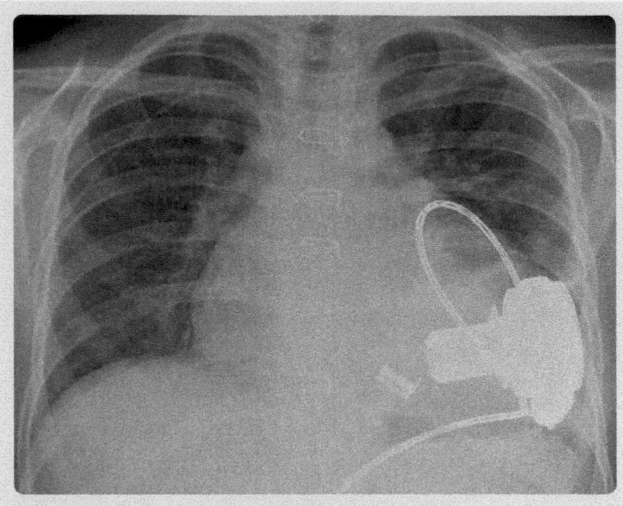

Figure 7.11 Chest X- ray from a patient with Heart Ware™.

Despite her international normalized ratio (INR) being on the therapeutic range, 2 months after being on the Berlin Heart™, she had an acute embolic stroke in the right middle cerebral territory, affecting her left upper and lower limbs. No obvious clots were seen in the Berlin Heart™ circuit or in any cardiac chamber on echocardiography. Fortunately, she recovered almost completely, with only mild residual left upper limb weakness.

Three months after being on the Berlin Heart™, a donor heart from a 10-year-old child who had suffered a severe head injury from a road traffic accident was offered to our centre. No contraindication to organ donation was found. Blood group of donor and recipient matched and no donor-specific HLA antibodies were noted. Following the usual consent procedures, the donor organ retrieval was coordinated in order to minimize the ischaemic time.

Expert comment Organ donation

Donation after diagnosis of death by neurological criteria

Donation after brain death is considered if there is evidence of irreversible cessation of brainstem function. Enough time must be given for all reversible causes, such as sedation, muscle relaxation, hypothermia, and other potentially reversible circulatory, metabolic, and endocrine conditions, to be excluded. Brain death is confirmed in the absence of brainstem reflexes and no respiratory response to hypercarbia.

Donation after circulatory determination of death

Donation after circulatory determination of death is performed in patients who are not brain-dead but have a severe brain or other unsurvivable injury justifying a planned withdrawal of intensive care. After termination of care leading to cardiopulmonary arrest, the patient continues to be fully monitored for 5 minutes. Following this period, the patient is checked for absence of pulse, apnoea, and absent brainstem reflexes. Following that, organs are immediately retrieved in order to minimize warm ischaemic damage.

Learning point

General indications for cardiac transplantation

- Refractory cardiogenic shock, heart failure requiring continuous intravenous inotropic or mechanical circulatory support
- Peak oxygen consumption (VO_2) of 14 ml/kg/min (without a beta-blocker) or VO_2 of 12 ml/kg/min (with a beta-blocker) or VO_2 ≤50% of predicted
- Progressive deterioration of cardiac function or functional capacity despite maximal medical treatment
- Unacceptable quality of life, inability to perform daily activities
- Congenital heart disease unsuitable for surgical palliation or repair
- Malignant life-threatening arrhythmias resistant to medical treatment, catheter ablation, surgery, or implantable cardioverter–defibrillator
- Progressive pulmonary hypertension that could potentially become a contraindication to heart transplantation in the future [1]

Contraindications to cardiac transplantation

- Non-reversible elevation of pulmonary vascular resistance to >6 WU/m^2 (normal upper limit <1.5 WU/m^2) or a transpulmonary gradient of >15 mmHg (normal upper limit <12 mmHg), both presenting a major risk for post-operative right ventricular failure
- Active or recently diagnosed malignancy
- Major brain pathology with poor or uncertain neurological prognosis
- Severe progressive metabolic disorder with multi-organ involvement
- Significant dysmorphism or genetic syndrome with poor or uncertain prognosis
- Severe irreversible end-organ failure (pulmonary and/or renal and/or hepatic)
- Small size, prematurity
- Major risk for drug non-compliance, lack of family support
- Mental illness, drug, tobacco, alcohol abuse
- Severe active infection or sepsis
- Relative contraindications: HIV, chronic hepatitis B and C infection

Surgical technique

She underwent orthotopic cardiac transplantation (Figure 7.12) and Berlin Heart™ removal. The total ischaemic time was just under 3 hours. Transient DDD pacing was required for complete heart block and a perioperative transoesophageal echocardiogram performed in theatre showed mild left ventricular systolic dysfunction, and the patient was transferred to the intensive care unit on milrinone and adrenaline. She was extubated on the third post-operative day with normal ventricular function.

Immunosuppression consisted of basiliximab given pre-transplant and on day 4 post-transplantation; high-dose intravenous methylprednisolone was changed to oral prednisolone. Long-term immunosuppression was with mycophenolate mofetil and tacrolimus (monitored with drug levels). The first cardiac biopsy showed no cellular or antibody-mediated rejection.

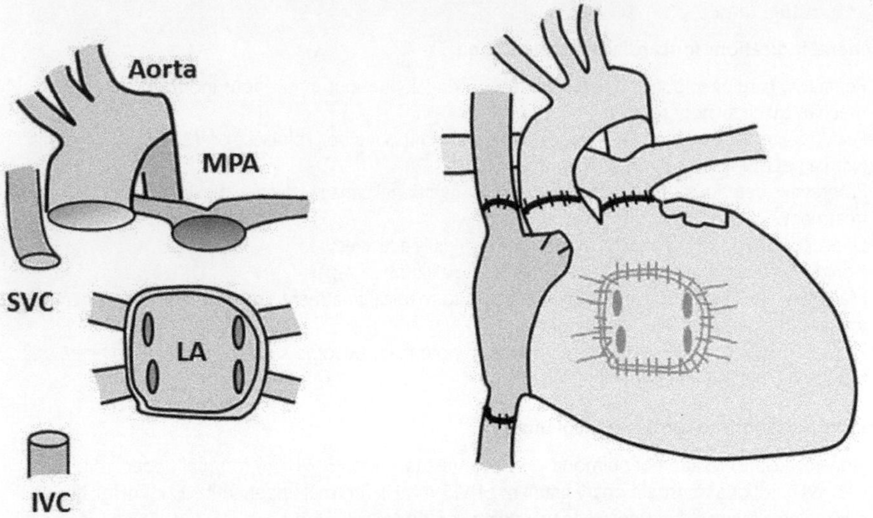

Figure 7.12 Orthotopic heart transplant: the bicaval technique. The recipient's cardioectomy is performed first, leaving a left atrial cuff with pulmonary vein orifices. The donor's heart is subsequently implanted, and left atrial, inferior vena cava, superior vena cava, aortic, and pulmonary anastomoses are carried out. IVC, inferior vena cava; LA, left atrium; MPA, main pulmonary artery; SVC, superior vena cava.

Learning point Immunosuppression after transplantation

There is no agreed international protocol for immunosuppression in paediatric transplantation.

Immunosuppressive treatment consists of an induction phase and a maintenance phase. Cellular rejection is most likely immediately after transplant and decreases with time. The intensity of treatment is decreased over a period of several months to maintenance therapy. It uses the lowest level of immunosuppression that is able to prevent rejection whilst minimizing drug toxicities. Over-immunosuppression should also be avoided as it increases the risk of malignancy and infection.

Immunosuppressive drugs

- **Corticosteroids**, such as prednisolone and methylprednisolone, cause a reduction in peripheral blood lymphocytes. If there is no rejection detected on routine biopsy, doses are progressively weaned to a maintenance dose and subsequently stopped. Adverse effects include electrolyte imbalances, hypertension, hyperglycaemia, growth retardation, osteoporosis, and myopathy.
- **Antiproliferative agents**, such as mycophenolate mofetil (MMF) and azathioprine (AZA), inhibit purine metabolism, resulting in the synthesis of dysfunctional DNA in lymphocytes. The use of MMF may be limited by adverse gastrointestinal symptoms (such as diarrhoea and abdominal pain). The major side effects of AZA include myelosuppression and hepatotoxicity.
- **Calcineurin inhibitors** include tacrolimus and ciclosporin. There is a lower incidence of rejection with tacrolimus, compared to ciclosporin, and therefore, tacrolimus is the preferred agent. Tacrolimus inhibits transcription of genes encoding interleukin 2 (IL-2) and IL-2 receptors. Toxicity usually presents as nephrotoxicity, hypertension, and encephalopathy with seizures.
- **mTOR (mammalian target of rapamycin) inhibitors**, such as sirolimus and everolimus, also block IL-2 (but different mechanism of action to calcineurin inhibitors). mTOR inhibitors are often used in patients with chronic renal dysfunction as they have low nephrotoxicity.
- **Immunosuppressive antibodies** are used as induction agents and lead to a high degree of T-cell suppression immediately after transplant, when the risk of rejection is highest. They allow calcineurin inhibitors to be introduced when renal function is stable and thus reduce their nephrotoxicity.

Clinical tip

Post-transplant immunosuppression has a vital importance in graft survival. Various factors can influence plasma drug concentrations and can lead to subtherapeutic drug levels or cause drug toxicity. Therefore, addition of a new drug with the potential for interaction should always be discussed with a transplant cardiologist.

Other commonly used drugs

Post-transplant hypertension is common and many patients require at least one blood pressure-lowering agent. CMV, fungal, and pneumocystis prophylaxis is needed for several months after transplant. Lipid-lowering drugs, such as pravastatin, are used in some institutions before discharge from hospital.

She suffered from early post-transplant hypertension, which was partly due to the side effects of tacrolimus and steroids, and was treated with antihypertensive medication.

On day 10, she was transferred to the cardiac ward and her parents were carefully instructed on how to administer transplant medications. A 24-hour ECG tape showed sinus rhythm with no evidence of atrioventricular block. She was discharged home on day 15, with follow-up in the heart transplant clinic. She returned back to school 3 months later and restarted her ballet classes.

Learning point Prognosis after cardiac transplantion

The overall survival of paediatric patients post-cardiac transplantation is determined by several conditions listed below. The survival rates are shown in Figure 7.13.

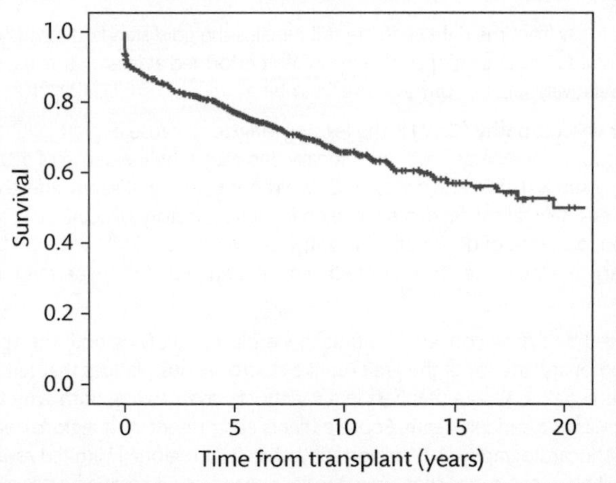

Figure 7.13 Survival after cardiac transplantation (in years) in paediatric patients from Great Ormond Street Hospital.

Primary graft failure (PVG) is a major cause of mortality within the first 30 days. It manifests with severe cardiac dysfunction early after surgery. Nowadays transplant centres face a significant organ shortage with progressively longer waiting lists. Therefore, in very sick patients with little alternatives and no reserves, some institutions accept hearts from donors that are not ideal (marginal hearts). This represents an additional risk for PVG.

It is believed that PVG is likely to be the result of ischaemic–reperfusion injury, causing calcium overload and oxidative stress [4]. Release of catecholamines triggered by brain death in the donor, use of high inotropic support, and prolonged storage times all lead to ischaemia. Additionally, unrecognized pulmonary arterial hypertension in the recipient can also lead to right ventricular dysfunction [5]. In general, organs from younger donors are expected to have more reserves and are less likely to fail [6]. **Infections** are a significant cause of death within the first year post-transplant. Several factors have an impact on the incidence and type of infectious complications. Firstly, the intensive care unit setting increases nosocomial infections (catheter sepsis, ventilator-acquired pneumonia, etc.). Secondly, immunosuppression makes patients more susceptible not only to common bacteria and viruses, but also to rare opportunistic pathogens. In particular, CMV can be transmitted through the transplanted organ from a CMV-positive donor to a CMV-negative recipient. Therefore, patients are routinely provided with viral, pneumocystis, and fungal prophylaxis for several months. Vaccinations should be given as early as possible in the course of disease. Inactivated vaccines are generally safe, but live vaccines must be avoided after transplant.

Cardiac allograft rejection is an immune response directed against the donor's heart recognized as non-self. It may ultimately lead to graft destruction [7]. The process is most common a few months after transplantation but can also develop anytime later. There are several types of rejection [7]. Acute cellular rejection is the most prevalent form, affecting patients in the first year after transplant. Donor HLA molecules presented by antigen-presenting cells (APCs) to the recipient's T-cells trigger an inflammatory response and graft infiltration by mainly effector T-cells. This leads to cell-mediated myocyte injury.

Antibody-mediated rejection occurs in the presence of antibodies reactive against donor HLA molecules (also called donor-specific antibodies). The recipient becomes sensitized through previous blood transfusions [8], pregnancies, and use of foreign materials (homografts, VADs). Binding of those antibodies to the allograft leads to complement activation, inflammation, and cell lysis. Therefore, the presence of donor-specific antibodies is routinely monitored after transplantation. Hyperacute rejection is rare nowadays and happens only when a patient is highly sensitized to the donor (positive donor-specific cross-match).

Endomyocardial biopsy from the right ventricle still remains the gold standard for the diagnosis of rejection, and several surveillance biopsies are routinely performed at least in the first 6–12 months [9]. The procedure is relatively safe but carries a small risk for a serious complication [10].

Cardiac allograft vasculopathy (CAV) is the leading long-term cause of graft failure [11]. Although the new immunosuppressive drugs have dramatically decreased the incidence of acute rejection and improved early survival, the occurrence of CAV has not been significantly affected. Despite an unclear pathogenesis, several risk factors have been identified: history of acute cell- or antibody-mediated rejection, presence of donor-specific anti-HLA antibodies, CMV infection [12], endothelial activation, coronary artery disease (donor or recipient), hyperlipidaemia, hypertension, and donor age.

CAV is characterized by diffuse concentric intimal hyperplasia, involving both the epicardial and intramyocardial coronary arteries of the graft (unlike atheromatous plaques that tend to be focal and non-circumferential). CAV can manifest in a variety of ways, ranging from symptoms of heart failure to arrhythmias and sudden death. Some patients can present with regional wall motion abnormality on echocardiography [13]. Importantly, absent or regionally limited re-innervation of the transplanted heart can cause silent myocardial ischaemia, with patients not experiencing chest pain. Routine surveillance coronary angiographies are therefore performed at 1- or 2-yearly intervals (Figure 7.14). In older children, angiography can be combined with intravascular ultrasound (IVUS). Escalation in immunosuppression does not slow the progress of CAV. Revascularization is rarely successful in the longer term. Re-transplantation is the only effective treatment for advanced disease.

The **development of malignancy** also has a major impact on long-term survival in transplanted patients. Chronic immunosuppression decreases the ability of the immune system to detect neoplastic cells and represents probably the most important risk factor. The peak of incidence of cancer is usually in the first year after transplantation when more potent immunosuppression is used to prevent rejection, but the risk is lifelong. Among solid organs, the heart requires one of the highest degrees of immunosuppression. This is reflected in higher malignancy rates in cardiac graft recipients. Infection with oncogenic viruses can be seen in cutaneous carcinomas (human papilloma virus infection) or in post-transplant lymphoproliferative disorder [14] (EBV infection). In children, post-transplant lymphoma accounts for virtually all cases of malignancy and, in most cases, responds to a reduction in immunosuppression and rituximab therapy.

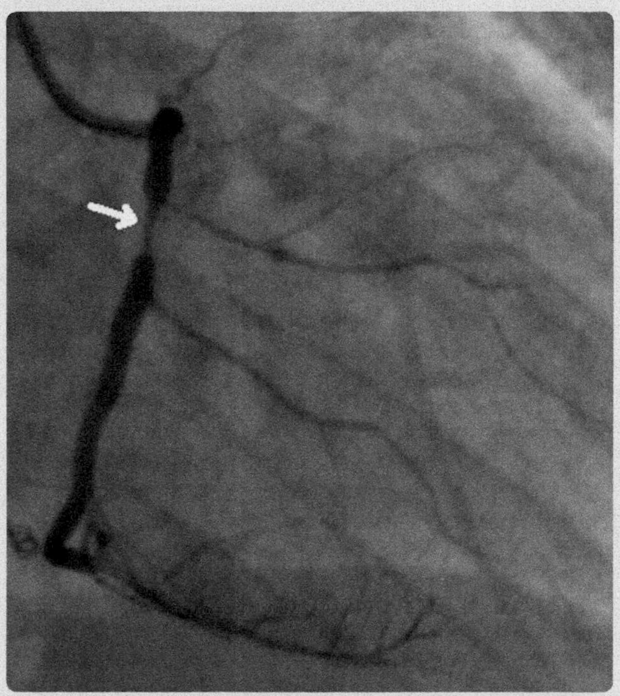

Figure 7.14 Focal right coronary artery (RCA) stenosis (arrow) and diffuse narrowing of distal RCA branches in a patient with CAV.

A final word from the expert

This case is a good example of complex decision-making in patients with terminal heart failure. With advances in surgical technique, post-operative care and immunosuppression heart transplantation has become an accepted therapy of end-stage heart failure. In the last decade, approximately 4000–4500 heart transplants were performed every year in the world, including 450–500 paediatric cases. Survival can reach, in most cases, 15–20 years.

Increasing waiting lists resulting from a significant shortage of donor organs is a major limitation. One of the reasons for the increasing demand in children is a growing number of patients with heart failure after surgical palliation for congenital heart disease, especially following palliation with a single-ventricle strategy.

Despite recent advances in mechanical circulatory support, the incidence of major complications, such as stroke, bleeding, or infection, remains relatively high. In current practice, mechanical circulatory support is not used as destination therapy in children, but only to bridge patients to heart transplantation.

References

1. Mehra MR, Canter CE , Hannan MM, et al. The 2016 International Society for Heart Lung Transplantation listing criteria for heart transplantation: a 10-year update. *J Heart Lung Transplant* 2016;35:1–23.
2. Brunner A, Dubois N, Rimensberger PC, Karam O. Identifying prognostic criteria for survival after resuscitation assisted by extracorporeal membrane oxygenation. *Crit Care Res Pract* 2016;2016:9521091.

3. Cassidy J, Dominguez T, Haynes S, et al. A longer waiting game: bridging children to heart transplant with the Berlin Heart™ EXCOR device—the United Kingdom experience. *J Heart Lung Transplant* 2013;32:1101–6.
4. Iyer A, Kumarasinghe G, Hicks M, et al. Primary graft failure after heart transplantation. *J Transplant* 2011;2011:175768.
5. Hoskote A, Carter C, Rees P, Elliott M, Burch M, Brown K. Acute right ventricular failure after pediatric cardiac transplant: predictors and long-term outcome in current era of transplantation medicine. *J Thorac Cardiovasc Surg* 2010;139:146–53.
6. Conway J, Chin C, Kemna M, et al.; Pediatric Heart Transplant Study Investigators. Donors' characteristics and impact on outcomes in pediatric heart transplant recipients. *Pediatr Transplant* 2013;17:774–81.
7. Lammers AE, Roberts P, Brown KL, et al. Acute rejection after paediatric heart transplantation: far less common and less severe. *Transpl Int* 2010;23:38–46.
8. Kotter JR, Drakos SG, Horne BD, et al. Effect of blood product transfusion-induced tolerance on incidence of cardiac allograft rejection. *Transplant Proc* 2010;42:2687–92.
9. Dixon V, Macauley C, Burch M, Sebire NJ. Unsuspected rejection episodes on routine surveillance endomyocardial biopsy post-heart transplant in paediatric patients. *Pediatr Transplant* 2007;11:286–90.
10. Zhorne D, Petit CJ, Ing FF, et al. A 25-year experience of endomyocardial biopsy safety in infants. *Catheter Cardiovasc Interv* 2013;82:797–801.
11. Kindel SJ, Law YM, Chin C, et al. Improved detection of cardiac allograft vasculopathy: a multi-institutional analysis of functional parameters in pediatric heart transplant recipients. *J Am Coll Cardiol* 2015;66:547–57.
12. Simmonds J, Fenton M, Dewar C, et al. Endothelial dysfunction and cytomegalovirus replication in pediatric heart transplantation. *Circulation* 2008;117:2657–61.
13. Dedieu N, Greil G, Wong J, Fenton M, Burch M, Hussain T. Diagnosis and management of coronary allograft vasculopathy in children and adolescents. *World J Transplant* 2014;4:276–93.
14. Haynes SE, Saini S, Schowengerdt KO. Post-transplant lymphoproliferative disease and other malignancies after pediatric cardiac transplantation: an evolving landscape. *Curr Opin Organ Transplant* 2015;20:562–9.
15. Secnikova Z, Gopfertova D, Hoskova L, et al. Significantly higher incidence of skin cancer than other malignancies in patients after heart transplantation. A retrospective cohort study in the Czech Republic. *Biomed Pap Med Fac Univ Palacky Olomouc Czech Repub* 2015;159:648–51.

CASE

8 Supraventricular tachycardia

Will Regan

Expert commentary Jasveer Mangat

Case history

A mother attended a planned review at 35 weeks' gestation with perinatal presentation of supraventricular tachycardia (SVT). The pregnancy had been low-risk, with normal antenatal scans and normal serology, to a mother with no past medical history. On arrival, the fetal heart rate was noted to be 200 bpm, and due to a recent history of minor trauma, the mother underwent an emergency Caesarean section. The baby was born in fair condition, weighing 2.8 kg, but continued to show signs of respiratory distress. As such, the baby was taken to the special care baby unit (SCBU), placed on positive pressure respiratory support for 12 hours, and covered with empirical antibiotics. During this time, short paroxysms of tachycardia, brief pauses, and periods of bradycardia were noted. The 12-lead electrocardiograms (ECGs) on days 1, 2, and 4 of life were felt to be normal. The respiratory distress improved, and initial sepsis concerns resolved.

On day 5 of life, the baby developed a narrow complex tachyarrhythmia, which was managed as an SVT. Ice and intravenous (IV) adenosine did not cardiovert the baby, and therefore, IV amiodarone was commenced with a loading dose, resulting in successful cardioversion after 1 hour. The baby was placed on continuous infusion of 1 mg/kg/hour for 36 hours, after which he was converted to oral amiodarone (Figures 8.1 and 8.2).

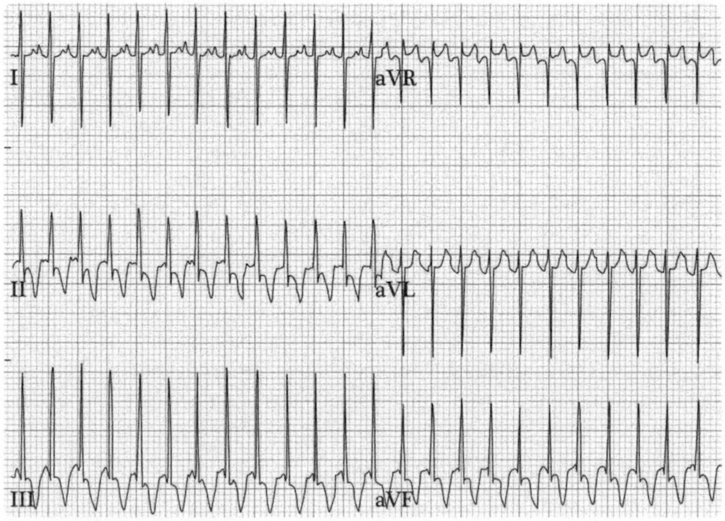

Figure 8.1 ECG recorded at 25 mm/s.

Expert comment Narrow complex tachycardia in neonates

Neonates can often tolerate narrow complex tachycardia well for short periods. However, at presentation, tachycardia may have been ongoing for several hours. A diagnosis based on the ECG is important. Management plans need two main components: firstly, immediate plans for support in the event of haemodynamic insufficiency or collapse; and secondly, a systematic approach that minimizes distress to the infant and is mindful of complications such as hypotension associated with a rapid amiodarone bolus and extravasation injury.

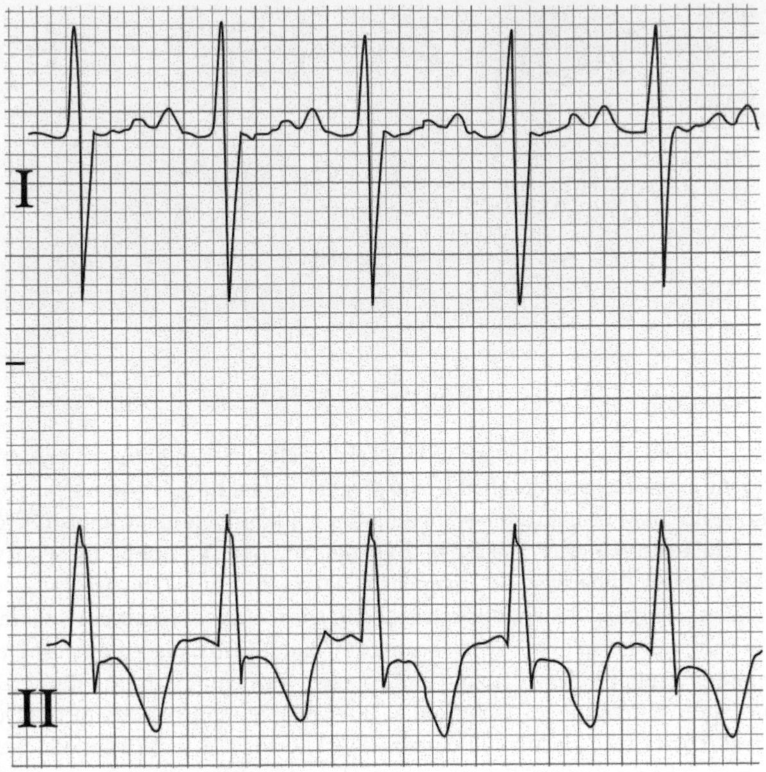

Figure 8.2 ECG recorded at 50 mm/s.

Expert comment Review of electrocardiograms

Reviewing the ECG, it represents a regular, narrow complex tachycardia at 300 bpm. The QRS axis is appropriate for a neonate. The p wave is in the terminal portion of the t wave, rendering it a long RP interval. The p wave morphology is positive in lead I, likely negative in leads II, III, and aVF. Determining the relationship of ventricular (QRS) and atrial depolarization (p) during tachycardia, at onset, and at termination aids the diagnosis. The p wave morphology indicates the area of the atria that is depolarized first. For instance, a focal atrial tachycardia initiating in the left upper pulmonary vein will be associated with a negative p wave in lead I and positive in the inferior leads. The first beat of tachycardia will be a p wave, and termination likely seen as a QRS deflection. A more common pattern is seen in atrial flutter where the p wave is broad and negative in the inferior leads and V1. In atrial flutter, the circuit of tachycardia is independent of the atrioventricular (AV) node and ventricle, and thus there may be more p waves than QRS complexes. A more common arrhythmia in infants is one mediated by an accessory pathway (AP), and this is outlined in Learning point, p. 110. The atria, ventricles, AV node, and AP are involved in the circuit of this form of SVT. If p wave morphology can be determined, it can lead to an observation as to which side of the heart the AP is located.

Learning point Acute management of narrow complex tachyarrhythmia

National and intensive care unit (ICU) transport guidelines should be followed in the treatment of a child presenting with a narrow complex tachyarrhythmia [1, 2]. In the stable child, sequential steps of assessment, followed by treatment with vagal manoeuvres, then, if required, increasing doses of adenosine, should be administered to restore sinus rhythm. The initial assessment is crucial to identify the child presenting in cardiogenic shock. The focus should be on peripheral perfusion, blood pressure, signs of heart failure (gallop rhythm or hepatomegaly), and signs of end-organ perfusion (mental status and urine output). In a decompensated child, the focus shifts towards supportive care, with early involvement of anaesthetic or ICU colleagues to consider electrolyte corrections and the need for airway and inotropic support. This supportive care is delivered in parallel with the anticipated need for urgent synchronized direct current (DC) cardioversion.

Clinical tip The use of amiodarone in refractory SVT

Mode of action

Amiodarone is a class III anti-arrhythmic (blocking potassium channels and prolonging repolarization), as per the Singh–Vaughan Williams classification. However, it also acts on sodium and calcium channels, as well as alpha- and beta-adrenoreceptors, meaning it shows all four electrophysiological classes of action [3, 4].

Practical points

- Screen for: renal, thyroid, and liver function tests (if possible at time of commencement).
- Advantages: minimal negative inotropic effect, effective on broad range of arrhythmias.
- Side effects [3]: hypotension and cardiovascular collapse (with quick IV doses), QTc prolongation (but rarely torsades de pointes), and fast ventricular conduction of atrial tachyarrhythmia via AP (blocking of AV node).
- Longer-term systemic side effects: hypothyroidism, liver dysfunction, corneal microdeposits, photosensitivity, and grey facial pigmentation.

Loading doses

- Advanced Paediatric Life Support (APLS) recommends 5 mg/kg loading dose over 20 minutes [1].
- Children's Acute Transport Service (CATS) guidelines, assuming cardiac dysfunction, recommend a slower infusion rate of 15–25 mcg/kg/min over 4 hours [2] (NB: 25 mcg/kg/min = 6 mg/kg total over 4 hours).

Evidence for IV amiodarone loading and maintenance dosing

A prospective study of the pharmacokinetics in children has shown adequate serum concentrations (as compared to adult data) with the 5 mg/kg loading dose over 30 minutes, followed by 10 mg/kg/day maintenance dose (approximately 7 mcg/kg/min) [5]. A previous randomized, double-blind therapeutic trial of IV amiodarone in 61 children with a range of tachyarrhythmias [6] compared three dosing regimes and followed time-to-success, as well as adverse events. The three regimes were:

1. Low = 1 mg/kg loading dose, then 2 mg/kg/day maintenance (= 1.4 mcg/kg/min maintenance)
2. Medium = 5 mg/kg loading dose, then 5 mg/kg/day maintenance (= 3.5 mcg/kg/min maintenance)
3. High = 10 mg/kg loading dose, then 10 mg/kg/day maintenance (= 7 mcg/kg/min maintenance).

The authors of these studies found that both time-to-success and side effects were dose-related. Common side effects included: hypotension, bradycardia, AV block, nausea, and vomiting. It therefore seems reasonable to follow a loading dose of 25 mcg/kg/min over 4 hours, with a 5 mcg/kg/min maintenance dose and close monitoring of heart rate, blood pressure, and repeat measurements of QTc. This initial dose can then be increased or decreased accordingly, depending on response and side effects. Finally, in refractory cases, it may be that a second agent is required to achieve conversion to sinus rhythm.

Expert comment Use of amiodarone in neonates and children

Neonates presenting with SVT that are maintaining adequate end-organ perfusion are often finely balanced, in particular if the tachycardia has persisted for several hours. Reducing some of the metabolic demands by withholding feeds, providing IV hydration, sedating, and ventilating is important. In the event amiodarone therapy is being considered, the clinical status of the infant must be considered. A slow infusion of amiodarone in this setting can both prove effective and prevent further morbidity. The more rapid bolus of amiodarone intravenously can result in hypotension, which can precipitate cardiac arrest. This is largely due to the effects of the solvent (Polysorbate 80). Amiodarone is only weakly negatively inotropic and this particular effect is transient. In addition to this acute clinical judgement, amiodarone efficacy has been shown to be dose-related.

On day 9 of life, whilst on oral amiodarone, the baby had sustained SVT (see Figure 8.3). This was cardioverted with 300 mcg/kg of adenosine. The baby was re-started on IV amiodarone, then 48 hours later converted to an oral preparation. At this stage, oral propranolol was added. On day 26 of life, he was discharged home on amiodarone 20 mg once daily (= 6.5 mg/kg) and propranolol 1 mg three times daily (= 0.33 mg/kg per dose).

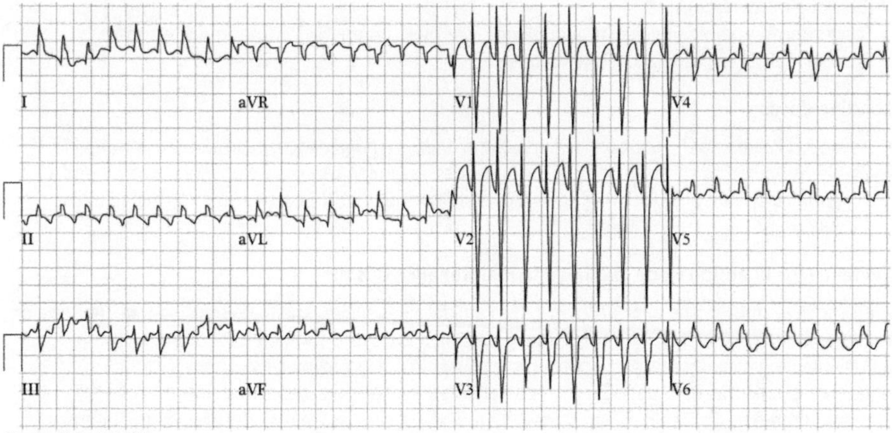

Figure 8.3 ECG at 9 days of age, showing tachycardia at around 200 bpm with a widened QRS duration (~110 ms). There is a non-specific intraventricular conduction delay, more in keeping with the left bundle branch block pattern, whilst the baby is on amiodarone at a maintenance dose. The P wave again is suggestive of long RP tachycardia and negative in leads II, III, and aVF. On this occasion, it may be negative in aVL and aVR and positive in the initial precordial leads, becoming negative between V3 and V4.

Expert comment Use of beta-blockers in acute setting

Beta-blockers are highly effective for the treatment of SVT. After a short episode of paroxysmal SVT is terminated, in an otherwise well child with no signs of heart failure, beta-blockers can be safely started as first-line therapy. However, in the acute setting when myocardial function is impaired or if there is cardiomyopathy, beta-blockade can precipitate acute decompensation. Hence, a complete assessment, including echocardiography, is recommended.

Learning point Comparison of propranolol and digoxin as secondary preventative treatment for neonates and infants with SVT

Two of the most commonly used medications that prevent recurrent SVT in neonates and infants have been digoxin and propranolol. Propranolol has an ease of use due to its side effect profile and ease of monitoring as an outpatient or in peripheral hospitals [7, 8]. Its side effects (namely bradycardia, hypotension, and hypoglycaemia) are easier to identify and manage. In comparison, due to the narrow therapeutic range of digoxin and concern of its side effects and for patients with pre-excitation, digoxin is no longer recommended. We review three important studies set out to compare the effectiveness of both treatments.

Two recent large retrospective studies [7, 9] compared outcomes of infants treated with either propranolol or digoxin. Again both of these studies excluded those with pre-excitation on the baseline ECG, but one of the two included those infants with coexisting congenital heart disease [9]. Hornik et al. showed a higher rate of recurrence in those treated with propranolol, but higher rates of hypotension in those treated with digoxin (although perhaps related to infants being sicker at the time of initiation). On the other hand, Moffett et al. showed similar success rates when comparing both medications.

The SAMIS Trial [10], reported in 2012, was a randomized, double-blind prospective trial designed to compare the efficacy and safety profile of digoxin and propranolol when used as treatment of infants with SVT. Unfortunately, the final analysis of 61 infants meant the study was underpowered. Their findings, however, showed no significant difference in SVT recurrence between the two groups.

These studies suggest that either propranolol or digoxin can be considered as first-line preventative therapy in neonates presenting with SVT without pre-excitation on baseline ECG. The data also give some evidence to support the concept of weaning, then stopping the anti-arrhythmic medication within the first year of life (or 3–6 months with no recurrence), hoping that the infant has 'grown out' of the pathway or substrate underlying the arrhythmia. However, we still have insufficient trial evidence to confidently conclude that secondary treatment of a first presentation of SVT in neonates or infants (currently favoured by most centres) is warranted to prevent recurrences or indeed is the ideal choice or length of initial therapy.

Learning point Review of current practice: treatment choices for SVT in infants

Infants under 1 year of age are at a higher risk for the development of SVT [11]. This is a challenge for several key reasons. Firstly, the neonate or infant presents differently, compared to an older, verbal child, meaning the arrhythmia may be incessant until symptoms of heart failure develop. Secondly, the underlying mechanisms are harder to define; in children under 1 year of age, certain mechanisms such as atrioventricular re-entry tachycardia (AVRT), atrial ectopic tachycardia (AET), and atrial flutter are more common; the faster ventricular rates and the lack of electrophysiological studies (EPS) result in empiric treatment, as opposed to mechanism-specific decisions. Finally, whilst in older children (generally above 20 kg), an EPS and catheter ablation become an attractive treatment option for a wide range of arrhythmias, these are reserved only for the most incessant cases in infants and small children.

Two recent reviews of current practice give insight into current trends in the treatment of neonates and infants [8, 12]. A majority (around 90%) of the infants in these two studies with a principal diagnosis of SVT were being treated with secondary preventative therapy on their discharge from the unit.

The larger of the two study groups (with 2848 infants across 348 neonatal units) [8] showed the most commonly used medications for secondary prevention were:

1. Digoxin (62%)
2. Beta-blockers (47%)
3. Amiodarone (7%)
4. Flecainide (3%)
5. Sotalol (4%).

This study showed a clear trend over time (1998–2012) of decreased use of digoxin and increased use of beta-blockers. Multidrug therapy was required in almost 20% of infants in this larger study (most commonly beta-blockers and digoxin, but almost all combinations of the above five drugs being used). They found that smaller weight and gestational age were risk factors for a significant number (18% of all infants) having adverse events whilst on secondary preventative therapy, the most common of which were hypotension, hyperkalaemia, hypoglycaemia, elevated liver enzymes, and bradycardia. The relatively favourable side effect profile of beta-blockers (e.g. lower incidence of hypotension and hepatoxicity) may again explain their increased use over time.

Finally, the study by Sesler et al. [12] showed, in a breakdown of diagnoses, a change in treatment preference for infants with a diagnosis of Wolff–Parkinson–White (WPW) or coexisting cardiomyopathy. In cardiomyopathy, more digoxin and amiodarone were used, in comparison to WPW where none of the 27 infants received digoxin, but instead favouring propranolol (81%) and amiodarone (41%).

Expert comment Side effects of medications

Clinicians should be aware of some of the common side effects and relative contraindications of anti-arrhythmic medications. Sodium channel blockers, such as flecainide or propafenone, are particularly effective in changing the refractory period of accessory pathways and an effective agent in treating AVRT or atrioventricular nodal re-entry tachycardia (AVNRT). However, flecainide can slow the cycle length of atrial flutter, resulting in a dangerous sustained 1:1 conduction to ventricles. Digoxin predominantly slows nodal conduction and may, in WPW syndrome—in theory—predispose to rapid conduction across the accessory pathway in the event that there is atrial fibrillation or flutter. Other pro-arrhythmic side effects, including QRS duration-prolonging effect of flecainide and QT interval-prolonging effects of sotalol and amiodarone, should always be considered.

He was well and asymptomatic for 9 months. Amiodarone was stopped, whilst continuing propranolol as monotherapy. Three weeks later, following 9 hours of diarrhoea, vomiting, and increasing floppiness, he presented to hospital. Assessment in the emergency department showed signs of dehydration, with a heart rate of 266 bpm, normotension, and a temperature of 38.5°C. SVT was diagnosed on 12-lead ECG, and a bolus of 10 ml/kg of normal saline and five doses of adenosine were administered (150–500 mcg/kg), with a brief reversion to sinus rhythm after the last dose. He was then given an IV bolus of amiodarone, which successfully converted him to sinus rhythm He was transferred to PICU where he required IV fluid rehydration He was later found to be both rotavirus- and norovirus-positive but had normal electrolytes throughout.

Clinical tip Practical guidance on the use of adenosine

Key points for administration:

1. Monitoring and frequent reassessment of child.
2. A 12 lead-ECG preferable (or at least a 3-lead monitor strip).
3. Repeat vagal manoeuvres (if any delay in IV access/adenosine).
4. Upper limb, large IV access preferable (take blood gas, sugar, and electrolyte sample).
5. Warn child and/or parents about side effects.
6. Give adenosine using 3-way tap, with quick saline flush and continuous ECG/rhythm strip running [100 mcg/kg starting dose (max 6 mg), at 2-minute intervals, with no cardioversion, up to a maximum dose of 500 mcg/kg (12 mg maximum dose or 300 mcg/kg in neonate)] (Figure 8.4).

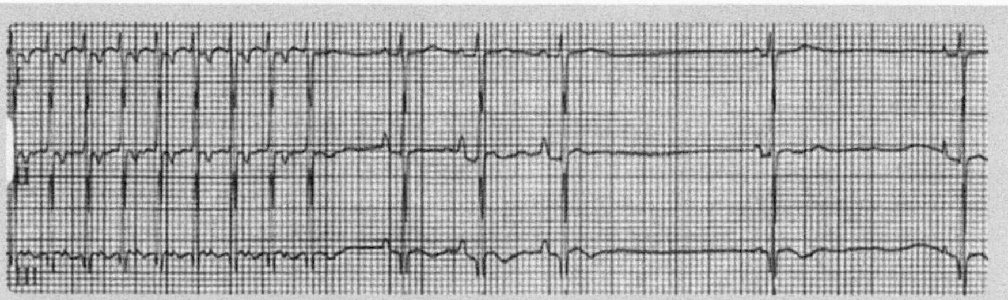

Figure 8.4 Rhythm strip example.

Adenosine—key points:

- A purine nucleoside (belonging to class V anti-arrhythmics).
- Given intravenously, it has a rapid effect primarily on the AV node, meaning it has the most effect on terminating SVT where the AV node forms part of re-entry circuit (commonly AVRT and AVNRT).
- Shown to be safe to use in children [13–15], with a very quick half-life of around 2 s.
- Although APLS guidelines state starting dose of 100 mcg/kg [1], it may well be that higher doses are needed to cardiovert. A recent study of 44 children showed only 24% converted to sinus rhythm after one dose and a mean dose of 173 mcg/kg was required [16]. Furthermore, an analysis of five available studies in children concluded that an initial higher dose (200–250 mcg/kg) significantly reduces the risk of unsuccessful cardioversion [17].
- Short-lived, but common and unpleasant, side effects: flushing, chest and jaw pain, and dyspnoea.
- Cardiovascular side effects: due to the transient block at the AV node and the potential to shorten the refractory time of antegrade conduction across certain accessory pathways, there is a potential to increase the ventricular rate (e.g. in atrial fibrillation in WPW or atrial flutter with bystander accessory pathway). Caution should also be taken in children with known sinus node disease due to a potential risk of prolonged asystole [18, 19].
- Other side effects: although rare, inducing bronchospasm in children with a history of significant reactive airway disease is a concern [20]. Interestingly, however, case reports also exist of adenosine used for cardioversion in SVT secondary to beta-agonists in children with asthma [21, 22].

Expert comment Adenosine

When used with simultaneous ECG monitoring, adenosine bolus infusions can be helpful both diagnostically and therapeutically. Potential side effects that need consideration include bronchospasm, atrial fibrillation, and short periods of asystole.

In addition, we would advocate an adenosine bolus is considered when reviewing a child in whom peripheral perfusion is stable and the presenting rhythm is a regular broad complex tachycardia. The QRS morphology and axis, as well as the relationship of the QRS and the P wave (VA relationship), need to be considered. Often in paediatric practice, the broad complex QRS is as a result of rate-related bundle branch block. The QRS morphology and axis should thus resemble a right or left bundle branch block pattern. Clinicians should be aware of common normal heart ventricular tachycardia (VT) presentations, such as fascicular re-entry (also referred to as Belhassen's and verapamil-sensitive VT) and right ventricular outflow tract VT, when giving adenosine as it can offer diagnostic and therapeutic utility.

Whilst in PICU, his anti-arrhythmic medications were optimized—**oral** propranolol was increased, and he was started on an amiodarone infusion (25 mcg/kg/min), which resulted in successful cardioversion. Prior to discharge, amiodarone was discontinued and converted to flecainide. He was discharged from PICU on propranolol 5 mg (= 0.5 mg/kg) three times daily and flecainide 25 mg (= 2.5 mg/kg) three times daily.

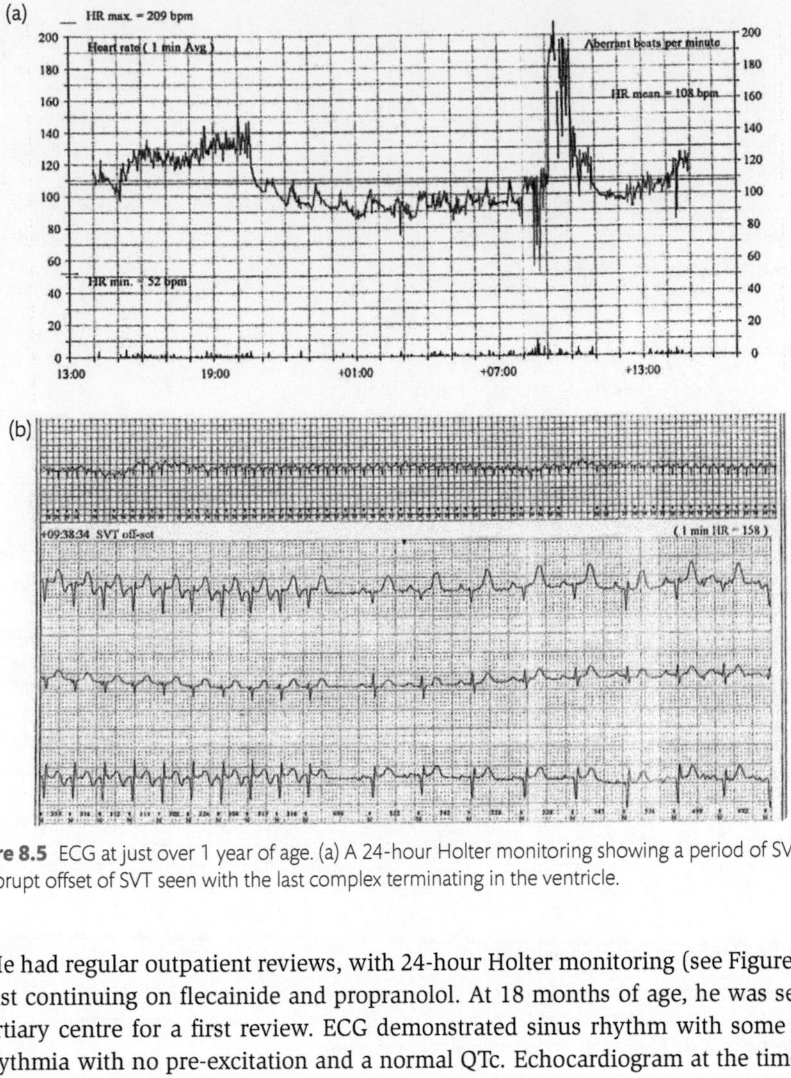

Figure 8.5 ECG at just over 1 year of age. (a) A 24-hour Holter monitoring showing a period of SVT. (b) Abrupt offset of SVT seen with the last complex terminating in the ventricle.

He had regular outpatient reviews, with 24-hour Holter monitoring (see Figure 8.5), whilst continuing on flecainide and propranolol. At 18 months of age, he was seen at a tertiary centre for a first review. ECG demonstrated sinus rhythm with some sinus arrhythmia with no pre-excitation and a normal QTc. Echocardiogram at the time was normal.

Expert comment Monitoring arrhythmias

Ambulatory monitors can offer several benefits to neonatal patients presenting with SVT. For those receiving medical therapy, they can help monitor the dose response (i.e. heart rate variability and bradycardia whilst on beta-blockers, and PR prolongation for those on digoxin). In addition, they can help sample for silent events, which, for a neonate, can help guide prescribing. Monitors worn for over 24 hours for small children can be a challenge to manage, in particular due to concerns over skin inflammation. The frequency and period of monitoring should be based on the likelihood the result will influence treatment decisions.

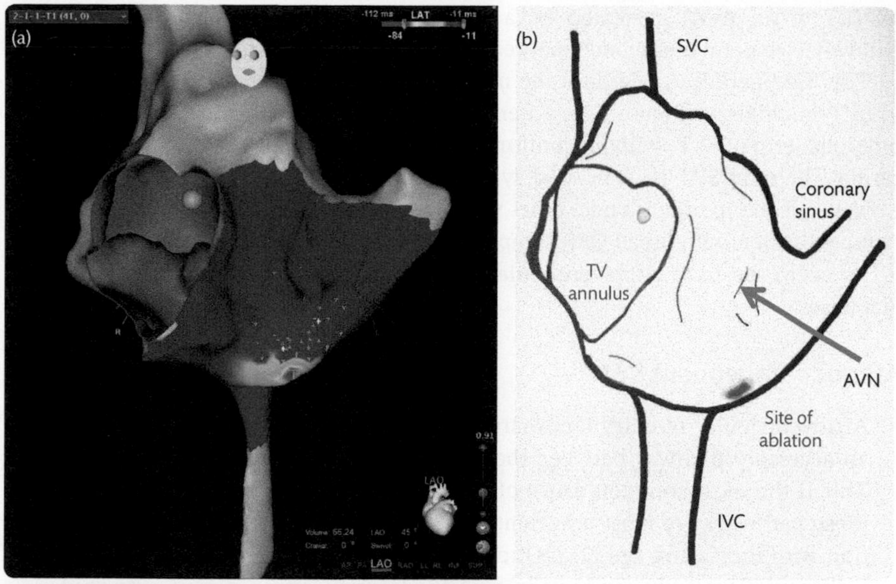

Figure 8.6 Three-dimensional map of the right atrium presented in the left anterior oblique (LAO) view. Cryoablation was used in the marked site of earliest activation (red area on colour map) of the first accessory pathway within the os of the coronary sinus. The yellow dot marks the exit from the AV node to the His–Purkinje system, and the arrow the site of the AV node (AVN).

Propranolol and flecainide were adjusted for his weight gain. At nearly 5 years of age (weighing 20 kg), despite his anti-arrhythmic therapy, he had a recurrence of SVT lasting 5 hours. The multidisciplinary team decision was for an EPS and catheter ablation.

This was carried out under general anaesthesia with catheters placed in the atria, ventricle, and coronary sinus and along the exit of the AV node (bundle of His). A three-dimensional mapping system was used without fluoroscopy (CARTO, Biosense Webster). The findings were of intermittent pre-excitation (interestingly not noted before) and inducible orthodromic AVRT mediated by two distinct posteroseptal accessory pathways. These were reached from within the coronary sinus and successfully cryoablated (Figure 8.6).

Discussion

The case represents a child who presented in a narrow complex tachyarrhythmia, with occasional presentation with broad tachyarrhythmia with a 'long' interval between the R and P wave. Ultimately, an EPS confirmed the diagnosis of AVRT, with successful ablation of two accessory pathways. These pathways were slowly conducting, resulting in the R-to-P relationship seen on the ECG. On initial presentation, the diagnosis was thought to be a focal atrial tachycardia, with a differential diagnosis including atypical

AVNRT or an AVRT mediated by a decremental or slowly conducting accessory pathway (see permanent junctional reciprocating tachycardia further below).

This case perhaps underlines the need for a pragmatic approach in the treatment of SVT in children (Figure 8.7). Often the child is diagnosed and treated under the umbrella term of **SVT**, without confirmation of the underlying substrate for the tachycardia. The term SVT is often used synonymously with narrow complex tachycardia. However, it is important to note other variations, including SVTs presenting with aberrant conduction with broad QRS complexes.

As such, the term **supraventricular tachycardia (SVT)** covers the following key diagnoses.

AV node-dependent SVT

- **Atrioventricular re-entry tachycardia (AVRT).** The substrate for tachycardia is an accessory pathway between the myocardium of the atrium and the ventricle. This is the most common cause of SVT in all age groups of children. However, these pathways are most prevalent in neonates, tending to decrease in proportion with increasing age [23]. Often commencing with an atrial ectopic, the tachycardia typically conducts in an orthodromic circuit—passing antegrade down the AV node and conduction fibres into the ventricle, followed by retrograde conduction across the accessory pathway back into the atria. Without pre-excitation on the resting ECG, these are termed 'concealed accessory pathways'. It is important to note that **Wolff–Parkinson–White (WPW) syndrome** is a form of AVRT, defined by symptoms and/or proven tachycardia, combined with ventricular pre-excitation (or delta wave) on the resting 12-lead ECG. Without symptoms, an incidental finding of pre-excitation can be termed a **WPW pattern**.
- **Atrioventricular nodal re-entry tachycardia (AVNRT).** The substrate for tachycardia involves a dual pathway of specialized myocardium proximal to the AV node within the right atrial tissue. The relatively different speeds of conduction and refraction (termed **slow** and **fast** pathways) allow an electrical impulse to pass antegrade through one pathway and passing back retrograde through the other, thus setting up a re-entry circuit (more typically slow–fast conduction). The likelihood of an SVT being an AVRNT increases with age in children, with proportionally 12- to 21-year-old females more likely to have AVNRT than AVRT [23].
- **Permanent junctional reciprocating tachycardia (PJRT).** A rarer form of AVRT with a concealed accessory pathway, which shows slow retrograde conduction. This sets up a form of orthodromic AVRT which is often incessant in nature,

with 18% of infants or children found to have tachycardia-induced cardiomyopathy in a recent retrospective review [24]. The long RP interval and negative P wave in the inferior leads are characteristic features. Our case had all of these ECG features, as well as a typical accessory pathway located in the right posteroseptal space. With optimal medical therapy, sinus rhythm was predominant.

SVTs originating in the atria

- **Atrial ectopic tachycardia** (AET). The substrate is a focus of abnormal electrical activity in the atria, often showing automaticity, and therefore not dependent on the AV node. Acting as an ectopic pacemaker above the rate of the sinus node, it can show varying atrial rates (higher in neonates) and varying degrees of conduction through the AV node (1:1, 2:1, or variable block). It can also show a 'warm-up period' on commencing the tachycardia
- **Atrial flutter.** A macro-re-entry circuit within the atrium, typically around the tricuspid valve annulus, and therefore not dependent on the AV node. The atrial rate varies between 300 and 400 (higher in neonates), and similarly to AET, it can show varying degrees of conduction through the AV node. It is most common in neonates or in older children following surgery for congenital heart disease.

Others

- **Junctional ectopic tachycardia** (JET). Broadly composed of two different forms: a rarer **congenital** or **permanent** form of incessant narrow complex tachycardia, and the more common **transient** form frequently presenting after surgery for congenital heart disease. The substrate for tachycardia is an area of automaticity within (or near) the bundle of His, hence its previous name of **His-bundle tachycardia**.

Not all forms of SVT are covered in this chapter such as atrial fibrillation (relatively rare in children, although important to recognize, especially in the presence of WPW or bystander accessory pathways due to the risk of fast antegrade conduction to the ventricles, with a consequent risk for sudden death), other forms of accessory pathways, and multifocal AET.

Learning point

(See Figure 8.7.)

	AVRT (including WPW) Orthodromic (usual)	Antidromic (rare)	AVNRT Typical (slow–fast) Atypical (fast–slow)		AET	Flutter	PJRT
Diagram	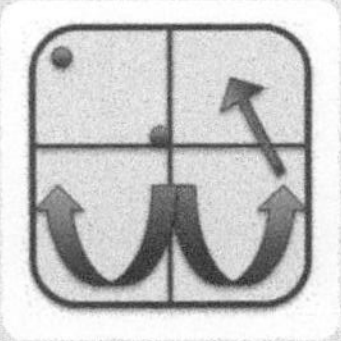	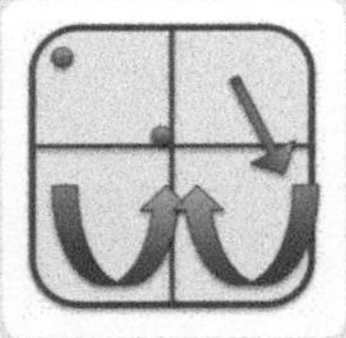	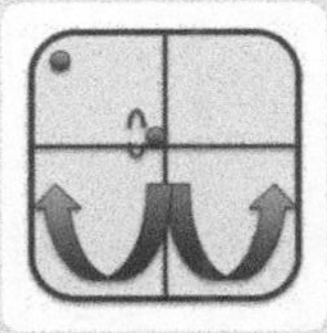	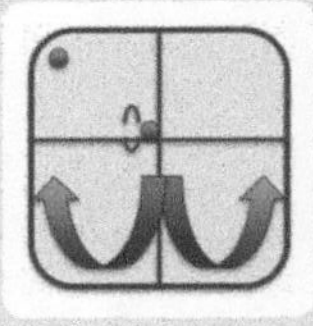	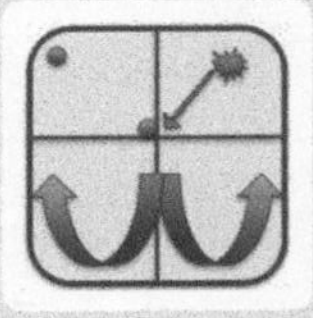	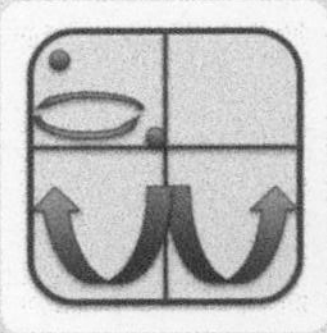	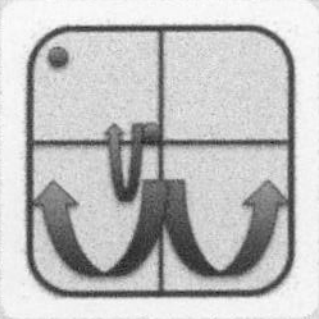
Mechanism	**Accessory pathway (AP)** **Circuit:** atrium, antegrade AV node, ventricle, retrograde AP to recommence	**AP Circuit:** atrium, antegrade AP, ventricle, retrograde AV node to recommence	**Slow–fast circuit adjacent to AV node** **Circuit:** antegrade slow AV node to ventricle, retrograde fast AV node, to recommence in atria	**Fast–slow circuit adjacent to AV node** **Circuit:** antegrade fast AV node to ventricle, retrograde slow AV node, to recommence in atria	Usually automatism of **ectopic atrial pacemaker** Not dependent on AV node or ventricle	**Macro-re-entry circuit in atrium** (usually around tricuspid valve) **Circuit:** clockwise or anticlockwise across the atria, with the tissue between inferior caval vein and tricuspid valve as the area of slow conduction Not dependent on AV node or ventricle	**AP (slow-conducting)** **Circuit:** atrium, antegrade AV node, ventricle, retrograde slow AP to recommence
Frequency and age groups	Common More frequent to find APs in neonates and younger children	Rare	Classically more frequently seen in older children and more common in females Rare in infancy		Any age	More common in neonates or later in children with congenital heart disease	Rare Can occur at any age, but more in infants
Rate of SVT and conduction	Ventricular rate: **200–300 bpm** (slower with age) **1:1 AV conduction**		Ventricular rate: **150–250 bpm** (slower with age) **1:1 AV conduction (rarely 2:1 AV conduction)**		Ventricular rate: **150–250 bpm** (slower with age)—showing **considerable variability in both rate** and **AV conduction (often 1:1)**	**Atrial rate: 300–400/min** (slower with age) **AV node conduction:** can be 1:1, 2:1, or variable	Ventricular rate: **150–300 bpm** (slower with age) **1:1 AV conduction**

ECG in SVT	Usually narrow QRS	Usually broad QRS (left AP mimics right bundle branch block, right AP mimics left bundle branch block)	Usually narrow QRS	Usually narrow QRS	Usually narrow QRS	Usually narrow QRS	Usually narrow QRS
	P waves: short RP, retrograde, and dependent on AP location	**P waves:** short RP and likely negative in inferior leads (II, III, and aVF)	**P waves:** either absent P waves (buried in QRS) or very short RP interval with P wave seen just after QRS (compare with resting ECG to distinguish)	**P waves:** longer RP interval (compared with typical AVRNT) and likely negative in inferior leads (II, III, and aVF)	**P waves:** long RP interval with abnormal P wave morphology (depends on site of ectopic, e.g. left-sided ectopic negative in aVL)	**P waves:** absence of isoelectric line with sawtooth pattern	**P waves:** long RP interval usually deep, negative in inferior leads (II, III, and aVF)
Adenosine	Usually **stops SVT** If transient AV block: tachycardia finishes on retrograde P wave before restarting	Usually **stops SVT** If transient AV block: tachycardia finishes on broad QRS before restarting	Usually **stops SVT**	Usually **stops SVT**	**Transiently slows ventricular rate, terminates approximately 30%** **Diagnostic info:** slowing AV conduction (>1:1), may unmask atrial tachycardia. Ventricular rate may then show 'warm-up' when restarting. If sinus beats conduct when slowed, can compare P wave morphology	**Transiently slows ventricular rate** **Diagnostic info:** slowing of AV node conduction should unmask typical sawtooth pattern	Usually stops SVT, but often only **transient effect** and SVT resumes
Resting ECG	Usually normal (concealed APs) **WPW:** review of QRS axis may help determine location of AP; left-sided pathways may have more subtle pre-excitation but show a right bundle branch block pattern, whereas right-sided pathways often show more overt pre-excitation with a left bundle branch block pattern		Usually normal Comparison is helpful to compare with tachycardia to distinguish retrograde P wave within the terminal portion of baseline QRS pattern		Usually normal	Usually normal	Usually normal

Learning point Treatment of paroxysmal supraventricular tachycardia

Treatment of paroxysmal SVT in childhood requires careful assessment to balance the symptom burden, the risks of side effects from drugs, and complications from invasive catheter procedures. Indeed it may be reasonable for patients and their families to choose no treatment at all, e.g. in an older child who experiences infrequent, brief episodes of SVT which are well tolerated and who has no pre-excitation in their resting ECG. Additionally, for young children who have presented in the newborn period and have been controlled on anti-arrhythmic medication initially, it is accepted practice to trial weaning off the medication by 6–12 months of life. This is based on a rationale that a high proportion of accessory pathways regress and focal atrial tachyarrhythmia recurrence in this age group is low.

In addition, when considering treatment strategies, it is important to understand which patient factors can be used to help risk-stratify children with SVT. A review in the United States [25] found overall fatality in SVT to be 4% (in-hospital mortality across *n* = 1755 children), with the following important risk factors for mortality:

1. <1 month old (odds ratio = 2.41)
2. Congenital heart disease (odds ratio = 2.67)
3. Cardiomyopathy (odds ratio = 6.72).

For those presenting after the age of 1 or with recurrent symptoms, treatment options broadly consist of anti-arrhythmic medications and/or an EPS and catheter ablation (largely reserved for children above 20 kg). Individualization of treatment is again based on the patient's symptom burden, severity, age, weight, and the suspected underlying aetiology of the SVT. In practice, many children are treated empirically under the umbrella term of 'paroxysmal SVT' without clear proof of the underlying mechanism. However, a key distinguishing feature is the presence of pre-excitation on the baseline ECG, with WPW syndrome having different assessment and treatment considerations.

Targeted treatment choices based on European Heart Rhythm Association (EHRA) consensus statement from 2013 [26]

AVNRT:

- Current treatment commonly use anti-arrhythmic medications, including beta-blockers (such as atenolol), class Ic agents, and non-dihydropyridine calcium channel blockers (however, these are not regularly used in the UK in the treatment of SVT in children). Class Ic agents, such as flecainide, can be combined with beta-blockers in poor responders and with no congenital heart disease.
- Catheter ablation offered as first line in older children or in treatment failure.

AVRT, with no pre-excitation on baseline ECG:

- Managed as per AVRNT, with preference for non-AV nodal-blocking anti-arrhythmic medications such as beta-blockers and class Ic agents.

WPW syndrome:

- All should be referred to a paediatric cardiologist for evaluation due to risk of life-threatening arrhythmias [27].
- Older children should generally be reviewed by an electrophysiology consultant, with a view to considering EPS and ablation of accessory pathway.
- Generally, in children aged <4 years or weighing <15–20 kg: anti-arrhythmic medication therapy is indicated; aim to slow conduction through the atrium and accessory pathway, i.e. class IC (flecainide) or class III (sotalol). Amiodarone should only be considered as second-line therapy.
- Anti-arrhythmics that primarily block the AV node conduction (e.g. digoxin, verapamil, and beta-blockers) are contraindicated in patients with pre-excitation, due to concerns of blocking the AV node and allowing fast antegrade conduction of atrial tachycardia down the accessory pathway.

AET:

- In infants: digoxin is a common first-line choice and adding a beta-blocker or a class IC agent as second line. Amiodarone can be considered in treatment failure.
- For older children, consider catheter ablation or anti-arrhythmic medications.

Atrial flutter:

- Synchronized DC cardioversion is the first-line treatment in neonates. It is unlikely to recur, and following conversion to sinus rhythm, no prophylaxis is usually needed.
- If considering anti-arrhythmic medication therapy, commence on digoxin. Consider flecainide or amiodarone if initial treatment fails (in our experience, the initial use of amiodarone may reduce the need to combine medications).

JET:

- Most frequently encountered in the post-operative period following congenital heart disease surgery and is usually self-limiting. Careful intensive care management (electrolyte correction, cooling, and weaning of pro-arrhythmic inotropic medication) can help speed recovery. If anti-arrhythmics are considered, amiodarone is used as first-line therapy to slow the heart rate.

PJRT:

- Risk of progression to tachycardiomyopathy: indicates for drug treatment or catheter ablation. Consider use of amiodarone or verapamil (may need combination with digoxin), or consider class IC agents such as flecainide (in our experience, single agents are often not effective and a trial of agents may be required to find the most effective and best tolerated combination. Common combinations are beta-blockers with either flecainide or amiodarone).

Catheter ablation in children with SVT

Increasingly, EPS and catheter ablation in children offer a safe and effective treatment for SVT without the continued need for anti-arrhythmic therapy. Overall, success rates are high, in terms of both the initial success rate and longer-term recurrence rates, with some variation between SVT substrates. The Prospective Assessment after Pediatric Cardiac Ablation (PAPCA) study showed initial success rates of 93%, combining all radiofrequency ablation data for 2761 patients with SVT [28–30]. Recurrence rates varied with the underlying substrate, e.g. with right-sided accessory pathways having a high recurrence rate (up to 24.6% for right septal accessory pathways at 12 months), compared to lower rates in AVRNT (4.8% at 12 months). Longer follow-ups across a 5-year period show overall recurrence-free success rates of 83% [31], with significantly more recurrences in younger age groups.

It is essential to discuss the safety and complications of catheter interventions when considering the balance of risks in the treatment of SVT in children. Broadly speaking, the risks of cardiac catheterization and ablation therapy fall into:

- Vascular complications: mostly at the site of access (bleeding, haematoma, vessel injury, thrombosis, and discomfort following the procedure)
- Less frequent, but major, complications: transient or permanent AV block (including subsequent need for pacemaker insertion), perforation with cardiac catheter (including need for emergency pericardiocentesis), and thrombi/emboli (including risk for stroke in left-sided procedures or those with potential for right-to-left shunt).

A review of the registry data from paediatric catheter radiofrequency ablations in the United States showed an overall mortality risk of 0.22% across 4651 cases [32]. The data showed higher mortality rates in children with structural heart disease (0.89% versus 0.12% in those with a structurally normal heart). In those with a structurally normal heart, lower weight, left-sided procedures, and an increased number of radiofrequency applications were risk factors for increased mortality. Although the overall risk is low, these factors should certainly be considered when risk-stratifying the treatment approach in children with arrhythmias. Comparison of data from Michigan and Utah University Hospitals [33] showed no statistically significant difference between the major complications of two weight groups (group 1, <15 kg = 8% versus group 2, 15–20 kg = 2%), but with a low incidence of major complications, it was difficult to obtain adequate statistical power.

For indications for catheter ablations, review the EHRA/Association for European Pediatric and Congenital Cardiology (AEPC) consensus statement [26] from 2013 and the more recent 2016 Heart Rhythm Society (HRS)/Pediatric and Congenital Electrophysiology Society (PACES) consensus statement for children and patients with congenital heart disease [34].

A final word from the expert

SVT provides a clinician several challenges, making a diagnosis when paroxysms are short-lived, and conversely when tachycardia is sustained or incessant, achieving cardioversion and maintaining sinus rhythm. Acutely, most children can be managed quickly and effectively in primary or secondary care. However, as highlighted, when there is impairment of myocardial contractility, as well as tachycardia, patients can be at risk of decompensation or cardiac arrest. The treatment options for patients in this state can range from intubation to bolus infusion of amiodarone, and it needs to be managed with care.

In the longer term, the outcomes are excellent from catheter ablation and continue to improve, giving a favourable outlook for this group of patients.

References

1. Advanced Life Support Group. *Chapter 10. The child with an abnormal pulse rate or rhythm.* Available at: http://www.alsg.org/en/files/Ch10_Abnormal_rate_or_rhythm2006.pdf
2. Ramnarayan P; NHS Children's Acute Transport Service. *Clinical guidelines: supraventricular tachycardia.* 2018. Available at: http://site.cats.nhs.uk/wp-content/uploads/2018/01/cats_svt_2018.pdf
3. Ali KM. Collateral effects of antiarrhythmics in pediatric age. *Curr Pharm Des* 2008;14:782–7.
4. Goldschlager N et al. Practical guidelines for clinicians who treat patients with amiodarone. Practice Guidelines Sub-committee, North American Society of Pacing and Electrophysiology. *Arch Intern Med* 2000;160:1741–8.
5. Ramusovic S, Läer S, Meibohm B, Lagler FB, Paul T. Pharmacokinetics of intravenous amiodarone in children. *Arch Dis Child* 2013;98:989–93.
6. Saul JP et al. Intravenous amiodarone for incessant tachyarrhythmias in children: a randomized, double-blind, antiarrhythmic drug trial. *Circulation* 2005;112:3470–7.
7. Hornik CP et al. Comparative effectiveness of digoxin and propranolol for supraventricular tachycardia in infants. *Pediatr Crit Care Med* 2014;15:839–45.
8. Chu PY, Hill KD, Clark RH, Smith PB, Hornik CP. Treatment of supraventricular tachycardia in infants: Analysis of a large multicenter database. *Early Hum Dev* 2015;91:345–50.
9. Moffett et al. Efficacy of digoxin in comparison with propranolol for treatment of infant supraventricular tachycardia: analysis of a large, national database. *Cardiol Young* 2015;25:1080–5.
10. Sanatani S et al. The study of antiarrhythmic medications in infancy (SAMIS): a multicenter, randomized controlled trial comparing the efficacy and safety of digoxin versus propranolol for prophylaxis of supraventricular tachycardia in infants. *Circ Arrhythm Electrophysiol* 2012;5:984–91.
11. Tripathi A, Black GB, Park YM, Jerrell JM. Factors associated with the occurrence and treatment of supraventricular tachycardia in a pediatric congenital heart disease cohort. *Pediatr Cardiol* 2014;35:368–73.
12. Seslar S et al. A multi-institutional analysis of inpatient treatment for supraventricular tachycardia in newborns and infants. *Pediatr Cardiol* 2013;34:408–14.
13. Till J et al. Efficacy and safety of adenosine in the treatment of supraventricular tachycardia in infants and children. *Br Heart J* 1989;62:204–11.
14. Losek J et al. Adenosine and pediatric supraventricular tachycardia in the emergency department: multicenter study and review. *Ann Emerg Med* 1999;33:185–91.
15. Paul T, Pfammatter JP. Adenosine: an effective and safe antiarrhythmic drug in pediatrics. *Pediatr Cardiol* 1997;18:118–26.

16. Díaz-Parra S et al. Use of adenosine in the treatment of supraventricular tachycardia in a pediatric emergency department. *Pediatr Emer Care* 2014;30:388–93.
17. Quail MA, Till J. Does a higher initial dose of adenosine improve cardioversion rates in supraventricular tachycardia? *Arch Dis Child* 2012;97:177–9.
18. Tan B-H et al. Sinus slowing caused by adenosine-5′-triphosphate in patients with and without sick sinus syndrome under various autonomic states. *J Electrocardiol* 2004;37:305–9.
19. Fragakis N et al. Sinus nodal response to adenosine relates to the severity of sinus node dysfunction. *Europace* 2012;14:859–64.
20. DeGroff CG, Silka MJ. Bronchospasm after intravenous administration of adenosine in a patient with asthma. *J Pediatr* 1994;125:822–3.
21. Trachsel D et al. Adenosine for salbutamol-induced supraventricular tachycardia. *Intensive Care Med* 2007;33:1676.
22. Cook P et al. Adenosine in the termination of albuterol-induced supraventricular tachycardia. *Ann Emerg Med* 1994;24:316–19.
23. Anand RG. Is the mechanism of supraventricular tachycardia in pediatrics influenced by age, gender or ethnicity? *Congenit Heart Dis* 2009;4:464–8.
24. Kang KT et al. Permanent junctional reciprocating tachycardia in children: a multicenter experience. 2014;11:1426–32.
25. Salerno JC. Case fatality in children with supraventricular tachycardia in the United States. *PACE* 2011;34:832–6.
26. Brugada J et al.; European Heart Rhythm Association; Association for European Paediatric and Congenital Cardiology. Pharmacological and non-pharmacological therapy for arrhythmias in the pediatric population: EHRA and AEPC-Arrhythmia Working Group joint consensus statement. *Europace* 2013;15:1337–82.
27. Cohen MI et al. PACES/HRS expert consensus statement on the management of the asymptomatic young patient with a Wolff-Parkinson-White (WPW, ventricular preexcitation) electrocardiographic pattern: developed in partnership between the Pediatric and Congenital Electrophysiology Society (PACES) and the Heart Rhythm Society (HRS). Endorsed by the governing bodies of PACES, HRS, the American College of Cardiology Foundation (ACCF), the American Heart Association (AHA), the American Academy of Pediatrics (AAP), and the Canadian Heart Rhythm Society (CHRS). *Heart Rhythm* 2012;9:1006–24.
28. Van Hare GF et al. Pediatric Electrophysiology Society. Prospective assessment after pediatric cardiac abla- tion: design and implementation of the multicenter study. *Pacing Clin Electrophysiol* 2002;25:332–41.
29. Van Hare GF. Prospective assessment after pediatric cardiac ablation: demographics, medical profiles, and initial outcomes. *J Cardiovasc Electrophysiol* 2004;15:759–70.
30. Van Hare GF et al. Prospective assessment after pediatric cardiac ablation: recurrence at 1 year after initially successful ablation of supraventricular tachycardia. Participating Members of the Pediatric Electrophysiology Society. *Heart Rhythm* 2004;1:188–96.
31. Buddhe S et al. Radiofrequency and cryoablation therapies for supraventricular arrhythmias in the young: five-year review of efficacies. *PACE* 2012; 35:711–17.
32. Schaffer MS et al. Mortality following radiofrequency catheter ablation (from the Pediatric Radiofrequency Ablation Registry). Participating Members of the Pediatric Electrophysiology Society. *Am J Cardiol* 2000;86:639–43.
33. Aiyagari R et al. Radio-frequency ablation for supraventricular tachycardia in children ≤15 kg is safe and effective. *Pediatr Cardiol* 2005;26:622–6.
34. Saul PJ et al. PACES/HRS expert consensus statement on the use of catheter ablation in children and patients with congenital heart disease: Developed in partnership with the Pediatric and Congenital Electrophysiology Society (PACES) and the Heart Rhythm Society (HRS). *Heart Rhythm* 2016;13:e251–89.

CASE

9 Solitary indeterminate single ventricle with aortic atresia

James Wong

Expert commentary Reza Razavi

Case history

A newborn baby was found to be cyanosed and tachypnoeic a few days after birth. The baby was a first child, born at full term by normal vaginal delivery. The pregnancy had progressed uneventfully and antenatal scans were all normal. The parents were not related. Initial assessment showed a 2.3-kg baby with significant respiratory distress, including grunting and subcostal and intercostal recessions. There was tachycardia and poor peripheral perfusion with a capillary refill time of 5 s. The chest was clear on auscultation. Heart sounds were normal, with no murmur, and femoral pulses were not easily felt. Right arm transcutaneous saturations were 85% on air. A blood gas showed metabolic acidosis: pH 7.1, pCO_2 4.5, base excess −8, lactate 6.

The child was resuscitated with two 10 ml/kg fluid boluses, followed by a dose of intravenous antibiotics. Administration of oxygen did not improve the saturations. A chest radiograph (Figure 9.1) revealed a large heart shadow, with plethoric lungs. ECG showed mild right axis deviation. The paediatric cardiology team were contacted for further advice. Given the suspicion of duct-dependent congenital heart disease, it was advised to start a prostaglandin infusion at 5 ng/kg/min and arrange urgent transfer to the cardiac centre.

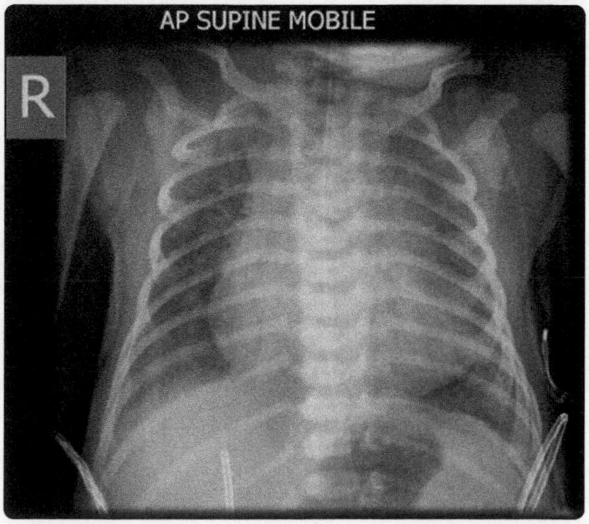

Figure 9.1 Chest radiograph on admission, showing an enlarged abnormal cardiac silhouette.

Learning point

Typically, infants with hypoplastic left heart syndrome (HLHS) have very subtle examination findings. These consist of feeble peripheral pulses, poor systemic perfusion, a single loud second heart sound, and often no murmur. Signs of heart failure may also be present.

Clinical tip

Prostaglandin E1 is a potent vasodilator of smooth muscle. It additionally causes inhibition of platelet aggregation. It is administered with an aim to reopen and/or maintain patency of the ductus arteriosus. The dose range is 5–40 ng/kg/min. The lowest dose is started and then titrated upwards to achieve an effect. Prostin has a number of undesirable side effects, which are more common in small infants (<2 kg in weight) and tend to occur most often in the first hour after administration. These include apnoeas, fevers, flushing, and hypotension. Once good flow has been demonstrated echocardiographically, the minimum possible dose to maintain patency is then administered.

The child arrived, and initial blood gas on the paediatric intensive care unit showed an improvement in the blood lactate to 3. An echocardiogram demonstrated situs solitus, absent right atrioventricular connection (the left atrium connected to a solitary indeterminate ventricle), and single outlet ventriculo-arterial connection with aortic atresia (Figure 9.2). There was depressed ventricular function, a large unrestrictive interatrial communication, normal-sized branch pulmonary arteries, and a large patent ductus arteriosus (PDA) measuring 5 mm in diameter with bidirectional shunting. The ascending aorta and transverse arch were severely hypoplastic. There was a good-sized descending aorta The child was placed on continuous positive airway pressure (CPAP). Umbilical lines were sited, and a prostin infusion of 5 ng/kg/min maintained. There was no difference in upper and lower limb blood pressures or saturations.

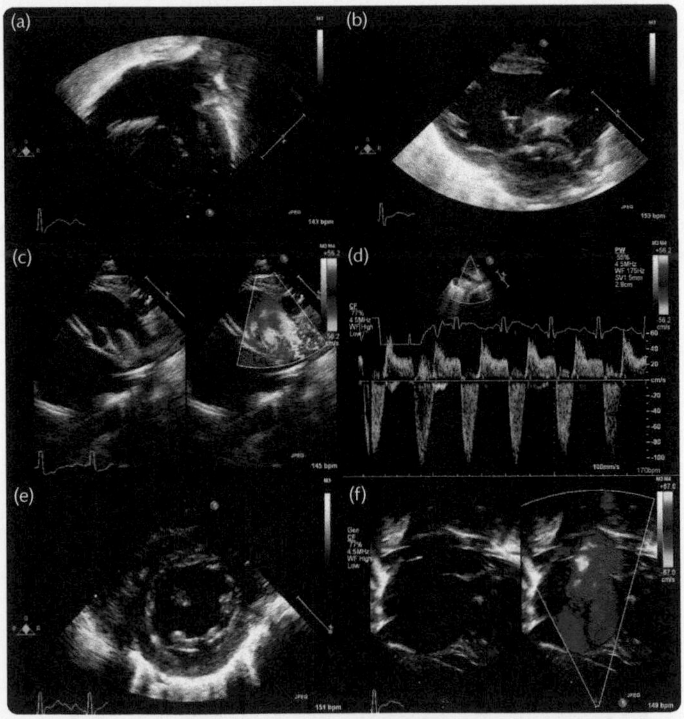

Figure 9.2 Transthoracic echocardiographic images demonstrating a solitary single ventricle of indeterminate morphology. (a) Apical view demonstrating a single apex forming a ventricle of indeterminate origin. (b) Parasternal long axis view showing a severely hypoplastic ascending aorta. (c) Ductal cut demonstrating the three-legged view of the branch pulmonary arteries and a widely patent ductus arterious. (d) Ductal Doppler showing a bidirectional flow pattern. Right-to-left in systole and left-to-right in diastole. (e) Parasternal short axis view showing a single ventricle. (f) Subcostal imaging of interatrial communication. There is unrestricted left-to-right flow across the defect.

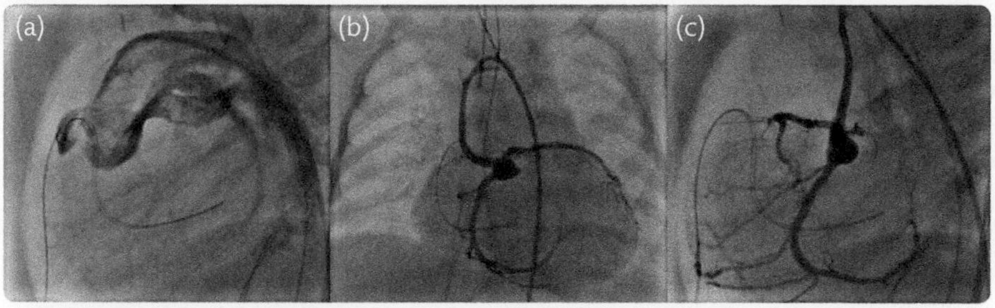

Figure 9.3 Angiographic images demonstrating important findings after bilateral pulmonary artery banding. (a) Pulmonary arteriogram. The catheter has been advanced retrogradely through the descending aorta, across the PDA into the branch pulmonary arteries. The site of the pulmonary artery bands can be seen. (b) Native aortogram (anteroposterior projection). The ascending aorta is severely hypoplastic. It measures a similar size to the coronary arteries. (c) Native aortogram (lateral projection). The coronary arteries are well visualized.

Findings were presented at the multidisciplinary meeting, and a recommendation was made for the baby to undergo bilateral branch pulmonary artery banding as an interim procedure before undergoing a Norwood operation at a later date.

Bilateral branch pulmonary artery bands were placed on day 4 of life via a midline sternotomy. There was an improvement in systemic blood pressure and a reduction in oxygen requirement. The PDA was not stented as there was good flow across a widely patent duct. The child remained in the high dependency unit to allow monitoring of ductal patency and saturations and to promote growth. At 2 months of age, the child's weight reached 3.7 kg and he underwent cardiac catheterization to delineate the cardiac anatomy. He was found to have low distal pulmonary artery pressures; there was good flow across the PDA and retrograde perfusion of the coronary arteries (Figure 9.3).

Expert comment

The hybrid approach was introduced by Galantowicz in 2008. It consists of: (1) bilateral pulmonary artery bands to provide adequate pulmonary blood flow, but without pulmonary hypertension; and (2) stent insertion into the ductus arteriosus to maintain patency and ensure systemic perfusion. In this instance, a decision was made by the surgeon and interventionalist not to stent the duct. This was not usual practice. However, echocardiographic imaging demonstrated a large duct with no restriction to flow. It was therefore proposed that placement of a stent within the PDA could be performed at a later date if any restriction to blood flow developed and this would minimize the risk for damage to the valves or vessels of the heart. This was felt to be particularly important, as at the point of surgery, the baby was haemodynamically unstable and required large amounts of inotropic support.

At 2.5 months of age, a 5-mm Sano conduit was inserted between the right ventricle (RV) and the branch pulmonary arteries. The distal main pulmonary artery (MPA) was disconnected. A Damus–Kaye–Stensel (DKS) anastomosis was made between the proximal MPA and the hypoplastic aorta. The interatrial communication was enlarged and the PDA was ligated.

The patient required mediastinal, pericardial, and bilateral chest drains. The chest was left open for 7 days to reduce intracardiac pressure and improve cardiac output. Inotropic support was required to maintain perfusion for 10 days. Drain and pacing wires were removed on the twelfth post-operative day due to initial sinus node dysfunction. The child remained intubated for 13 days and then was weaned to CPAP for a further 2 days. Oral feeds were introduced on day 7 post-operatively. Captopril was introduced with feeds. The child was discharged home with home monitoring at 3.5 months of age.

Learning point

There is growing evidence of a reduction in inter-stage mortality following the Norwood procedure after the introduction of home monitoring. Common illnesses, including fever, dehydration, or diarrhoea, can adversely affect the haemodynamic stability, contributing to mortality. Through a programme of monitoring feeds, weight, and transcutaneous oxygen saturations, survival to stage II has been greatly improved.

Learning point

Captopril is an angiotensin-converting enzyme inhibitor. It acts to produce vasodilatation by inhibiting angiotensin II formation. It has potential beneficial effects on the heart: (1) reduction in afterload, which enhances stroke volume and function; (2) reduction in pre-load with a decrease in pulmonary congestion; (3) reduced sympathetic activation and reduced myocardial work; and (4) reduction of deleterious remodelling of the myocardium through inhibition of angiotensin II. The evidence for a benefit is still to be proven, but many centres still give captopril in the hope of preserving cardiac function.

Discussion

Hearts with a functionally single ventricle comprise a wide spectrum of uncommon malformations, representing 2–3 % of all cases of congenital heart disease (CHD). This spectrum includes HLHS, tricuspid atresia, pulmonary atresia with an intact ventricular septum, unbalanced atrioventricular septal defect, and double inlet ventricle. The common feature is only one ventricle of sufficient size to adequately support the circulation. In this case, the ventricular morphology was of a solitary indeterminate ventricle. The characteristics of the left and right ventricles are shown in Table 9.1. A solitary indeterminate ventricle is a specific morphological variant with an extremely coarse trabecular pattern, quite distinct from a left or right ventricle and found in 2–3 % of cases.

Table 9.1 Characteristics of the left and right ventricles

Anatomic features	Right ventricle	Left ventricle
Trabeculations	Coarse Few Straight	Fine Numerous Oblique
Papillary muscles	Numerous Small Septal and free wall	Two Large Free wall origins only
Atrioventricular valve leaflets	Three Approximately equal depth	Two Very unequal depths
Infundibulum	Well developed	Absent
Semi-lunar-atrioventricular fibrous continuity	Absent	Present
Coronaries	Right coronary artery	Left anterior descending + circumflex
Conduction system	One	Two

The correct morphological diagnosis does not change the surgical strategy but is important for determining the prognosis. Children with systemic left ventricle have better function than those with systemic right ventricular physiology and, as a result, better prognosis.

The surgical approach involved palliating with a Norwood procedure (Figure 9.4). The first stage is performed soon after birth, with the aim of reconstructing the native aorta and arch, maintaining pulmonary perfusion via a shunt, and promoting mixing of blood with an atrial septectomy. Two available strategies exist. The use of a modified Blalock–Taussig shunt was first suggested by Norwood et al. [1]. The procedure uses a tube made of polytetrafluoroethylene (PTFE) to connect the innominate or subclavian artery to the pulmonary arteries. Early mortality following the Norwood procedure performed via a modified Blalock–Taussig shunt was initially 30–35%, primarily due to the rapid, unpredictable fall in pulmonary vascular resistance (PVR), resulting in systemic hypoperfusion and reduced coronary perfusion due to diastolic run-off of blood into the low-pressure pulmonary circulation [2]. Improved experience of managing patients with HLHS is now reflected by some centres reporting a 30-day survival rate of 85–90% [3]. Other factors related to outcome following stage 1 surgery include low birthweight and length of time on circulatory arrest or bypass [4].

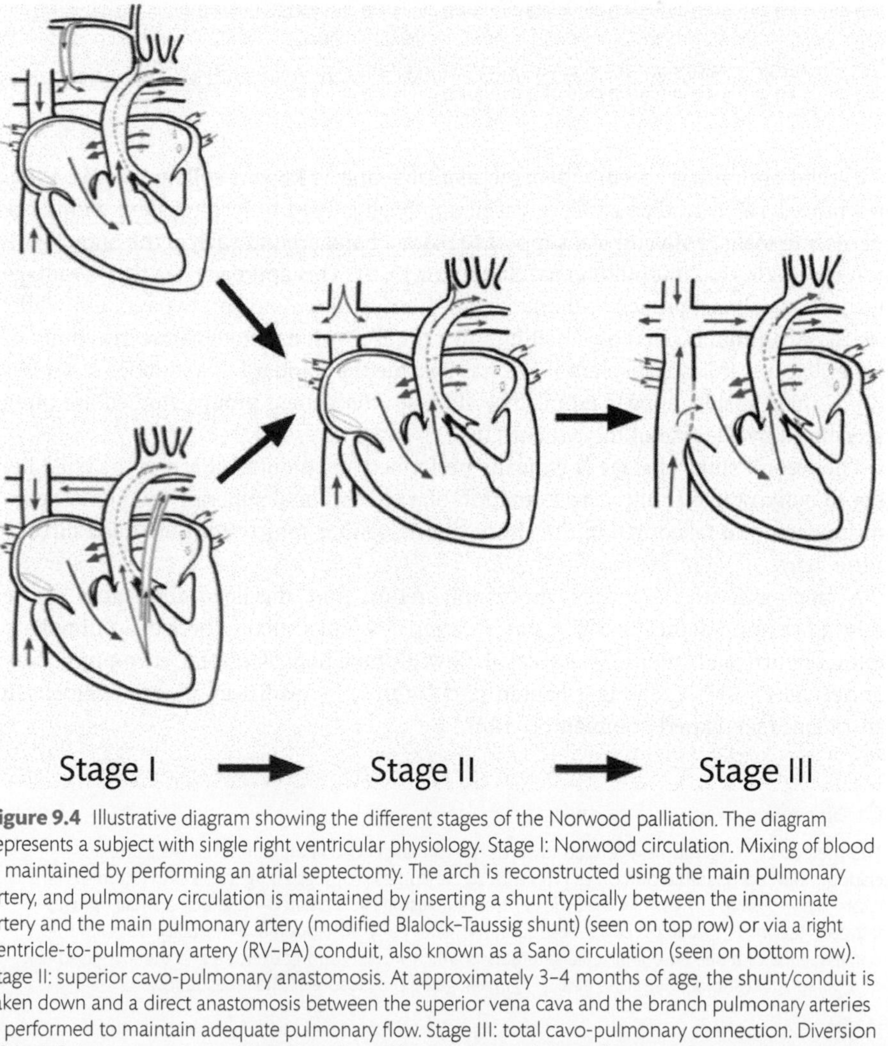

Figure 9.4 Illustrative diagram showing the different stages of the Norwood palliation. The diagram represents a subject with single right ventricular physiology. Stage I: Norwood circulation. Mixing of blood is maintained by performing an atrial septectomy. The arch is reconstructed using the main pulmonary artery, and pulmonary circulation is maintained by inserting a shunt typically between the innominate artery and the main pulmonary artery (modified Blalock–Taussig shunt) (seen on top row) or via a right ventricle-to-pulmonary artery (RV–PA) conduit, also known as a Sano circulation (seen on bottom row). Stage II: superior cavo-pulmonary anastomosis. At approximately 3–4 months of age, the shunt/conduit is taken down and a direct anastomosis between the superior vena cava and the branch pulmonary arteries is performed to maintain adequate pulmonary flow. Stage III: total cavo-pulmonary connection. Diversion of the inferior vena cava, via either a lateral tunnel or an extracardiac conduit, at 3–4 years of age maintains pulmonary blood flow. A small fenestration is shown. This circulation is also known as a Fontan circulation.

In response to early high mortality rates, Sano et al. helped to develop an alternative method to the modified Blalock–Taussig shunt, consisting of a right ventricle-to-pulmonary artery (RV–PA) conduit [5]. Sano's initial data reported greater haemodynamic stability with improved short-term survival rates, as although blood could regurgitate into the ventricle through the valveless conduit, systemic perfusion was maintained. However, there has been concern regarding the effect of a residual scar on the function of the ventricle.

Expert comment

The Single Ventricle Reconstruction Trial, a large randomized North American study [6], found the RV–PA conduit was superior to the modified Blalock–Taussig shunt for the primary endpoint of death or transplant at 12 months. However, the RV–PA conduit had significantly more interventions and complications. At the close of the study (3 years), there were no differences in transplantation-free survival between the two groups. Echocardiographic measures of function found right ventricular end-diastolic volume and ejection fraction both superior for the RV–PA group up to stage 2, but this had equalized between groups by 14 months. However, comparisons between those undergoing a Sano conduit versus a Blalock–Taussig shunt have demonstrated clear differences in the shape of the ventricle, presumably due to volume loading from regurgitation through the RV–PA conduit and the function of the ventricle due to the effects of a ventriculotomy scar. Currently, institutional preference and experience determine the choice of procedure.

A third option has recently become available and is known colloquially as a 'hybrid procedure'. A cardiac catheter-based approach is used to insert a stent within the ductus arteriosus, with surgical support to place a band around each of the branch pulmonary arteries to limit pulmonary blood flow [7, 8]. This approach has the advantage of a less invasive approach without the need for cardiopulmonary bypass, and whilst it is most commonly used on small infants or those with haemodynamic instability or as a bridge to cardiac transplant [9], it has become the standard in a number of centres [10]. Current results appear promising, although the patient groups studied are often determined by the size of the patient [11].

The second surgical stage is typically performed at 4 months of age as the child begins to outgrow the shunt. The formation of a bidirectional superior cavo-pulmonary anastomosis and takedown of the shunt directs venous return from the head directly to the lungs.

At approximately 3–4 years, the venous return from the head diminishes as the body grows, and saturations dip due to arterial–venous mixing between pulmonary venous return and inferior vena caval flow. Completion of a total cavo-pulmonary connection (TCPC), creating a Fontan circulation [14], results in an improvement in saturations (see Expert comment, p. 122).

Expert comment

The ventricle of a functionally univentricular heart has been described as 'dilated, hypertrophic and hypocontractile' [12]. Stage 2 surgery reduces the volume overload on the dilated RV, leading to improved ejection fraction [13]. It reduces the work of pulmonary blood flow and increases efficiency by directing desaturated venous blood flow to the lungs, in comparison to the previous arterial–venous mixture [2].

Expert comment

The method of TCPC has now tended towards the formation of a lateral tunnel or extracardiac conduit, with comparable outcomes [15], with some studies [16] suggesting those with a tunnel were more likely to have arrhythmia. In some centres, a fenestration is created—in effect, a small right-to-left connection. The addition of a fenestration mitigates early post-operative mortality, but with the consequence of a decrease in arterial saturations which worsen during exercise and the increased risk of a paradoxical stroke. Meadows et al. [17] investigated the closure of the fenestration in

20 patients and found improvements in arterial saturations, but with decreased cardiac output and no improvement in exercise tolerance. However, minute ventilation–carbon dioxide (CO_2) extraction improved during exercise, reducing the work of breathing as CO_2 extraction was improved by a reduction in ventilation–perfusion mismatching. As our experience of Fontan surgery has grown, so too have survival rates. In 1997, a study by Gentle et al (JCTVS) showed 5-year survival to be 70–84% [18]. By 2007, the 20-year survival had risen to 84% [19].

Assessing children with CHD at first presentation is tricky, and a strong suspicion is needed by the attending physician. The most common cause of an unwell infant remains sepsis, but in those with tachycardia out of proportion to tachypnoea, weak pulses, an enlarged liver, or other signs of heart failure—either clinically or on imaging—then management should additionally be tailored towards cardiac pathology. Echocardiography is the mainstay of diagnosis; however, it may not be available at first presentation. Therefore, stabilization, including potential intubation and ventilation and use of prostin, needs to be considered.

Learning point

In the majority of cases, the cardiac anatomy is adequately demonstrated by echocardiography. Occasionally, additional imaging might be required to delineate structures such as complex arch anatomy or venous pathways. Cardiac catheterization provides both haemodynamic and anatomical data but is invasive. Computed tomography (CT) and cardiac magnetic resonance (CMR) provide anatomical data but can be difficult to gain diagnostic imaging quality in those that are small or have fast heart rates. The choice of imaging modality is often determined by the facilities available and the level of expertise in each field.

Patients with single ventricle physiology have a guarded medium- to long-term prognosis. Heart failure contributes significantly towards mortality [18]. The Fontan circulation exposes patients to high systemic venous pressures and relative pulmonary hypotension due to the lack of a subpulmonary ventricle. This leaves them exposed to a wide range of complications, with progressive deterioration in function over time [19]. The long-term morbidity for those with a single ventricle circulation includes reduced exercise tolerance [1, 17, 20], increasing cyanosis, protein-losing enteropathy [21], plastic bronchitis, arrhythmias, and thromboembolic events [2, 18]. Many complain of breathlessness and fatigue [22].

Expert comment

The incidence of exercise intolerance following Fontan has been measured at 55–63%, comparably less than in univentricular left ventricular, compared to univentricular right ventricular, circulation [23]. It is inversely related to age at Fontan completion [24]. Exercise intolerance in this group is multifactorial. The lack of a subpulmonary ventricle to drive blood through the pulmonary bed, alongside abnormalities in cardiac function and systemic vascular resistance [25, 26], contributes to diminished exercise capacity. During exercise, patients with a Fontan circulation exhibit diminished peak oxygen consumption (VO_2 max), decreased heart rate response, and lower stroke volumes, leading to reduced cardiac output [27, 28].

Learning point

The transpulmonary gradient is the difference in mean pressures between the main pulmonary artery and the left atrium. It provides a driving force for blood flow across the lungs. In those with single ventricle circulation, the transpulmonary gradient is reduced due to the absence of a subpulmonary ventricle. A low driving force reduces pre-load on the systemic ventricle, which, in turn, can reduce stroke volume.

Expert comment

In one large study, Anderson et al. [29] found that the systemic RV has worse systolic function, compared to the systemic left ventricle, and diastolic dysfunction exists in 81% of patients, as measured by echocardiography. However, inadequate pre-load can induce similar effects, making these differences difficult to tease out. The systemic right ventricular function may be impaired by underfilling and inadequate pre-load, as the circulation of those with HLHS is affected by the absence of a subpulmonary ventricle [25]. A low PVR and low ventricular filling pressures are essential for augmenting cardiac output, especially during exercise [30]. Altered PVR as a cause of lowered pre-load has been proposed as a limitation to blood flow [31] and may be related to downregulation of endogenous pulmonary vasodilators, chronic pulmonary microemboli, loss of passive recruitment of capillaries, and loss of pulsatile blood flow [32]. The transpulmonary gradient should increase in exercise [33], mediating a fall in PVR. The absence of a subpulmonary ventricle means that those with a Fontan circulation are not able to increase pulmonary pressures accordingly. The use of sildenafil, a pulmonary vasodilator, has been shown to improve ventilatory efficiency during exercise, but without improvements in peak VO_2 max [34, 35]. However, the direct effects on the PVR are unknown, though estimations suggest that, in older groups, a fall in PVR occurs [36].

Strategies to improve outcomes for patients with single-ventricle palliation are ongoing. Patient numbers in individual centres are often small, and large multi-centre studies are required.

A final word from the expert

HLHS is a rare, but serious, condition that is challenging to manage. It requires an experienced team to work closely to deliver high-quality care to extremely sick patients. Despite improvements in our peri-operative management at each of the three stages of surgery, patients continue to experience a serious burden of morbidity. The focus on care now involves how we can continue to keep these children healthy and well as they grow into young adults. Advanced imaging techniques are now providing us with a greater understanding of the complex pathophysiology and the hope that, in the future, targeted interventions can be developed to help preserve the function of their cardiovascular system.

References

1. Norwood WI, Lang P, Hansen DD. Physiologic repair of aortic atresia-hypoplastic left heart syndrome. *N Engl J Med* 1983;308:23–6.
2. Feinstein JA, Benson DW, Dubin AM, et al. Hypoplastic left heart syndrome: current considerations and expectations. *J Am Coll Cardiol* 2012;59:S1–42.
3. Tweddell JS, Ghanayem NS, Mussatto KA, et al. Mixed venous oxygen saturation monitoring after stage 1 palliation for hypoplastic left heart syndrome. *Ann Thorac Surg* 2007;84:1301–10; discussion 1310.
4. Nilsson B, Mellander M, Sudow G, Berggren H. Results of staged palliation for hypoplastic left heart syndrome: a complete population-based series. *Acta Paediatr* 2006;95:1594–600.
5. Sano S, Ishino K, Kawada M, et al. Right ventricle–pulmonary artery shunt in first-stage palliation of hypoplastic left heart syndrome. *J Thorac Cardiovasc Surg* 2003;126:504–9.
6. Ohye RG, Sleeper LA, Mahony L, et al. Comparison of shunt types in the Norwood procedure for single-ventricle lesions. *N Engl J Med* 2010;362:1980–92.
7. Gibbs JL, Rothman MT, Rees MR, Parsons JM, Blackburn ME, Ruiz CE. Stenting of the arterial duct: a new approach to palliation for pulmonary atresia. *Br Heart J* 1992;67:240–5.

8. Gibbs JL, Wren C, Watterson KG, Hunter S, Hamilton JR. Stenting of the arterial duct combined with banding of the pulmonary arteries and atrial septectomy or septostomy: a new approach to palliation for the hypoplastic left heart syndrome. *Br Heart J* 1993;69:551–5.
9. Ruiz CE, Gamra H, Zhang HP, Garcia EJ, Boucek MM. Stenting of the ductus arteriosus as a bridge to cardiac transplantation in infants with the hypoplastic left-heart syndrome. *N Engl J Med* 1993;328:1605–8.
10. Bacha EA, Daves S, Hardin J, et al. Single-ventricle palliation for high-risk neonates: the emergence of an alternative hybrid stage I strategy. *J Thorac Cardiovasc Surg* 2006;131:163–71.e2.
11. Galantowicz M, Cheatham JP, Phillips A, et al. Hybrid approach for hypoplastic left heart syndrome: intermediate results after the learning curve. *Ann Thorac Surg* 2008;85:2063–71.
12. Gewillig M. The Fontan circulation. *Heart* 2005;91:839–46.
13. Bellsham-Revell HR, Tibby SM, Bell AJ, et al. Serial magnetic resonance imaging in hypoplastic left heart syndrome gives valuable insight into ventricular and vascular adaptation. *J Am Coll Cardiol* 2013;61:561–70.
14. Fontan F, Baudet E. Surgical repair of tricuspid atresia. *Thorax* 1971;26:240–8.
15. Fiore AC, Turrentine M, Rodefeld M, et al. Fontan operation: a comparison of lateral tunnel with extracardiac conduit. *Ann Thorac Surg* 2007;83:622–9; discussion 629.
16. Robbers-Visser D, Miedema M, Nijveld A, et al. Results of staged total cavopulmonary connection for functionally univentricular hearts; comparison of intra-atrial lateral tunnel and extracardiac conduit. *Eur J Cardiothorac Surg* 2010;37:934–41.
17. Meadows J, Lang P, Marx G, Rhodes J. Fontan fenestration closure has no acute effect on exercise capacity but improves ventilatory response to exercise. *J Am Coll Cardiol* 2008;52:108–13.
18. Gentles TL, Mayer JE Jr, Gauvreau K, et al. Fontan operation in five hundred consecutive patients: factors influencing early and late outcome. *J Thorac Cardiovasc Surg* 1997;114:376–91.
19. d'Udekem Y, Iyengar AJ, Cochrane AD, et al. The Fontan procedure: contemporary techniques have improved long-term outcomes. *Circulation* 2007;116(1 Suppl):I157–64.
18. Khairy P, Poirier N, Mercier LA. Univentricular heart. *Circulation* 2007;115:800–12.
19. van den Bosch AE, Roos-Hesselink JW, Van Domburg R, Bogers AJ, Simoons ML, Meijboom FJ. Long-term outcome and quality of life in adult patients after the Fontan operation. *Am J Cardiol* 2004;93:1141–5.
20. Connor JA, Thiagarajan R. Hypoplastic left heart syndrome. *Orphanet J Rare Dis* 2007;2:23.
21. Feldt RH, Driscoll DJ, Offord KP, et al. Protein-losing enteropathy after the Fontan operation. *J Thorac Cardiovasc Surg* 1996;112:672–80.
22. Takken T, Tacken MH, Blank AC, Hulzebos EH, Strengers JL, Helders PJ. Exercise limitation in patients with Fontan circulation: a review. *J Cardiovasc Med (Hagerstown)* 2007;8:775–81.
23. Ohuchi H, Yasuda K, Hasegawa S, et al. Influence of ventricular morphology on aerobic exercise capacity in patients after the Fontan operation. *J Am Coll Cardiol* 2001;37:1967–74.
24. Nakamura Y, Yagihara T, Kagisaki K, Hagino I, Kobayashi J. Ventricular performance in long-term survivors after Fontan operation. *Ann Thorac Surg* 2011;91:172–80.
25. Gewillig M, Brown SC, Eyskens B, et al. The Fontan circulation: who controls cardiac output? *Interact Cardiovasc Thorac Surg* 2010;10:428–33.
26. Sundareswaran KS, Kanter KR, Kitajima HD, et al. Impaired power output and cardiac index with hypoplastic left heart syndrome: a magnetic resonance imaging study. *Ann Thorac Surg* 2006;82:1267–75; discussion 1275.
27. Moller P, Weitz M, Jensen KO, et al. Exercise capacity of a contemporary cohort of children with hypoplastic left heart syndrome after staged palliation. *Eur J Cardiothorac Surg* 2009;36:980–5.
28. Durongpisitkul K, Driscoll DJ, Mahoney DW, et al. Cardiorespiratory response to exercise after modified Fontan operation: determinants of performance. *J Am Coll Cardiol* 1997;29:785–90.

29. Anderson PA, Sleeper LA, Mahony L, et al. Contemporary outcomes after the Fontan procedure: a Pediatric Heart Network multicenter study. *J Am Coll Cardiol* 2008;52:85–98.
30. Redington A. The physiology of the Fontan circulation. *Progr Pediatr Cardiol* 2006;22:179–86.
31. Khambadkone S, Li J, de Leval MR, Cullen S, Deanfield JE, Redington AN. Basal pulmonary vascular resistance and nitric oxide responsiveness late after Fontan-type operation. *Circulation* 2003;107:3204–8.
32. Presson RGJ, Baumgartner WAJ, Peterson AJ, Glenny RW, Wagner WWJ. Pulmonary capillaries are recruited during pulsatile flow. *J Appl Physiol (1985)* 2002;92:1183–90.
33. Stickland MK, Welsh RC, Petersen SR, et al. Does fitness level modulate the cardiovascular hemodynamic response to exercise? *J Appl Physiol (1985)* 2006;100:1895–901.
34. Goldberg DJ, French B, McBride MG, et al. Impact of oral sildenafil on exercise performance in children and young adults after the fontan operation: a randomized, double-blind, placebo-controlled, crossover trial. *Circulation* 2011;123:1185–93.
35. Giardini A, Balducci A, Specchia S, Gargiulo G, Bonvicini M, Picchio FM. Effect of sildenafil on haemodynamic response to exercise and exercise capacity in Fontan patients. *Eur Heart J* 2008;29:1681–7.
36. Van De Bruaene A, La Gerche A, Claessen G, et al. Sildenafil improves exercise hemodynamics in Fontan patients. *Circ Cardiovasc Imaging* 2014;7:265–73.

CASE

10 Challenges of percutaneous pulmonary valve implantation

Robin HS Chen and Salim Jivanji

Expert commentary Sachin Khambadkone

Case history

An ex-35-weeker female infant with a birthweight of 2.95 kg was born via spontaneous vaginal delivery to a gestational diabetic mother as the first child in the family. After initial stability during establishment of feeds, she deteriorated on day 9 of life with low saturations and respiratory distress. She was transferred to the tertiary paediatric cardiology unit where she was subsequently reviewed by a paediatric cardiologist and was diagnosed with type I truncus arteriosus. Echocardiography demonstrated the pulmonary artery coming off the posterior surface of the aorta with confluent branch pulmonary arteries. The truncal valve was trileaflet, non-stenotic, and non-regurgitant. There was muscular outlet ventricular (VSD) and a secundum atrial septal defect (ASD). Blood test confirmed a negative 22q11 status.

On day 23 of life, at 3.1 kg, she underwent complete repair, including VSD closure, direct ASD suture, and a 12-mm right ventricle-to-pulmonary artery (RV–PA) Contegra® conduit. During the procedure, it was noted that the heart was volume-loaded and her truncal valve was bileaflet and overriding a large muscular VSD.

She progressed well and was regularly reviewed in her local joint paediatric cardiology clinic. However, 11 years post-surgery, she reported worsening exercise tolerance, increasing shortness of breath, and palpitations. Although she was previously reviewed for palpitations with a normal 24-hour Holter, her symptom of breathlessness was new. On examination, she was noted to have a grade 4/6 ejection systolic murmur (ESM), with a thrill in the left upper sternal edge (LUSE). Her lung fields were clear, with no hepatomegaly and easily palpable peripheral pulses.

Echocardiography showed good biventricular function with no residual VSD. The truncal valve was competent, but there was narrowing of the RV–PA conduit, with a peak velocity of 4 m/s and free pulmonary regurgitation (PR). There was good flow to the branch pulmonary arteries. To further investigate her anatomy, she was referred for a non-general anaesthetic magnetic resonance imaging (MRI) and cardiopulmonary exercise testing (CPEX).

The MRI demonstrated severe proximal stenosis and mild regurgitation of the conduit. Additionally, there was mild hypoplasia of the right pulmonary artery (RPA), limiting flow to the right lung. The right-to-left flow ratio was noted to be 41:59. As described by the surgeon, the truncal valve was bicuspid, but dilated, with mild regurgitation. The biventricular chambers had normal volumes and function (Table 10.1). The right ventricular indexed volume was 72 ml/m^2.

Table 10.1 Right ventricular outflow tract dimensions

Area	Dimension
RV–PA conduit	7 × 14 mm (proximally) and 17 × 21 mm (distally)
Right pulmonary artery	7 × 9 mm (proximally) and 9 × 15 mm (distally)
Left pulmonary artery	19 × 21 mm (proximally) and 20 × 23 mm (distally)

Following discussion in the multidisciplinary meeting, she was listed for a percutaneous pulmonary valve implantation (PPVI).

Expert comment

Common arterial trunk is one of the cono-truncal anomalies that require the creation of a non-existent right ventricular outflow tract (RVOT). The operation is performed at the time of primary repair in the neonatal period or early infancy. This limits the size of the conduit used to create the RVOT. Most often, valved conduits are used—the common types being homografts (human pulmonary or aortic valve graft) or composite porcine valved bioprosthesis (Hancock®) and bovine jugular vein graft (Contegra®). As the size of the patient limits the size of the conduit, these patients often require multiple interventions in childhood for early degeneration or patient prosthesis mismatch in a growing child. This can often result in multiple sternotomies during the lifetime of the patient. As such, these patients are ideal candidates in exploring transcatheter interventions to reduce the operative burden.

Learning point Indication for PPVI

As with most medical innovations, the indication for PPVI has been ever expanding since its first description at the turn of the century [1]. The indication and timing of the procedure remain incompletely defined, and not uncommonly, it is an extrapolation of pre-existing controversial guidelines for surgical pulmonary valve replacement (PVR) (Table 10.2).

Table 10.2 Inclusion and exclusion criteria for PPVI

Inclusion criteria	Exclusion criteria [2–6]

• >5 years* [6]
• >30 kg [6] (some centres will accept down to >20 kg* [7]
• Existence of a full circumferential RV–PA conduit diameter# OR BPV
• RV–PA conduits:
  ○ >16 mm [4–6] (down to >14 × 14 mm [2, 3])
  ○ <22 × 22 mm [2, 3]
• BPV:
  ○ Inner diameter >16 mm
  ○ Melody® valve implantation has been reported to be successful in stenotic BPVs of up to 33 mm (outer diameter of prosthesis) [8]
• Dysfunctional RVOT
	• Active endocarditis
	• Active infection/sepsis
	• Pregnancy
	• IV drug use
	• Central venous occlusion/significant obstruction
	• Coronary anatomy at risk for compression at time of implant [3]

BPV, bioprosthetic pulmonary valve.
* Although age and weight criteria were initially arbitrary, it is now generally accepted that one should focus on whether the patient can accept a large (22-Fr) delivery sheath.
# Primarily for studies involving Melody® valves. Also highly dependent on the characteristics of the conduit (see separate Learning point, p. 132 and Expert Comment, p. 136–137).

Further assessment is based on the clinical condition of the patient. PPVI is indicated if:

- **New York Heart Association (NYHA) class I plus:**
  - Echocardiography*:
    - Doppler mean gradient >40 mmHg and/or [5, 6, 9]
    - Moderate/severe PR + either of the following [2, 3, 6, 7, 9]:
      - Severe right ventricular dysfunction (right ventricular area change ≤40%) [6]
      - Severe right ventricular dilatation [tricuspid valve (TV) annular Z-score ≥2] [6]
      - Impaired exercise capacity (peak oxygen consumption <65% predicted)

* In current practice, rarely is a decision for PPVI based solely on the echocardiogram. However, these parameters are widely used in the initial clinical studies.

  - MRI [10] (for patients with PR) with either of the following:
    - Right ventricular end-diastolic volume (RVEDV) >150 ml/m^2 or Z-score >4
    - Right ventricular end-systolic volume (RVESV) >80 ml/m^2
    - RV/LV volume ratio ≥2 [11]
    - Right ventricular ejection fraction (RVEF) <47%
    - Left ventricular ejection fraction (LVEF) <55%
    - Large RVOT aneurysm
  - Holter ECG (for patients with moderate or severe PR):
    - Sustained tachyarrhythmia [7] attributable to right ventricular volume overload + QRSd >140 ms [10]
  - Invasive haemodynamics [2, 10]:
    - RVOT obstruction (RVOTO) with right ventricular systemic pressure (RVSP) ≥3/4 systemic pressure
- **≥ NYHA class II plus:**
  - Echocardiography:
    - Doppler mean gradient >35 mmHg [4–6, 9] and/or
    - Moderate PR [2, 5, 6]
  - Invasive haemodynamics [2, 3]:
    - RVOTO with RVSP ≥2/3 systemic pressure
  - MRI [11]:
    - RV/LV volume ratio ≥1.5.

The summary described is generated mainly from the literature on PPVI with the Melody® transcutaneous pulmonary valve, since it has the longest history and has, as such, been extensively studied. However, readers are reminded to refer to Table 10.3 for various implantable pulmonary valves being developed—though the list is non-exhaustive.

Table 10.3 Types of percutaneous valves

Name	Minimum diameter of conduit (mm)	Maximum diameter of conduit (mm)	Sheath size (Fr)	Frame	Type	Size range of valve (mm)
Melody valve®	Variable and depending on the conduit	22	22	Platinum iridium	Bovine	18, 20, and 22
Edwards Sapien XT Pulmonic®	Variable and depending on the conduit	29	16–20	Cobalt chromium	Bovine	23, 26, and 29 XT

(continued)

Table 10.3 Continued

Name	Minimum diameter of conduit (mm)	Maximum diameter of conduit (mm)	Sheath size (Fr)	Frame	Type	Size range of valve (mm)
Alterra Adaptive Prestent®	Self-expandable, but designed for larger outflow tracts	40	16	Nitinol frame assembly and polyethylene terephthalate (PET) fabric covering. Has designated inflow and outflow ends	Bovine*	29 (*used with Edwards Sapien 3)
Pulsta®	Self-expandable valve with flared ends; minimum 18 mm	28	18	Knitted nitinol	Trileaflets made from treated porcine pericardial tissue	18–28 (2-mm increments) 38 mm in length 4 mm wider outer flares
Venus P valve®	Self-expandable with flared ends	34	18–26	Nitinol	Porcine	22–36 mm, with lengths of 25 mm and 30 mm

Expert comment

The guidelines for intervention are influenced by the nature of the studies. For example, for the US Investigational Device Exemption (US IDE) studies, the regulatory requirements are as important as the clinical criteria. As with any new techniques, the safety, feasibility, and efficacy studies have provided increasing confidence in undertaking this procedure well before cardiac decompensation manifests either on investigations (echocardiogram or MRI) or clinically. This has become the standard of care for most valvular heart diseases.

The lack of evidence for the timing of intervention on isolated regurgitant lesions in asymptomatic patients and the lack of criteria for interventions on mixed lesions—stenosis and regurgitation—remain as confounding factors. As such, every patient needs meticulous investigations to customize treatment, based on evolving guidelines.

Increasing experience has led to expanding the inclusion criteria, but these should be applied by experienced teams only [12, 13].

Learning point Pre-procedural workup

Clinical perspective

History:

- Functional status—NYHA class
- Symptoms suggestive of arrhythmia:
  - Consider Holter ECG or other investigation
- Exercise-related symptoms, e.g. chest pain—not uncommon in patients with severe RVOTO:
  - Consider exercise stress ECG/CPEX
- Any other exclusion criteria as stated
- Background history:
  - Primary diagnosis
  - Previous surgeries—types/size of RV–PA conduit
  - Previous interventions/possible other residual lesions:
    - Issue of limited venous access
    - Lesions that need to be dealt with simultaneously
- Physical examination.

Echocardiogram

Echocardiography has important limitations in reproducibility and accuracy in quantitative assessment of right ventricular volume and function, especially in patients with predominant regurgitant conditions. However, in general, patients with predominantly obstructive disease require less supportive evidence from pre-procedural workup to qualify for a PPVI, in which case a good-quality transthoracic echocardiogram will often be adequate to substantiate the need for intervention.

Echocardiographic parameters should include, but not be limited to, the following:

- Biventricular systolic and diastolic function
- Semi-quantitative assessment of right ventricular volume:
  - Role of right ventricular volume assessment has been replaced largely by CMR
  - TV annular dimension Z-score:
    - TV annular Z-score correlates poorly with RVEDV from CMR [14]
  - Area–indexed right ventricular apical end-diastolic area:
    - Correlates closely with RVEDV values of CMR [14, 15]
    - In one study [14], all patients with indexed right ventricular end-diastolic area ≥30 cm^2/m^2 will have a CMR RVEDV ≥160 ml/m^2
- Presence and degree of tricuspid regurgitation (TR)
- TR jet velocity—estimate RVSP
- RVOT flow velocity—estimate RVOT obstruction:
  - Doppler estimate of mean pressure gradient (versus peak gradient) correlates best with peak-to-peak gradient from catheterization data [14, 16]
- Qualitative assessment of degree of PR
- Residual anatomical lesions other than RVOT dysfunction:
  - Branch pulmonary artery (PA) stenosis:
    - Severity—warrants intervention?
    - Need detailed pre-procedural planning, e.g. significant bilateral proximal branch PA stenosis
  - Lesions that are possibly better dealt with by surgical repair.

ECG and Holter ECG

Controversies remain surrounding the useful cut-off point for QRS duration in patients with a history of RVOT surgery where intervention is required. Nonetheless, they might still be useful in terms of risk stratification in patients eligible for PPVI.

A study showed significant reduction in QRS duration in patients who had PPVI. This suggests important electrical remodelling following treatment of PR after an interventional technique [17].

Cardiopulmonary exercise testing

In patients with clear-cut symptomatology or poorer functional class, performing pre-procedural CPEX probably is not warranted. CPEX is probably more valuable in patients who are otherwise well (NYHA class I), with or without suspicious symptoms, in order to consider eligibility for PPVI. In a number of the larger series reported, a peak oxygen consumption of <65% predicted has been used as a supporting criterion for PPVI in asymptomatic patients with moderate/severe PR [3, 6, 7].

Expert comment

Echocardiography is useful in screening for patients with RVOTO. The importance of meticulous attention to TR measurement in the apical four-chamber view and the parasternal right ventricular inflow view to estimate RVSP with concomitant measurement of the cuff blood pressure provides the best haemodynamic assessment of right ventricular hypertension. In this same context, in most cases, it also provides a reliable estimation of RVOTO. The pitfall is to overly depend on RVOT Doppler gradients, as there are limitations to the application of the modified Bernoulli equation to long-segment stenosis in conduits, and the estimation of TR gives a more realistic estimation of RVOTO.

Clinical tip Cross-sectional imaging

MRI has evolved as an important tool providing quantitative assessment in patients with dysfunctional RVOT. Despite the controversy surrounding the optimal cut-off for MRI parameters, which essentially being an extrapolation of the surgical PVR counterpart, it is believed that, for PPVI, a less stringent criteria should be adopted in light of the relatively less invasive nature of the procedure [18]. One should be aware, however, that there are important variations in the methodology of obtaining CMR data in different centres, especially in right ventricular volume assessment (e.g. inclusion/exclusion of right ventricular trabeculation/muscle band in volumetric assessment). Hence, it is important to work closely with a centre's CMR specialist to ensure data consistency.

Learning point Cross-sectional imaging

Other than quantitative assessment, cross-sectional imaging also provides important morphological information. One of the greatest challenges in managing patients with dysfunctional RVOT with PPVI is the vast variability of the morphology of the RVOT. Even for patients with a circumferential RV–PA conduit, a peculiar RVOT/conduit morphology could render PPVI difficult, if not impossible. Cross-sectional imaging, including CT and CMR, hence becomes an essential assessment tool for these patients.

There are a number of important roles for cross-sectional imaging:

1. Size and distensibility of the RVOT/RV–PA conduit
2. Morphology of the RVOT/RV–PA conduit
3. Proximity of the RVOT/conduit with the coronary arteries
4. Degree of conduit calcification.

1. Size and distensibility of the RVOT/RV–PA conduit

Due to size limitations of the currently available percutaneous implantable pulmonary valves, the dimension of the target RVOT/conduit is of great importance. Small non-distensible RVOT/conduits may preclude complete opening of the device, leaving important stenosis—though some conduits may be stretched, as in the patient we have described (see separate Expert Comment p. 136–137). By contrast, large aneurysmal RVOTs/conduits may predispose to device instability and run the risk for device embolization. It is important to bear in mind that one should not rely solely on the dimension of the conduit documented in operative records to make decisions on PPVI procedures, as they quite often show progressive aneurysmal dilatation (Contegra® and pulmonary homograft). CMR or CT hence provide important measurement of the actual RVOT.

2. Morphology of the RVOT/RV-PA conduit

Dysfunctional RVOT/RV-PA conduit can exhibit a wide range of morphology, some being more amendable to PPVI than others. Attempts were made to classify them into different subgroups, based on three-dimensional CMR, as depicted in Figure 10.1 [19].

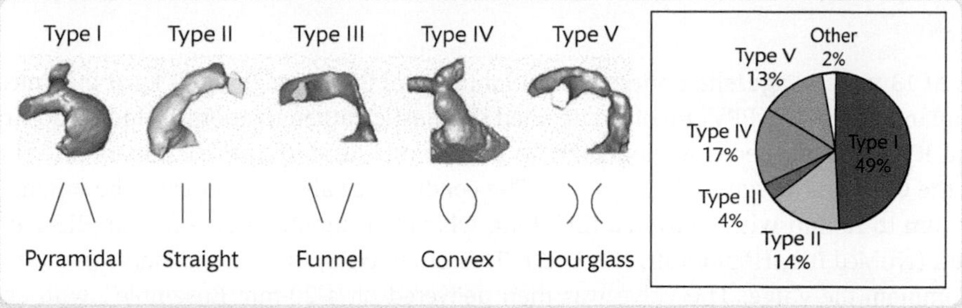

Figure 10.1 Classification of various shapes of right ventricular outflow tracts. Type I: pyramidal shape–wide proximally and narrow distally. Type II: straight—constant diameter. Type III: funnel shape (or known as the inverted funnel)—narrowed proximally and wide distally. Type IV: convex—wide centrally, but narrowed proximally and distally. Type V: hourglass—narrowed centrally, but wide proximally and distally.

Source data from Schievano S, Coats L, Migliavacca F, et al. Variations in right ventricular outflow tract morphology following repair of congenital heart disease: implications for percutaneous pulmonary valve implantation. *J Cardiovasc Magn Reson* 2007;9:687–95.

Among the five types, straight, parallel RVOT/conduit walls (type II) and an hourglass appearance (type V) confer the best stability of an implanted device, hence are the most suitable for PPVI. By contrast, pyramidal RVOTs (type I), most commonly found in patients post-transannular patch repair of RVOT, are the least favourable, with a high risk for device embolization.

3. Proximity of the RVOT/conduit with the coronary arteries

Inadvertent coronary artery compression is one of the most catastrophic complications of PPVI [7, 20–24]. Cross-sectional images provide essential information on the proximity of the RVOT/conduit to the coronary arteries. Traditionally, CT coronary angiogram has the advantage over CMR in delineating the course of coronary arteries—though, in recent years, coronary arteries can be confidently traced most of the time by CMR with steady-state free precession (SSFP) three-dimensional whole heart sequences.

4. Degree of conduit calcification

Valvar calcification has been an important area of interest for transcatheter aortic valve implantation (TAVI), the degree of which may affect immediate post-procedural outcome and survival. However, conduit or RVOT calcification has been receiving much less attention, and certainly without a universally agreed way of assessing the degree of calcification. Albeit the limited information, a prospective observational study did show that significant calcification is the only significant risk factor for conduit rupture in multivariate logistic regression models [25]. Further studies are probably required to substantiate the finding and possibly to stratify the risk with quantitative assessment of calcification with CT scanning.

Clinical tip

Important caveats exist, as most CMR data are obtained using three-dimensional data from magnetic resonance (MR) angiogram or ECG-gated whole heart imaging at diastole, which often does not reflect the maximal dimension of the RVOT. Differences in RVOT dimensions of up to 20% exist when measurements are taken at systole [26]. Hence, it is important that the maximum dimensions are taken with combined assessment with two-dimensional cine sequence.

Expert comment

Cross-sectional imaging is mandatory with the development of experienced imaging teams that collaborate closely with interventional cardiologists. The limitations of cross-sectional imaging, particularly the absence of dynamic imaging and non-gated imaging strategies, should be recognized. The presence of prosthetic material within the conduit valves and metallic stents or valves in close proximity to the zone of implantation may create artefact precluding a robust assessment of the RVOT. The most important limiting factor remains the difficulty in predicting compliance characteristics of the RVOT for safe anchoring or complete relief of stenosis without compromising the surrounding structures. Balloon interrogation with simultaneous injection of coronary arteries or aortography should be mandatory until more robust imaging techniques are available. The use of three-dimensional rotational angiography provides real-time three-dimensional relationships between the coronary artery and the zone of implantation [27]. There remains a significant discrepancy between advanced imaging techniques and procedural testing, and if in doubt, one should rather not proceed with PPVI [28].

At 13 years of age, she underwent implantation of PPVI, weighing 51 kg at the time. Implantation of the PPVI involved detailed diagnostic catheterization, including aortic and RVOT simultaneous angiography, to see the relationship of the coronary arteries to the Contegra® conduit (Figure 10.2). The conduit was also dilated from the original 12 mm to 20 mm with a covered CP® stent, which was mounted on a 20-mm BIB balloon (NuMed Inc, Hopkinton, NY, USA). This provided a suitable and stable platform to implant the valve. The valve was then delivered on a 20-mm Ensemble®, with an excellent result [29, 30]. Her procedure was carried out without any complication and she made a good post-procedural recovery. She had a single 'Z' stitch to close her femoral venous access. Echocardiogram at discharge demonstrated good biventricular function, with a mildly reduced right ventricular function. It showed that the CP® stent protruded into the RVOT, however distal from the TV. There was mild turbulence across the RVOT, with a Vmax of 3.1 m/s, and no significant PR with good flow into branch pulmonary arteries. She was commenced on lifelong aspirin.

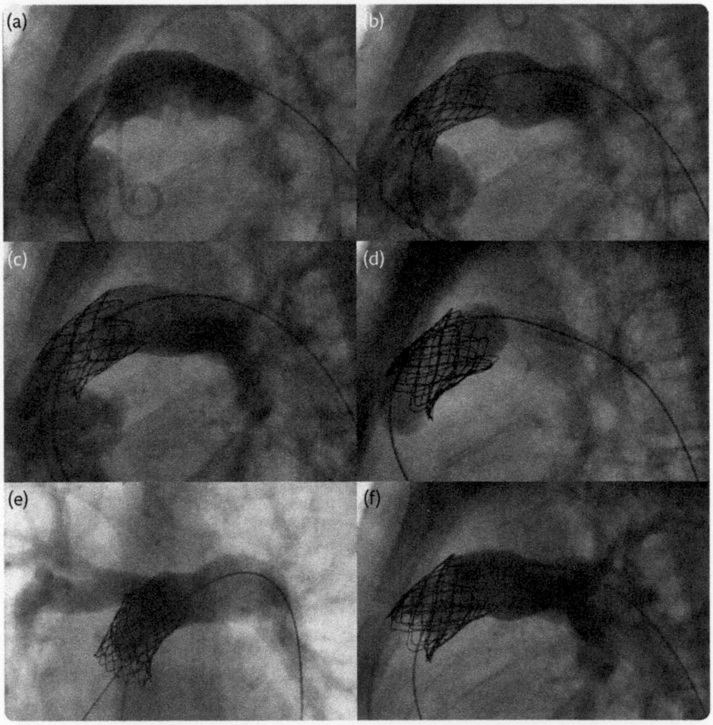

Figure 10.2 (a) to (d) Left lateral projection. (a) RVOT angiogram demonstrating a narrow Contegra® (12 mm) with a larger proximal RVOT and a distal pulmonary artery. (b) Angiogram after implantation of a 39-mm covered CP® stent with the waist measuring 14 mm. (c) Angiogram post-dilatation of the stent with a 20-mm Atlas® balloon to improve the RVOT calibre. (d) Implantation of a Melody® valve on a 22-mm Ensemble®. (e) Anteroposterior and (f) left lateral angiogram of the RVOT following implantation of a Melody® valve and post-dilatation with a 22-mm Atlas® balloon with a good-calibre valve with excellent competence.

Learning point What is the Melody® valve?

The Melody® Valve, manufactured by Medtronic, comprises a bovine jugular vein (BJV) valve sutured within a platinum iridium frame (Figure 10.3). In the late 1990s, Philipp Bonhoeffer, then in Paris, developed his first prototype for a stent-mounted biological valve intended for implant in the pulmonary position. This valve was initially developed for surgical implantation. However, over the years, it became clear that this would be the perfect valve for a transcutaneous application, and it underwent a series of modifications, resulting in what is now called the Melody® transcatheter pulmonary valve.

Following harvest of the valve, it undergoes a rigorous testing and quality control process. The valve tissue is then sutured to the stent frame—using blue suture at the distal end of the valve, ensuring correct orientation of the valve corresponding to the blue carrot tip on the end of the Ensemble® transcatheter delivery system. Following further inspection and testing of the valve, it is placed in a preservative solution for package and use (Figure 10.4).

It was important for the valve to function well in various sized conduits and be delivered in a catheter—after crimping to a diameter that is no more than 7 mm and be expandable from anywhere between 14 mm and 22 mm in diameter, without damaging the valve. The Ensemble® system used to implant the valve consists of an integrated balloon in balloon, a long-sheath, and an introducer, such that it can be introduced through the skin and delivered over a guidewire to the RVOT without any additional vascular sheaths or catheters. The system comprises two concentric balloons—an outer balloon and an inner balloon, which is half the diameter and shorter than the outer balloon. The delivery system is manufactured with outer balloon diameters of 18, 20, and 22 mm [30].

The valve is usually delivered from the femoral vein through fluoroscopic guidance. In 2000, the Melody® valve became the first transcatheter valve implanted in a human [1]. By 2006, it became the first commercially available transcatheter valve in the world [32].

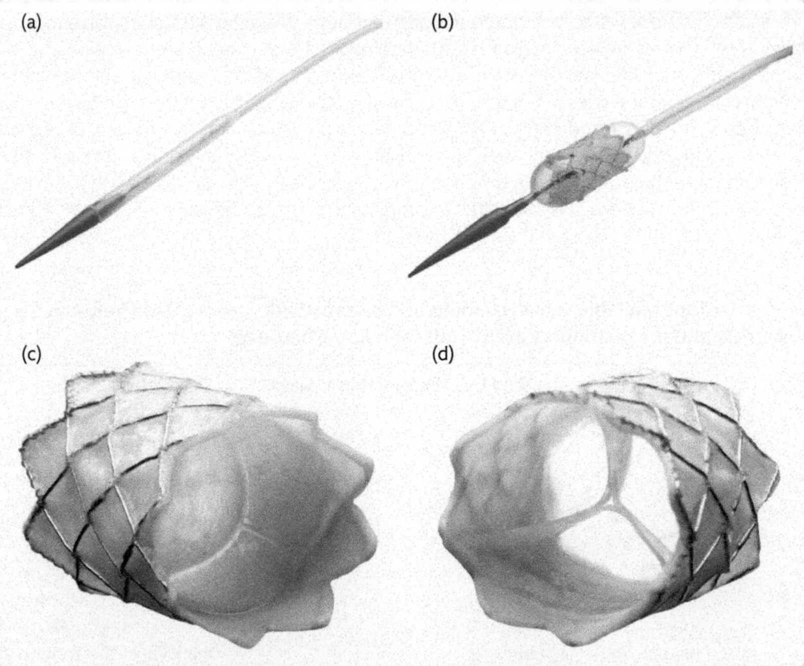

Figure 10.3 (a) Melody Ensemble® showing a fully assembled system with the valve covered. (b) Fully inflated BIB® balloon with a Melody® valve. (c) Melody® valve showing leaflets when closed from the underside. The flow direction is towards the blue stitching. (d) Closed Melody® valve demonstrating the trileaflet nature of the valve.
Images with permission from Medtronic®.

Expert comment

Aspirin is used to reduce the thrombotic burden around the biological tissue valve. Expecting endothelialization, early protocols used antiplatelet agents for a period of 6 months. Explanted valves showed poor endothelialization on the valve leaflets. Additionally, the perceived risk for endocarditis related to abrupt cessation of aspirin has led to continuation whilst the Melody® valve remains *in situ* [31].

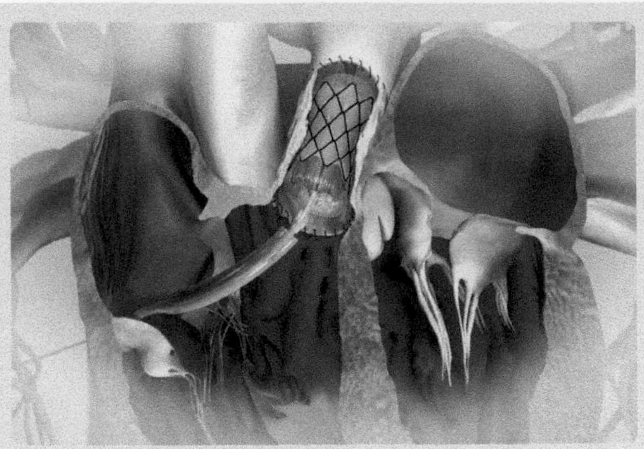

Figure 10.4 A Melody Ensemble® with the valve advanced from the inferior vena cava in the RVOT. The balloon is fully expanded to implant the valve.
Images with permission from Medtronic®.

Expert comment

It is absolutely mandatory for the interventional team to know the characteristics of bioprosthetic valves, conduits, and their morphological characteristics and material properties (see Table 10.4 for some examples). The manufacturer's information should be sought and published literature explored to understand how these valves or conduits respond to balloon dilatation or stent implantation. The bioprosthetic valves are now imaged in great detail with CT scans and three-dimensional echocardiography. The interventional teams also need to understand the mechanisms of device failure from pathological studies. The implant site within a failed bioprosthesis needs to be identified to improve good anchoring and as much as relief of stenosis. The bioprosthetic structure allows for good implantation zones and may not need pre-stenting. Valve-in-valve procedures are now well established for failed bioprosthetic valves not only in the pulmonary position, but also in the mitral, aortic, and tricuspid positions. It is also extremely important to go through the surgical notes of such implants.

Table 10.4 Various available valved conduits and bioprosthetic valves placed between the right ventricle and the pulmonary artery (this list is not exhaustive)

Valved conduits	Biomaterial	Attached to	Expandable	Sizes	Description
Aortic homograft	Aorta from human		Yes	Variable	
Pulmonary homograft	Pulmonary artery from human		Yes	Variable	
Contegra®	Bovine internal jugular vein	Can be with or without ring support	Yes	12–22 mm	Also known as xenograft The ring support can be at the level of the annulus and commissures Sizes go up in 2 mm. The smallest conduit of 12 mm is 7 cm long and the rest 10 cm. These are shortened as required

(continued)

Table 10.4 Continued

Valved conduits	Biomaterial	Attached to	Expandable	Sizes	Description
Gore-Tex®	Pericardial tissue to 'create' a valve	Gore-Tex	Very difficult	Variable	Soft and, as such, conforms to space in a limited chest wall cavity. Lasts a long time if luminal diameter can be maintained without stenosis or endothelialization
Carpentier Edwards® valved conduits	Three-cusp structure made from bovine pericardial tissue	Dacron cloth-covered titanium frame	No		
Dacron®	Pericardial tissue to 'create' a valve	Dacron	No	Variable	Prone to stenosis—not used much now
Hancock® bioprosthetic valved conduit	Porcine aortic valve	Woven fabric conduit	No	12–26	A ring support at the level of valve annulus

She was followed up a month after her procedure, which confirmed an improvement in her physical activity and energy overall. On auscultation, she had normal first heart sound, with exaggerated splitting of her second heart sound. She had a soft grade 2/6 ESM, with good distal pulses. Her groin access site was well healed. Her echocardiographic findings were reassuring, with findings similar to her post-procedural echocardiogram.

Evidence base Outcomes

PPVI has become an integral part in managing patients with dysfunctional RVOT. Despite the expanding indication and the rapid development of new implantable valves, the vast majority of the literature on PPVI still focus on Melody® valve implantation in dysfunctional RV–PA conduits. Hence, this outcomes review was largely based on this subgroup of patients.

Acute success

From various published prospective cohorts and series, PPVI has been demonstrated to be a safe and effective means for managing dysfunctional RV–PA conduits. The acute success rate ranges from 93.6% to 100%, resulting in excellent reduction in pulmonary stenosis, with none or minimal PR in the majority of patients.

Acute complications

The reported procedural complication rate spans a wide range, probably due to the interpreted definition and partly contributed by an era effect. The reported range is from 2.9% to 13.3% and included the following:

1. Complication requiring emergent surgery—1.5–2% [5, 9, 22]: conduit rupture and severe coronary compression
2. Contained conduit tear—5–11% [3, 4, 25]: usually managed conservatively or by covered stent

Expert comment

Procedural mortality from pulmonary valve insertion is related to either coronary compression or conduit rupture with severe internal bleeding (personal communication) [34]. Salvage techniques using coronary stenting, covered stenting of ruptured conduit, use of extracorporeal support, and emergent surgery have all been used as bail-out procedures. All centres performing such procedures should have robust supporting teams and mechanisms to counter unexpected complications despite meticulous testing during investigations.

3. Coronary compression (transient or on balloon interrogation)–5–6% [21, 24]: associated with abnormal coronary anatomy
4. Complete atrioventricular conduction block–1% [7]
5. Device embolization–1.5% [5]
6. Significant arrhythmia
7. Femoral vein thrombosis or trauma.

Medium-term mortality and morbidity

The 30-day mortality ranged from 0.7% to 1% and was mostly related to either underlying comorbidity or catastrophic coronary complications [7, 33].

A wide range of late mortality rates, understandably due to highly heterogenous patient groups, spanning from <1% to 4.7% have been reported. Higher mortality rates were observed from studies including frail patients, with deaths related to end-stage heart failure, malignant arrhythmia, or multi-organ failure [2, 10, 33].

Infective endocarditis (IE) was one of the important causes accounting for late morbidity and even mortality, whilst different degrees of Melody® valve stent fracture (MSF) also contribute to late morbidity.

Expert comment

Coronary compression and conduit rupture remain as two catastrophic procedural complications and need meticulous attention during procedure planning. Cross-sectional imaging helps in judging the spatial relationship of coronary arteries; however, it does not show clearly the proximity to the implantation zone. A CT angiogram probably shows better delineation of calcification than MRI. Balloon interrogation is necessary if there is any suspicion of coronary proximity to the implantation zone. Balloon interrogation should be done using a balloon size of at least the same diameter as, or a few millimetres more than, that to be used for final dilatation of the implanted pre-stent and Melody® valve complex. Failure to abolish the waist during balloon interrogation does not allow prediction of coronary compression. This leads to a dilemma of dilating a severely stenosed conduit in the absence of a 'protective' covered stent to control any potential conduit dissection or rupture against robust testing for coronary compression. The risk for coronary compression in this scenario outweighs the benefit of a transcatheter procedure over surgical PVR, and one should bail out unless there are clear contraindications for surgery.

There are experienced operators who would consider leaving a coronary wire down the coronary artery suspected to be at risk to perform coronary stenting to rescue coronary compression, and indeed this has been successfully performed soon after coronary compression is documented [35]. Late coronary compression is a rare event and the mechanism is not well understood [36].

If the coronary artery is a safe distance from the conduit, a covered stent could be deployed first and then dilated with a high-pressure balloon to create a suitable landing zone. This could be done in a graded fashion that may reduce the risk of major conduit disruption. The final diameter is determined by the implantation diameter of the conduit, the current diameter of the dilatable part of the conduit, if any, or the final intended diameter of the Melody® valve. The aim is to leave as little gradient as possible that provides longer freedom from re-intervention and, some believe, also reduces the risk for endocarditis.

Two years following PPVI, she was noted to be well, with no palpitations, chest pain, or syncope. Examination revealed a soft ESM, with delayed split of the second heart sound. Echocardiography confirmed good biventricular function, a well-functioning Melody® valve, and no evidence of stenosis.

Learning point Post-procedural follow-up

The currently available biological implantable pulmonary valves are subject to degeneration, similar to its surgical counterpart. Hence, it is important to monitor for potential valve dysfunction. The frequency and extensiveness of follow-up actions will be dependent on whether there are residual lesions or risk factors leading to premature valve dysfunction.

It is worth mentioning that any change in clinical signs and symptoms should prompt timely assessment to investigate for possible valve-related complications. For example, one should remain highly vigilant for possible subclinical IE in patients with unexplained malaise or a change in general condition or a rapid increase in gradient across the Melody® valve. This should initiate investigation with a CT scan to look for stent fractures (see separate Learning point, Melody valve stent fracture, p. 139).

Most centres will perform an MRI at 6–12 months following implant. This is a useful tool, as it allows objective assessment of the right ventricular function and remodelling. Follow-up MRI study also demonstrated improvements in terms of [37, 38]:

- Reduction in right ventricular dilatation: ↓ RVEDV and RVESV
- Improvement in right ventricular systolic function: ↑RVEF and RVSVI
- Improved left ventricular function: ↑ LVSVI.

Learning point Melody® valve stent fracture

MSF have been well reported, ranging from 5% to 25% [2, 7, 9, 39]. The wide range possibly was a result of the heterogeneity of patients, as well as the definition of MSF. MSF has been classified by Nordmeyer et al. [39], as shown in Figure 10.5.

Potential risk factors for MSF include [39–42]:

- Severe pre-procedural conduit obstruction
- Higher residual gradient post-PPVI
- Smaller angiographic diameter of the RVOT conduit
- Lack of calcification of the RVOT
- Implantation in native RVOT
- Stent compression or recoil after deployment
- Direct apposition of the transcatheter valve to the chest wall
- Younger age.

Protective factors include:

- Implantation in a pre-existing or newly implanted stent
- Implantation in a circumferential bioprosthetic valve.

Among all these factors, RVOT pre-stenting (or implanting in a pre-existing stent) seemed to have attracted the most attention. In a recent meta-analysis involving five studies and 360 patients, MSFs were significantly reduced in the pre-stenting group, as compared with the group of patients without pre-stenting [16.7% versus 33.5%, odds ratio (OR) 0.39; 95% confidence interval (CI) 0.22–0.69]. Pre-stenting was also associated with a lower incidence of type II/III MSF and the need for re-intervention. Despite this fact, questions remain—what the best pre-stenting strategy is, universal pre-stenting or selected group, single or multiple stenting, and the type of stent used. Multi-centre prospective trials are probably required to answer all these questions.

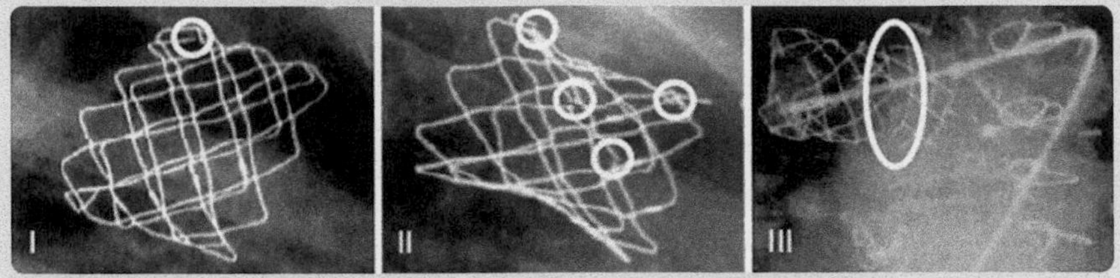

Figure 10.5 Melody® valve stent fractures. Type I: stent fracture of ≥1 strut, no loss of stent integrity. Type II: stent fracture of ≥1, with loss of stent integrity. Type III: embolization of the stent/separation of segments.

A few months later, she presented to her local hospital with a 2-day history of feeling generally unwell and fevers. Initial examination did not reveal a focus for her fevers, although she complained of central chest pain. Inflammatory blood markers were raised, whilst two separate blood cultures taken at that time were positive for *Streptococcus oralis*. In the absence of a focus and given that she had a PPVI, she was started on intravenous (IV) antibiotics. An echocardiogram done at the time showed no evidence of vegetations and a well-functioning truncal valve and Melody® valve in the pulmonary position.

She became afebrile 24 hours after starting IV ceftriaxone. However, she developed a fever again 10 days later. Initial suspicion was thought to be a line infection, as there was a modest increase in her C-reactive protein (CRP). However, the next dose of antibiotic resulted in her having an anaphylactic reaction requiring intramuscular adrenaline. Fortunately, she recovered well. Following discussion with the microbiologists, the antibiotic was changed to IV vancomycin.

She was reviewed regularly between her local hospital and the tertiary paediatric cardiology unit. Additionally, she also underwent cross-sectional imaging to look for evidence of IE. She made a good recovery with conservative treatment after completing 6 weeks of antibiotic treatment. On her most recent review, she was upbeat and although tired, she was slowly gaining her energy back and had returned back to school.

Clinical tip

Diagnosis of IE is already quite difficult and even more contentious in the setting of PPVI. It is worth noting the following points from the studies discussed:

- May have been overdiagnosed from loose inclusion
- Some of the IE cases did not involve the implanted valve
- Half of the patients responded to antibiotics alone
- Importantly, these episodes of IE were not acute. The subacute nature of the presentation makes it unlikely to be a procedural complication.

Learning point Infective endocarditis

The true incidence of IE in patients with PPVI is unknown, partly contributed by the lack of prospective data and the variable definitions used. The reported rate of IE among patients with Melody® valve PPVI ranges from 2% to 6% [4, 5, 10], which also accounted for some late mortality [10, 31, 43]. Data from a database of three prospective North American and European studies including 309 patients and 1660 [3] patient-years' follow-up recorded 46 patients with IE, of whom 35 were Melody® valve-related [44]. The annual incidence of IE and Melody® valve-related IE was 3.1% and 2.4% per patient-year, respectively. At 5 years post-Melody® valve implantation, freedom from IE and Melody® valve-related IE was 89% and 92%, respectively. Among the patients with IE, 32% required valve explantation at some point with or without prior catheter re-intervention, whilst 48% required antibiotics alone with no further interventions. These figures may appear alarming. However, due to the innate limitation from results generated from the database, there may be significant ascertainment bias. In turn, the true rate of Melody® valve-related IE might have been overestimated. Nonetheless, due to the significant morbidity associated with IE in this group of patients, clinicians should remain vigilant in detecting IE. Patient education is also of paramount importance.

Various potential risk factors have been reported, including:

- Post-implantation residual gradient ≥15 mmHg [44]
- Age ≤12 years at implant [44]
- History of IE prior to PPVI [2, 43]
- Discontinuation of aspirin [31, 45]
- Prior dental procedure
- Intravenous drug addict.

Learning point Need for re-intervention and re-intervention-free survival

Re-interventions are sometimes necessary, mostly for recurrent RVOTO secondary to MSF or inadequate gradient relief during the initial PPVI. A smaller proportion of re-interventions are secondary to IE. Re-interventions include: balloon valvuloplasty, second PPVI (valve-in-valve), valve explantation, and conduit revision [2, 3, 5, 7, 33].

Re-intervention-free survival varies from study to study due to variable follow-up periods. The recently published US IDE study reported 5-year re-intervention- and explantation-free survival rates of 76 ± 4% and 92 ± 3%, respectively. These results, however, may not be representative of contemporary best practice, as patients recruited included the initial experience in PPVI in the United States; hence, a learning curve effect exists. Furthermore, the first tertile of patients were prohibited from pre-stenting, a factor which is potentially protective from MSF and hence re-intervention. Hence, the true incidence of re-intervention should be lower.

As for longevity in otherwise MSF- and IE-free valves, short-term follow-up studies have demonstrated satisfactory valve function [2, 4–7, 9]. Regarding this aspect, the US IDE trial data have provided further support to the claim in the medium term. For the re-intervention-free patients in that study (113 out of 148 patients), the Melody® valve function remained unchanged from the early post-implantation echocardiogram. These results were undoubtedly encouraging, though longer-term follow-up will provide more information on the lifespan of these implantable valves.

Learning point Functional outcome

A substantial proportion of patients undergoing PPVI have been reported to enjoy an improvement in their functional class, almost immediately after the procedure, with the proportion of patients in NYHA class I rising from a baseline of 14–35% to 74–89% post-PPVI [4, 33]. However, data from objective measurements of exercise capacity were conflicting. Albeit reports of small improvement in maximum workload and minute ventilation to CO_2 production (VE/VCO_2) 6–12 months post-intervention, most studies failed to show a substantial improvement of other maximal or submaximal exercise parameters, including peak VO_2, which was discordant from the clinical improvement [6, 33, 46]. The discrepant findings, in part at least, may be accounted for by the heterogeneity of studied patients. One of the most notable variables is the different indications for PPVI. Improvement of objective exercise parameters were demonstrated only in patients with RVOTO as a primary indication for implantation, and not in those with primary PR, in a number of studies [47–49].

Clinical tip

It is important to note that PPVI does not replace surgery completely; rather its function primarily is to extend conduit life, to delay surgical conduit replacement or RVOT surgeries, and to reduce the number of lifetime open heart surgeries. It is noteworthy that transcatheter pulmonary valve implantation is not inferior to surgical procedures [50]. Nevertheless, the longevity of the valves remains to be seen.

A final word from the expert

Percutaneous pulmonary valve implantation has now matured as a first-choice procedure for stenotic, mixed, or regurgitant lesions of the operated RVOT in congenital heart disease. Various devices are available on balloon-expandable or self-expanding stents. Pre-stenting is mandatory to provide a good landing zone and to reduce the risk for stent fractures. Often it provides a safe anchoring site for the devices. Infection remains an important risk factor in these devices, whilst procedural mortality has been described from coronary compression or conduit rupture. This technique allows a reduction in the number of operations in the lifetime management of congenital heart disease.

References

1. Bonhoeffer P, Boudjemline Y, Saliba Z, et al. Percutaneous replacement of pulmonary valve in a right-ventricle to pulmonary-artery prosthetic conduit with valve dysfunction. *Lancet* 2000;356:1403–5.
2. Lurz P, Coats L, Khambadkone S, et al. Percutaneous pulmonary valve implantation: impact of evolving technology and learning curve on clinical outcome. *Circulation* 2008;117:1964–72.
3. Vezmar M, Chaturvedi R, Lee KJ, et al. Percutaneous pulmonary valve implantation in the young 2-year follow-up. *JACC Cardiovasc Interv* 2010;3:439–48.
4. Armstrong AK, Balzer DT, Cabalka AK, et al. One-year follow-up of the Melody transcatheter pulmonary valve multicenter post-approval study. *JACC Cardiovasc Interv* 2014;7:1254–62.
5. Butera G, Milanesi O, Spadoni I, et al. Melody transcatheter pulmonary valve implantation. Results from the registry of the Italian Society of Pediatric Cardiology. *Catheter Cardiovasc Interv* 2013;81:310–16.
6. Zahn EM, Hellenbrand WE, Lock JE, McElhinney DB. Implantation of the Melody transcatheter pulmonary valve in patients with a dysfunctional right ventricular outflow tract conduit early results from the US clinical trial. *J Am Coll Cardiol* 2009;54:1722–9.
7. Eicken A, Ewert P, Hager A, et al. Percutaneous pulmonary valve implantation: two-centre experience with more than 100 patients. *Eur Heart J* 2011;32:1260–5.
8. Cabalka AK, Asnes JD, Balzer DT, et al. Transcatheter pulmonary valve replacement using the Melody valve for treatment of dysfunctional surgical bioprostheses: a multicenter study. *J Thorac Cardiovasc Surg* 2018;155:1712–24 e1.
9. McElhinney DB, Hellenbrand WE, Zahn EM, et al. Short- and medium-term outcomes after transcatheter pulmonary valve placement in the expanded multicenter US melody valve trial. *Circulation* 2010;122:507–16.
10. Fraisse A, Aldebert P, Malekzadeh-Milani S, et al. Melody® transcatheter pulmonary valve implantation: results from a French registry. *Arch Cardiovasc Dis* 2014;107:607–14.
11. Chung R, Taylor AM. Imaging for preintervention planning: transcatheter pulmonary valve therapy. *Circ Cardiovasc Imaging* 2014;7:182–9.
12. Boshoff DE, Cools BL, Heying R, et al. Off-label use of percutaneous pulmonary valved stents in the right ventricular outflow tract: time to rewrite the label? *Catheter Cardiovasc Interv* 2013;81:987–95.
13. Malekzadeh-Milani S, Ladouceur M, Cohen S, Iserin L, Boudjemline Y. Results of transcatheter pulmonary valvulation in native or patched right ventricular outflow tracts. *Arch Cardiovasc Dis* 2014;107:592–8.
14. Brown DW, McElhinney DB, Araoz PA, et al. Reliability and accuracy of echocardiographic right heart evaluation in the U.S. Melody Valve Investigational Trial. *J Am Soc Echocardiogr* 2012;25:383–92 e4.
15. Greutmann M, Tobler D, Biaggi P, et al. Echocardiography for assessment of right ventricular volumes revisited: a cardiac magnetic resonance comparison study in adults with repaired tetralogy of Fallot. *J Am Soc Echocardiogr* 2010;23:905–11.
16. Silvilairat S, Cabalka AK, Cetta F, Hagler DJ, O'Leary PW. Outpatient echocardiographic assessment of complex pulmonary outflow stenosis: Doppler mean gradient is superior to the maximum instantaneous gradient. *J Am Soc Echocardiogr* 2005;18:1143–8.
17. Plymen CM, Bolger AP, Lurz P, et al. Electrical remodeling following percutaneous pulmonary valve implantation. *Am J Cardiol* 2011;107:309–14.
18. Tretter JT, Friedberg MK, Wald RM, McElhinney DB. Defining and refining indications for transcatheter pulmonary valve replacement in patients with repaired tetralogy of Fallot: contributions from anatomical and functional imaging. *Int J Cardiol* 2016;221:916–25.

19. Schievano S, Coats L, Migliavacca F, et al. Variations in right ventricular outflow tract morphology following repair of congenital heart disease: implications for percutaneous pulmonary valve implantation. *J Cardiovasc Magn Reson* 2007;9:687–95.
20. Biermann D, Schonebeck J, Rebel M, Weil J, Dodge-Khatami A. Left coronary artery occlusion after percutaneous pulmonary valve implantation. *Ann Thorac Surg* 2012;94:e7–9.
21. Fraisse A, Assaidi A, Mauri L, et al. Coronary artery compression during intention to treat right ventricle outflow with percutaneous pulmonary valve implantation: incidence, diagnosis, and outcome. *Catheter Cardiovasc Interv* 2014;83:E260–8.
22. Kostolny M, Tsang V, Nordmeyer J, et al. Rescue surgery following percutaneous pulmonary valve implantation. *Eur J Cardiothorac Surg* 2008;33:607–12.
23. Mauri L, Frigiola A, Butera G. Emergency surgery for extrinsic coronary compression after percutaneous pulmonary valve implantation. *Cardiol Young* 2013;23:463–5.
24. Morray BH, McElhinney DB, Cheatham JP, et al. Risk of coronary artery compression among patients referred for transcatheter pulmonary valve implantation: a multicenter experience. *Circ Cardiovasc Interv* 2013;6:535–42.
25. Boudjemline Y, Malekzadeh-Milani S, Patel M, et al. Predictors and outcomes of right ventricular outflow tract conduit rupture during percutaneous pulmonary valve implantation: a multicentre study. *EuroIntervention* 2016;11:1053–62.
26. Schievano S, Taylor AM, Capelli C, et al. First-in-man implantation of a novel percutaneous valve: a new approach to medical device development. *EuroIntervention* 2010;5:745–50.
27. Bruckheimer E, Rotschild C, Dagan T, et al. Computer-generated real-time digital holography: first time use in clinical medical imaging. *Eur Heart J Cardiovasc Imaging* 2016;17:845–9.
28. Bosi GM, Capelli C, Khambadkone S, Taylor AM, Schievano S. Patient-specific finite element models to support clinical decisions: a lesson learnt from a case study of percutaneous pulmonary valve implantation. *Catheter Cardiovasc Interv* 2015;86:1120–30.
29. Khambadkone S. Percutaneous pulmonary valve implantation. *Ann Pediatr Cardiol* 2012;5:53–60.
30. McElhinney DB, Hennesen JT. The Melody® valve and Ensemble® delivery system for transcatheter pulmonary valve replacement. *Ann N Y Acad Sci* 2013;1291:77–85.
31. Malekzadeh-Milani S, Ladouceur M, Patel M, et al. Incidence and predictors of Melody® valve endocarditis: a prospective study. *Arch Cardiovasc Dis* 2015;108:97–106.
32. Khambadkone S, Coats L, Taylor A, et al. Percutaneous pulmonary valve implantation in humans: results in 59 consecutive patients. *Circulation* 2005;112:1189–97.
33. Cheatham JP, Hellenbrand WE, Zahn EM, et al. Clinical and hemodynamic outcomes up to 7 years after transcatheter pulmonary valve replacement in the US Melody® valve investigational device exemption trial. *Circulation* 2015;131:1960–70.
34. Chatterjee A, Bajaj NS, McMahon WS, et al. Transcatheter pulmonary valve implantation: a comprehensive systematic review and meta-analyses of observational studies. *J Am Heart Assoc* 2017;6. pii:e006432.
35. Jimenez VA, Iniguez A, Baz JA, Sepulveda J, Zunzunegui JL. Extrinsic compression of the left anterior descending coronary artery during percutaneous pulmonary valve implantation. *JACC Cardiovasc Interv* 2014;7:224–5.
36. Dehghani P, Kraushaar G, Taylor DA. Coronary artery compression three months after transcatheter pulmonary valve implantation. *Catheter Cardiovasc Interv* 2015;85:611–14.
37. Romeih S, Kroft LJ, Bokenkamp R, et al. Delayed improvement of right ventricular diastolic function and regression of right ventricular mass after percutaneous pulmonary valve implantation in patients with congenital heart disease. *Am Heart J* 2009;158:40–6.
38. Secchi F, Resta EC, Cannao PM, et al. Four-year cardiac magnetic resonance (CMR) follow-up of patients treated with percutaneous pulmonary valve stent implantation. *Eur Radiol* 2015;25:3606–13.

39. Nordmeyer J, Khambadkone S, Coats L, et al. Risk stratification, systematic classification, and anticipatory management strategies for stent fracture after percutaneous pulmonary valve implantation. *Circulation* 2007;115:1392–7.
40. McElhinney DB, Bergersen L, Marshall AC. *In situ* fracture of stents implanted for relief of pulmonary arterial stenosis in patients with congenitally malformed hearts. *Cardiol Young* 2008;18:405–14.
41. McElhinney DB, Cheatham JP, Jones TK, et al. Stent fracture, valve dysfunction, and right ventricular outflow tract reintervention after transcatheter pulmonary valve implantation: patient-related and procedural risk factors in the US Melody® Valve Trial. *Circ Cardiovasc Interv* 2011;4:602–14.
42. Cardoso R, Ansari M, Garcia D, Sandhu S, Brinster D, Piazza N. Prestenting for prevention of Melody® valve stent fractures: a systematic review and meta-analysis. *Catheter Cardiovasc Interv* 2016;87:534–9.
43. McElhinney DB, Benson LN, Eicken A, Kreutzer J, Padera RF, Zahn EM. Infective endocarditis after transcatheter pulmonary valve replacement using the Melody® valve: combined results of 3 prospective North American and European studies. *Circ Cardiovasc Interv* 2013;6:292–300.
44. McElhinney DB, Sondergaard L, Armstrong AK, et al. Endocarditis after transcatheter pulmonary valve replacement. *J Am Coll Cardiol* 2018;72:2717–28.
45. Patel M, Iserin L, Bonnet D, Boudjemline Y. Atypical malignant late infective endocarditis of Melody® valve. *J Thorac Cardiovasc Surg* 2012;143:e32–5.
46. Batra AS, McElhinney DB, Wang W, et al. Cardiopulmonary exercise function among patients undergoing transcatheter pulmonary valve implantation in the US Melody valve investigational trial. *Am Heart J* 2012;163:280–7.
47. Coats L, Khambadkone S, Derrick G, et al. Physiological consequences of percutaneous pulmonary valve implantation: the different behaviour of volume- and pressure-overloaded ventricles. *Eur Heart J* 2007;28:1886–93.
48. Coats L, Khambadkone S, Derrick G, et al. Physiological and clinical consequences of relief of right ventricular outflow tract obstruction late after repair of congenital heart defects. *Circulation* 2006;113:2037–44.
49. Lurz P, Nordmeyer J, Giardini A, et al. Early versus late functional outcome after successful percutaneous pulmonary valve implantation: are the acute effects of altered right ventricular loading all we can expect? *J Am Coll Cardiol* 2011;57:724–31.
50. Caughron H, Kim D, Kamioka N, et al. Repeat pulmonary valve replacement: similar intermediate-term outcomes with surgical and transcatheter procedures. *JACC Cardiovasc Interv* 2018;11:2495–503.

CASE

11 Challenges in the management of coarctation of the aorta

Salim Jivanji and Robin HS Chen

Expert commentary Eric Rosenthal

Case history

A 17-month-old boy presented to his general practitioner (GP) with a viral upper respiratory tract infection (URTI). He was managed conservatively but was noted to have a murmur and was referred for a cardiology opinion. On review by the paediatric cardiologist, he was noted to be a well-grown toddler and essentially asymptomatic. His right arm pulse was less pronounced than his left arm pulse, whilst both his femoral pulses were easily palpable and there was no radiofemoral delay. His heart sounds were normal, with a grade 3/6 ejection systolic murmur, loudest in the apex and softly radiating to the back. The rest of the examination was normal.

Expert comment

Measurement of the blood pressure should be routine in all children, and the right arm is the limb of choice as it is closest to the heart. It is more representative of the true blood pressure in the unoperated child and after coarctation surgery. Only in the setting of an anomalous origin (rare) or surgical sacrifice of the right subclavian artery (RSCA) will it not be accurate. In this child, a four-limb blood pressure would have been required, as the **right** arm pulse was weaker than the **left**.

Echocardiography confirmed a normal abdominal and cardiac situs with normal connections. The heart was structurally and functionally normal, but the aortic arch appeared to have an abrupt angle just distal to the left subclavian artery (LSCA) towards the descending aorta. Although there was no discrete coarctation, there was an increase in velocity across the descending aorta of 3 m/s, with no diastolic continuation. There was no left ventricular hypertrophy.

Over the following years, he was reviewed regularly and was always noted to have good exercise tolerance, no cardiac symptoms, and consistent clinical examination findings. At the age of 7, he was noted to have bounding carotid pulses and slightly weaker right arm and femoral pulses, but a good left arm pulse. The systolic blood pressure in his right arm was 100 mmHg, whilst his left was 130 mmHg. Echocardiography showed mild left ventricular hypertrophy and there was the presence of a short diastolic tail in the Doppler profile of the descending aorta. The velocity on continuous-wave Doppler remained at 3 m/s. He was discussed at the multidisciplinary meeting at the time and was referred for diagnostic cardiac catheterization.

Angiography revealed a mild degree of ascending aortic dilatation with the arch, quite high up in the thorax (gothic arch) (see Figure 11.4 for different types of aortic arches). There was a small diverticulum of Kommerell with a ductal ampulla, and although not seen well on echocardiography, there was also a discrete coarctation (gradient of 20 mmHg under general anaesthesia; see Table 11.1), with an aberrant right subclavian artery (ARSCA) just inferior to the narrowing. There were no significant collateral vessels.

Table 11.1 Haemodynamics

Site	Pressure (mmHg)
RA	Mean 5
RV	20, EDP 6
PA	18/7, mean 12
PCW	Mean 8
LV	84, EDP 9
Asc aorta	80/40, mean 57
Desc Aorta	60/40, mean 50

No intervention was carried out, and on completion of the procedure, instructions were placed in the notes to ensure all future blood pressure measurements were from the left arm The patient was then re-discussed at the multidisciplinary meeting.

The multidisciplinary team consensus preferred balloon angioplasty ± stenting of the coarctation segment. It was felt that surgical repair would be high risk in view of poor collateral circulation, as the distal circulation would not be well protected during cross-clamping.

Expert comment

Spinal cord ischaemia with paraplegia is a devastating, but rare, complication of surgical repair of aortic coarctation. The risk is increased when there is a paucity of collaterals to the lower body segment. In older patients, it may be safer to perfuse the lower body segment with bypass cannulae, rather than just to cross-clamp the descending aorta for a prolonged period. During stent implantation, the aorta is blocked for less than a minute, and therefore, the risk of paraplegia is negligible. A covered stent in the usual coarctation site is unlikely to affect the spinal arteries, which arise much lower in the thoracic aorta at T9–T12 level.

Learning point Percutaneous balloon angioplasty versus surgical correction for native coarctation

Drs Crawford and Nylin performed the first coarctation surgery in 1944. Surgical repair remained the only treatment for coarctation of the aorta until the introduction of balloon angioplasty [1]. Although achieving comparable acute results, evidence showed a tendency for a higher rate of re-coarctation in up to 15–25% of patients [2–5], and even in up to 80% of neonates [6].

Despite the potential higher re-coarctation rate with balloon angioplasty, it still provides some advantage over traditional surgical repair, including shorter hospital stay [6] and lower rate of severe procedure-related complications [7]. A number of studies have addressed the potential use of balloon angioplasty as first-line management for native coarctation. A meta-analysis comparing surgical versus balloon angioplasty for native coarctation found no difference in the acute post-intervention gradient nor in the mid- and long-term re-coarctation rate [7]. There was, however, a significantly increased risk for early re-coarctation that required intervention, as well as a higher risk for aneurysm formation associated with balloon angioplasty. This could be explained by the mechanism of angioplasty, which involves 'controlled' disruption of the vessel wall, followed by healing remodelling, which was also the potential lead-point for aneurysm formation. In a large multicentre cohort of the Congenital Cardiovascular Interventional Study Consortium (CCISC) published in 2014, of the 76 patients who underwent balloon angioplasty for native coarctation, up to 11% suffered from acute aortic wall injury [8]. The incidence of post-angioplasty aortic aneurysm ranges from 5% to 45% in different small series [2–4, 9]. However, these were either retrospective series or observational studies without per-protocol follow-up and specific definitions for aortic aneurysm, making the detection rate questionable. The natural history of these post-procedural aortic aneurysms—if left untreated—is also unclear. Small aneurysms could be managed conservatively as long as other risk factors (e.g. hypertension) are well controlled.

Although there are many limitations to these studies, the apparent association of higher re-intervention rates and aneurysm formation led to balloon angioplasty falling gradually out of favour for native coarctation and it has largely been replaced by stenting in bigger children.

Learning point Comparison between surgical repair, balloon angioplasty, and stenting for delayed presentation of native coarctation of the aorta

There has been a long-standing debate on the optimal treatment modality for native coarctation. Existing evidence has been largely limited by the heterogeneity of patient groups, small sample sizes, and lack of randomization. In 2011, a multi-centre observational study (involving 350 patients across 36 institutions) was published by the CCISC group, describing the acute and long-term outcomes by comparing surgical repair, balloon angioplasty, and stenting in patients with native coarctation with a body weight of >10 kg [9]. The study was heavily skewed towards stenting, as 217 patients (62%) underwent stenting, whereas only 61 (17%) and 72 (21%) patients underwent balloon angioplasty and surgical repair, respectively. The study showed that all three methods achieved satisfactory short-term results in relieving obstruction. However, both surgery and stenting were superior to balloon angioplasty in achieving a lower gradient on follow-up. The stenting group also had significantly shorter hospital stay versus surgery and fewer complications as compared to the other two groups. The angioplasty group, not surprisingly, had the highest rate of aortic wall injury (up to 9.8%).

The groups, however, were quite heterogenous, with two obvious baseline differences being the age and body size of the patients at the time of intervention. The stenting group were significantly older and heavier, accounting for the larger sheaths required for stenting. Furthermore, a per-protocol follow-up was lacking, making head-to-head comparison of the three modalities difficult. This was reflected by missing data on aortic wall injury in the surgery group, as routine screening had not been performed on surgical patients—hence, the bias in picking up aortic wall injury in patients undergoing balloon angioplasty and aortic stenting.

A Cochrane review published in 2012, aiming to compare the effectiveness and safety of stenting versus surgical management for coarctation [10], failed to arrive at a conclusion since all the studies identified were excluded as none of them were randomized or quasi-randomized controlled to compare the two modalities.

Cardiac catheterization a few weeks later (26.4 kg and age 7 years) via a percutaneous right femoral artery (RFA) access with an 11-Fr sheath was carried out to stent the narrowing with a bare metal P308 Palmaz Stent (Cordis, Baar, Switzerland) on a 14-mm Cristal balloon (Pyramed, Queensland, Australia). The distal end was flared with a 16-mm Tyshak II balloon. There was an excellent angiographic result. There was no compromise of right upper limb perfusion, and the small right groin haematoma was managed conservatively. Post-procedural echocardiography showed good pulsatility of the descending aorta, and he was discharged the following day.

Learning point Pushing the limits—stenting in smaller children, infants, and neonates

To accommodate for somatic growth and re-dilating the stents later, many of the stents used for coarctation stenting have a large profile, hence necessitating large-calibre delivery sheaths. The vascular complications associated with large sheaths are non-negligible, even in adults, let alone in small children. Hence relatively few reports are available describing the outcome of aortic stenting in smaller patients. Kang et al. reported their single-centre experience of using a low-profile stent (Valeo stent) in managing patients of <30 kg with coarctation, achieving a 100% success rate with no aortic wall injury [11]. There are also other series involving children of <30 kg using various other stents (Palmaz Genesis, Genesis, JoStent, EV3 series, and CP® stent), which also showed excellent acute success rates [12–18]. As anticipated, the vascular complication rate was significantly higher, with up to 20% in selected studies. As many of these patients would also require a planned re-intervention for stent expansion to keep up with somatic growth, stenting in this group of patients remains debatable.

Stenting may be required in infants and even neonates, especially when complex aortic obstruction persists despite surgical interventions, or in certain cases where comorbidities would rule out surgical correction (Class IIb recommendation, level of evidence C—American Heart Association guideline) [19]. In the past decade, the development of growth stents and biodegradable stents in children has received much attention [20–22]. Despite being largely experimental at this stage, these technologies could make aortic stenting in infants and small children more plausible by negating the need for re-intervention.

Learning point Types of stents

(See Table 11.2.)

Table 11.2 Different types of stents used in congenital heart disease

Stent	Material	Design	Nominal diameter (potential)	Length (mm)	Sheath (Fr)	Guidewire (in)	Mounting	Common usage	Advantages	Disadvantages
Sinus Superflex-DS	N	O	7–9	12–20	4	0.018	Self-expandable	Neonate/infant lesion	Small sheath size	Low radial strength
Palmaz Blue	Cc	C	4–7 (12)	12–24	4–5	0.014–0.018	Aviator plus Slalom	Neonate/infant lesion		
Genesis Medium	Ss	C	4–8 (12)	12–24	5–6	0.018–0.035	Slalom Opta Pro Unmounted	Neonate/infant lesion		
Formula 535	Ss	O	5–8 (20)	12–30	5–6	0.035	High-pressure balloon catheter	PAs; atrial septum, RVOT	Small sheath size; used for smaller vessels	Cannot be inflated to large diameters
Genesis Large	Ss	C	5–10 (12)	19–79	5–6 6–7	0.018–0.035	Slalom Opta Pro Unmounted	PAs; atrial septum, RVOT		
Valeo Life Stent	Ss	O	6–10(20)	18–56	5–6	0.035	High-pressure balloon catheter	PAs; atrial septum, RVOT	Low profile, small sheath size	Low radial strength; cannot fracture easily
Genesis XD	Ss	C	10–12 (18)	19–59	8	Depends on balloon catheter	Unmounted	Pulmonary arteries		
Mega LD	Ss	O	9–12 (18)	16–36	9	Depends on balloon catheter	Unmounted	Pulmonary arteries	Good radial strength	Large sheath size
Maxi LD	Ss	O	12 (26)	16–36	11	Depends on balloon catheter	Unmounted	Coarctation; pulmonary arteries, pulmonary veins	Very good radial strength	
Advanta V12	Ss	O	12–16 (22)	29–61	9–11	0.035	High-pressure balloon catheter	Coarctation; pulmonary arteries, pulmonary veins		
Covered Cheatham Platinum	Pi	C	12–24 (26) (up to 30 mm for 10 Zig)	16–45	12–14	0.035	Unmounted or premounted on BIB catheter	Coarctation; pulmonary arteries, pulmonary veins	Covered; good radial strength Can be dilated to large diameters (10 Zig)	Shortens significantly in larger diameters

Cheatham Platinum 8 Zig	Pi	C	12–24 (26) (up to 30 mm for 10 Zig)	16–45	12–14	0.035	Unmounted or premounted on BIB catheter	Coarctation; pulmonary arteries, pulmonary veins	Good radial strength Can be dilated to large diameters (10 Zig) Available in long lengths	Shortens significantly in larger diameters
Andrastent XL	Cc	H	14–25	13–57	8–9	Depends on balloon catheter	Unmounted	Coarctation; pulmonary arteries, pulmonary veins	Good radial strength	
Andrastent XXL	Cc	H	30–32	17–57	10–11	Depends on balloon catheter	Unmounted	Coarctation; pulmonary arteries, pulmonary veins	Very good radial strength	
BeGraft	Cc	C—single stent	12–24	19–59	9–14	Mounted on medium-pressure balloon	Premounted	Coarctation; pulmonary arteries, pulmonary veins	Low profile; CE marked for aortic use Covering inside and outside stent	Less stability in overlapping stents

Potential diameters from reported experience—not confirmed by the manufacturer.
C, closed; Cc, chromium cobalt; H, hybrid; N, nitinol; O, open; Pi, Platinum-iridium; Ss, stainless steel.
Adapted from *Cardiac Catheterization for Congenital Heart Disease*. Butera et al. [23]

Learning point

Although some centres continue to use surgical cut-down as access for aortic stenting, which allows for subsequent haemostasis and repair, most centres use ultrasound access with the Seldinger technique. Haemostasis, especially in large-sheath access areas, remains inconsistent among various centres. Whilst an array of vascular closure devices are commonly used in the adult population, paediatric centres lean towards manual compression to achieve haemostasis due to relatively small sheath sizes.

Expert comment

Particularly when 12- to 16-Fr sheaths are required, a vascular occlusion device is invaluable in ensuring haemostasis after the procedure. In the past, when haemostasis was not achieved easily by manual pressure, external compression devices could be needed for several hours after the procedure. These were uncomfortable, impeded mobilization, and could also be accompanied by severe haematoma formation when used after initial manual compression had failed.

Clinical tip Access

Whilst it is important to be familiar with both methods of femoral access (ultrasound-guided and using landmarks and palpation), ultrasound-guided access has transformed the way we do cardiac catheterization since Seldinger first described a safe and consistent method of accessing central vessels [24]. The information available with the use of ultrasound, compared with the traditional landmark technique, is invaluable. Once skilled, the process allows for rapid access in the femoral artery or any other central vessels, even in the most difficult patients, and reduces morbidity significantly. The ability to see where the needle lies ensures that, whilst accessing the vessel, we do not transfix the vessel by going through to the posterior wall (reducing vessel morbidity), maintain future patency by reducing multiple attempts, clean central luminal position, and reduces anaesthetic time [25–27].

Expert comment

In spite of the advantages of ultrasound-guided access, it remains important to pay attention to the anatomical landmarks and not puncture exclusively based on the ultrasound. Femoral artery angiography is then essential to confirm the puncture site is in the superficial or common femoral artery, and not above the pelvic brim. Puncture of the profunda femoral artery prevents use of closure devices easily AND is commonly associated with femoral artery pseudoaneurysms and haematoma. Puncture above the pelvic brim makes manual compression difficult and may be associated with substantial retroperitoneal extravasation, especially with large-bore sheaths, when not using closure devices.

He was followed up regularly, making satisfactory progress. At 15 years of age, secondary to somatic growth, the echocardiography markers were suggestive of inadequacy of the stented area, relative to his body size. As such, he was referred for an exercise test and repeat cardiac catheterization to further dilate the stent.

Exercise testing showed excellent effort capacity of 230 W. Peak oxygen consumption was 51.4 ml/kg/min (normal 44–58 for age and gender), with a peak heart rate of 178 bpm There was a mildly hypertensive response with a maximum systolic blood pressure of 208 mmHg. Resting blood pressure in his left arm was 126/80 mmHg.

Expert comment

Hypertension after coarctation repair is the most important cause of late morbidity that includes left ventricular hypertrophy, coronary artery disease, cerebrovascular ischaemia, and aneurysm formation at the coarctation site [28]. The age and adequacy of repair are key factors in determining the presence of post-operative hypertension. Hypertension is increasingly common, the later the repair, and almost invariably when performed after early childhood. Impeccable blood pressure management is required to prevent the long-term morbidity that accrues without antihypertensive treatment.

A hypertensive response to exercise is not uncommon, even after a 'perfect' repair with normal resting blood pressure and no gradient across the coarctation site. Whilst it may reflect a suboptimal repair, it may also be due to a vasculopathy present from fetal life and is poorly understood.

He underwent cardiac catheterization the following year (16 years), with a view to dilating the stented coarctation site, but an aneurysm was noted in the anterolateral wall just proximal to the stent (Figure 11.1). Although a covered stent would have been indicated to simultaneously treat the aneurysm and the 're-coarctation', there was concern that the ARSCA would be compromised. The procedure was terminated, and he was re-discussed at the multidisciplinary meeting for further evaluation

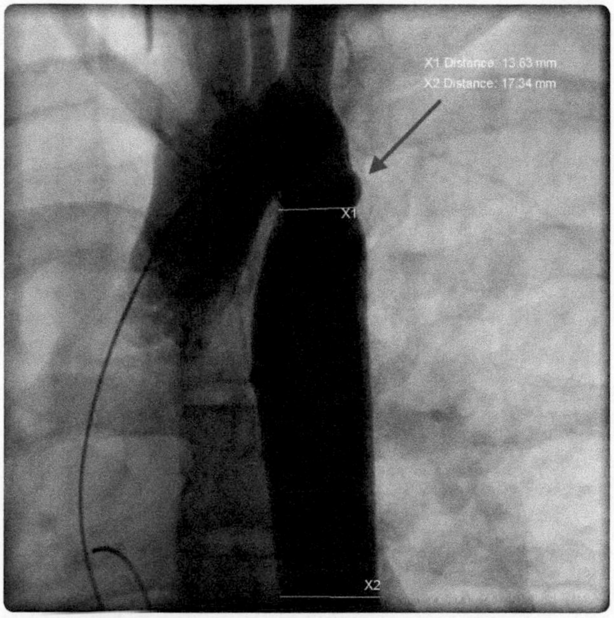

Figure 11.1 Left anterior oblique (LAO) view of an aortic angiogram. Red arrow shows the site of an aneurysm, with the narrowest (stented) region measuring 13 mm in diameter and the descending aorta at the level of the diaphragm 17 mm.

Learning point Issues on medium- to long-term follow-up: delayed presentation of aortic wall injury

Despite the reasonably low rate of acute injury, late presentation of aortic wall injury remains a significant concern. The reported rate of aortic aneurysm formation spans a wide range from 9% to 17% [13, 15, 29–32], but only 0–9% are lesions significant enough to require re-intervention [29–32]. In Forbes et al.'s study, among 578 patients with aortic stenting, a subgroup of 144 patients had follow-up aortic imaging in the form of CT or MRI or cardiac catheterization, with a median follow-up of 12 months. Up to 25.6% had abnormal imaging results, with intimal proliferation and aneurysm formation being the most common findings. In this group, 3.5% had aortic dissection, which was managed conservatively, and 9% had various degrees of aneurysm formation. The majority of these aneurysms were managed conservatively, with only 30% undergoing interventions. There were several factors identified to be associated with aortic injury, including pre-stent angioplasty, a larger percentage increase in coarctation diameter, and a balloon-to-coarctation ratio of >3.5.

A CT scan was performed, and the medical engineers created a rapid prototyping three-dimensional model of his aorta with an indwelling stent. This allowed analysis of the relationship of his indwelling stent with the aberrant subclavian artery and descending aorta (Figure 11.2). The engineers also performed computer modelling using finite element analysis and confirmed that there would be enough room to insert an 18-mm covered stent whilst protecting the origin of the RSCA with a small balloon.

Expert comment

The use of the three-dimensional computational technique was an elegant approach to re-dilating the stent, occluding the aneurysm, and simultaneously preserving patency of the ARSCA. Without this, it would have been necessary to deploy the covered stent only after obtaining right radial artery access. This would have allowed retrograde puncture through the side of the covered stent, with balloon dilatation to open the struts to the subclavian artery if the pressure was low after the covered stent had been placed.

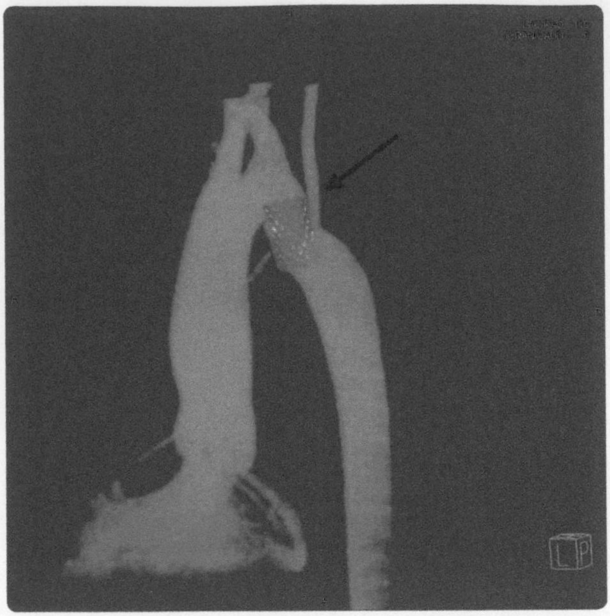

Figure 11.2 A volume-rendering technique (VRT) in left anterior oblique (LAO) 45° showing the stent and ARSCA (blue arrow).

He returned for cardiac catheterization when he was 17 years of age and approaching 70 kg in weight (Table 11.3).

Table 11.3 Cardiac catheterization

Pre-stent		Post-stent	
Site	Pressures (mmHg)	Site	Pressures (mmHg)
LVEDP	10		
Ascending to descending aorta (pullback gradient)	15	Ascending to descending aorta (pullback gradient)	3

A 14-Fr Mullins sheath (Medtronic, MN, USA) was used, through which a 29-mm covered CP® stent was advanced over an 18 mm × 45 mm BIB balloon to overlie the previous stent. To ensure patency of the RSCA, an additional balloon (Opta 7 mm × 20 mm) was placed at the proximal segment via a second femoral artery access. Both balloons were hand-inflated, with the secondary balloon in the RSCA protecting the vessel. The result was almost exactly as postulated by the medical engineers (Figure 11.3). The residual gradient was only 3 mmHg. His femoral artery access site was closed with a perclose vascular device.

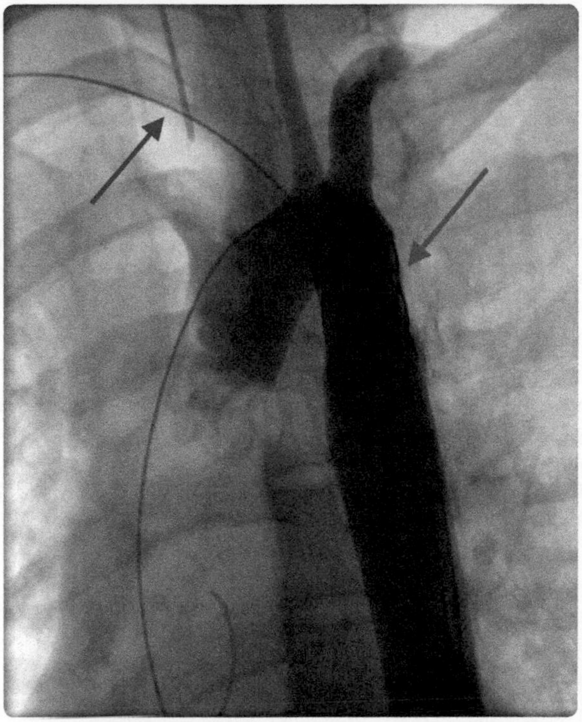

Figure 11.3 Image in left anterior oblique (LAO) 25°. Angiogram demonstrating the aneurysmal part (shown in figure 11.1) now covered with a covered CP stent (red arrow). The blue arrow shows the wire in the ARSCA to ensure patency following stenting.

The patient was discharged the following day. Subsequent reviews confirmed excellent progress. As he had almost reached adulthood, his care was transferred over to the grown-up congenital heart (GUCH) team.

Discussion

Coarctation of the aorta accounts for 4–5% of all congenital heart defects and has a male preponderance [33]. The prevalence of this condition is four per 10,000 but can increase significantly when associated with certain conditions such as Turner's syndrome.

Coarctation of the aorta was first described by Morgagni in 1760 as a zone of constriction in the aorta [34]. Bonnet, more than 200 years later, in 1903 proposed to classify the aorta into two types: 'adult' coarctation, a sharply localized zone of constriction, and 'infantile' coarctation—suggesting that this described a long and uniformly narrow segment [35]. It was not until 1948 when Edwards and his associates made a more exacting description of this condition by introducing the idea of hypoplasia of the arch as a separate entity from coarctation of the aorta [36].

The presentation of patients with coarctation of the aorta is variable. In this case, the described patient had equivocal symptoms after an incidental finding, but patients can present with failure to thrive, heart failure, and collapse in the newborn period and commonly older asymptomatic patients can present with hypertension. Associated lesions are common, with bicuspid aortic valve seen in as many as two-thirds of all patients with coarctation.

Treatment of coarctation of the aorta can be relatively straightforward. Younger patients are often treated surgically via a left-sided thoracotomy by excision and end-to-end anastomosis. Older (and resulting larger) patients are often treated with an interventional approach. Those with associated hypoplasia of the arch are often referred for surgical arch augmentation, together with repair on cardiopulmonary bypass. However, cases with concomitant 'mild' aortic arch hypoplasia often bring challenging conundrums when discussions take place at the multidisciplinary meeting.

Expert comment

Once considered to be 'cured' after surgical repair, it is now clear that patients with coarctation require lifelong follow-up. Imaging (echo, CT, and MRI) to review the coarctation site, as well as the complications of hypertension, is needed on at least a 2- to 5-yearly basis. Regular monitoring of blood pressure is essential and there is a role for self-monitoring at home.

Long-term outcome of patients after treatment

Long-term survival after coarctation repair (surgical or transcatheter) is excellent. Despite timely interventions, patients are still at risk for long-term morbidity; hence, lifelong follow-up is warranted. Long-term morbidity include:

- Re-intervention for primary lesion: re-coarctation, late aortic wall injury
- Associated cardiac/vascular conditions:
  - Morbidity from bicuspid aortic valve
  - Ascending aortic dilatation/dissection
  - Berry aneurysm and its complications
- Ventricular dysfunction
- Premature coronary disease
- Hypertension
- Impaired cardiopulmonary function/exercise tolerance.

Issues on long-term follow-up: aortic re-intervention and re-stenosis

Re-intervention is not uncommon, with a reported rate of up to 25% [37, 38], due to acute aortic wall injury (secondary to transcatheter treatment) or re-stenosis as a late morbidity. The reported rates of re-interventions for re-stenosis or re-dilatation of stents ranged from 4% to 25% [37, 39, 40]. The wide range is mainly due to the heterogeneity of the patients involved, namely with different disease substrates, treatment strategies, and follow-up durations. The re-intervention rate may be higher for a subgroup of patients who underwent aortic stenting early in life. These are mainly carried out to re-dilate stents to match the somatic growth of patients. Reasons accounting for re-stenosis included the presence of complex coarctations (e.g. associated hypoplastic arch), scarring from surgery, residual gradient post-stenting (> 10 mmHg), and intimal hyperplasia after stenting. Most re-interventions would be transcatheter interventions, including balloon angioplasty for smaller post-operative patients and stenting for those bigger children or adults.

Learning point Role of balloon angioplasty in re-coarctation

Balloon angioplasty has gained popularity in managing post-operative re-coarctation with a high success rate [8, 41]. The reported rate of aortic wall injury was around 1–17%, which is much lower than that of patients with native coarctation. Most of these were relatively mild and managed conservatively. Hence, this is now the preferred method of management in patients with re-coarctation, especially in the subgroup of patients with univentricular heart with ventricular dysfunction, as supported by the latest American Heart Association consensus statement (Class IC recommendation) [19].

Issues on long-term follow-up: hypertension

Hypertension remains a significant concern, affecting 35–69% of patients despite the absence of significant re-coarctation late after repair [42–45]. From the Coarctation Repair in Long-term Follow-Up (CoAFU) study, published in 2017, describing a cohort of patients with median post-operative follow-up of 31 years, 69% had hypertension and up to 27% required two or more antihypertensives. Many pathophysiological hypotheses have been suggested to account for the high prevalence of hypertension in this group of patients. These included dampened baroreceptor response, increased arterial stiffness, endothelial dysfunction, and increased muscle sympathetic nerve activity [42, 43, 46]. An abnormal arch geometry has also been advocated to be associated with hypertension Ou et al. described (Figure 11.4) a series of post-operative patients in whom an association was found between the presence of gothic arch (an aortic arch that is sharply angulated) with the development of hypertension, as in our index case [47]. However, there is as yet no well-described strategy to avoid such arch geometry, whilst arch reconstruction solely for an abnormal configuration is not advocated in light of the associated morbidity.

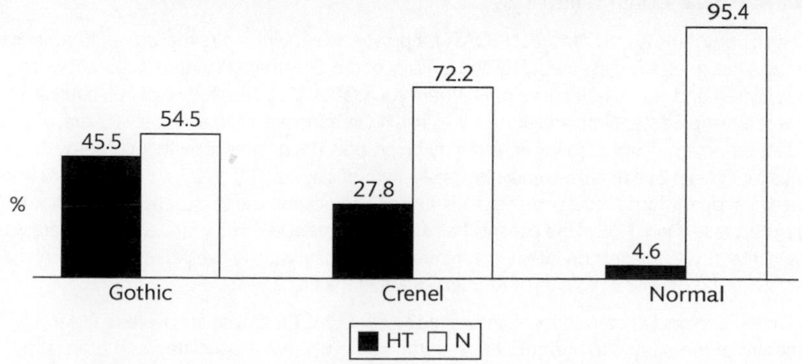

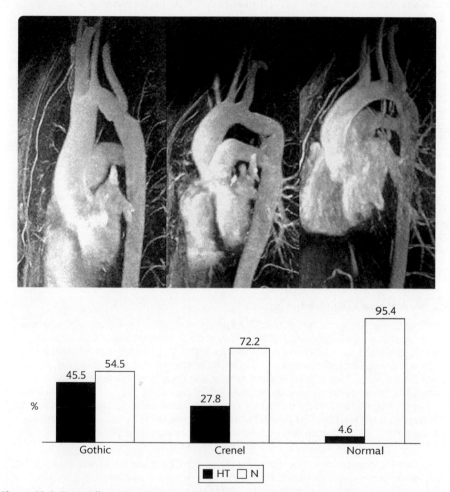

Figure 11.4 Three different morphologies of the aortic arch after coarctation repair. Left to right: gothic geometry, crenel form, and normal form. At the bottom, the percentage of patients with normal blood pressure (N in white) and hypertension (HT in black) in the three types of aortic arch geometry.
Reproduced from Ou P, Bonnet D, Auriacombe L, et al. Late systemic hypertension and aortic arch geometry after successful repair of coarctation of the aorta. *Eur Heart J* 2004;25:1853–9, with permission from Oxford University Press.

Even in patients without resting hypertension, exercise-induced hypertension is still prevalent. From a meta-analysis addressing issues on exercise and hypertension for patients with coarctation, up to 27% experience exercise hypertension associated with abnormal arch geometry and impaired ventricular function. Intriguingly, more younger patients, as compared to adults, were found to have exercise hypertension (43% versus 10%) [48]. Importantly, exercise-induced hypertension can predict future systemic hypertension, whilst hypertension is independently associated with early morbidity and mortality. Hence, blood pressure monitoring and exercise testing are vital during long-term follow-up.

Learning point Evolution of treatment for coarctation in older children and adults

Aortic stenting: performance and associated complications

Over the past two decades, endovascular stenting (first reported in 1991 [49]) has gradually evolved to be the treatment of choice in bigger children and adults. The acute success rate is excellent for both native and recurrent coarctation [15, 29–31]. Having a stent *in situ* has the advantage of a constant radial force applied to the aortic wall, reducing potential aortic wall recoil. Since disruption of the intima is not a prerequisite for successful stenting (as compared with angioplasty), theoretically, the risk for aortic wall injury should be much lower. This advantage has been difficult to prove, as most of the early case series were relatively small and heterogenous. In 2007, Forbes et al. reported the results of aortic stenting from a large 17-centre retrospective study involving 565 procedures performed on patients over the age of 4 years and showed an acute success rate of 98% [14]. Similarly, the CCISC in 2010 reported another large series with similar results and a 96% success rate [50]. Both these studies, however, were quite heterogenous with a wide range of ages (2–63 years), body sizes, and types of stent used. Both studies reported a low acute aortic wall injury rate of between 1% and 4% [14, 50]. However, some smaller series have reported a rate of up to 11%. Factors that were associated with acute wall injury included pre-stenting angioplasty and over-aggressive stent dilatation [13, 14, 32, 50]. Prolonged and repeated guidewire negotiation across the stenotic coarctation site has also been implicated in aortic wall injury [51].

Other acute complications were not negligible. Often a large delivery sheath would be required for the procedure; as such, the incidence of femoral vessel injury was reported at around 1–3%. Other complications associated with aortic stenting include haemorrhage and haematoma formation (2–3%), cerebrovascular events (around 1%), and other technical complications, including stent migration (3–5%) and balloon rupture (0.3–2.3%).

Evidence base COAST I and II trials

The Coarctation of the Aorta Stent Trial (COAST), a prospective multi-centre trial across 19 American centres, was designed to assess the safety and efficacy of the Cheatham Platinum (CP) stent when used in children and adults with native or recurrent coarctation [52]. The study had 105 patients who underwent attempted stent implantation, of which 104 were successful. In all patients, there was immediate reduction in upper to lower extremity blood pressure difference, with this improvement sustained for at least 2 years. The average hospital length of stay was 1.0 ± 0.3 days, and there were no procedural deaths or adverse complications. Overall medication use to treat hypertension was also noted to decrease. Only 10% of the patients had stent fractures noted at 2 years, although there was no loss in integrity. Complication rates were minimal, with aneurysms in five patients treated with a covered stent and only 10% requiring a re-intervention in the first 2 years.

Whilst COAST I looked at conventional uncovered stents, COAST II looked at covered CP stents (CCPS) [53]. The aim of the study is to prevent or treat aortic wall injury (AWI) associated with coarctation of the aorta trial. In effect, it is a continuation of the first study but allows the investigators to look at CCPS, which are so readily used in European centres. There lies the conundrum. Whilst the stent was designed and conceived in the United States, the Food and Drug Administration (FDA)'s stringent guidelines have resulted in significant delays of its use in North American centres, compared to

European centres and centres across the rest of the world. Of the 158 patients who underwent CCPS, 83 had pre-existing AWI. Like COAST I, all had a reduction in the gradient across the coarctation site and 93% of the 83 patients had complete coverage of the AWI. There were no acute AWI, repeat interventions, or deaths. The most common important complication was arterial injury at the access site, which was explained by the larger sheath size (compared to the uncovered CP stents) needed to accommodate the CCPS.

Learning point Covered versus bare metal stent

Despite a number of case series demonstrating the efficacy and safety of covered CP stent in managing coarctation [40, 54, 55], head-to-head comparison of covered versus bare stents remains scarce. Butera et al. described their single-centre experience in a large retrospective study (143 patients over 15 years) comparing bare and covered stents in managing native or post-operative coarctation [38]. A comparable success rate of 95% was demonstrated in both groups. However, procedural complications, on the other hand, were significantly higher in the bare stent group (21.3% versus 8.3%), of which aortic wall injury occurred in 7% in the bare stent group versus 0% in the covered stent group. These results were limited by the use of various stents during the study period, especially for the bare stent group. Some of these stents have relatively sharper struts, potentially increasing the risk for aortic wall injury. There was also a significant learning curve effect, with most of the patients from the bare stent group falling in the centre's early experience period. Additionally, despite having more complex coarctations* in the covered stent group, 44% of patients from the bare stent group also suffered from complex coarctation, which understandably would have a higher chance of aortic wall injury.

* Complex coarctation: aortic inflammatory disease, previous conduit or patch implantation, atretic or subatretic segments, severe lesions with a proximal aorta-to-coarctation segment ratio of >3, irregular aortic wall, or presence of aortic aneurysm.

Evidence base Bare versus covered CP stent in native coarctation

The first randomized trial comparing bare and covered CP stents was published in 2014 by Sohrabi et al. [51]. The study randomized 120 patients aged >10 years and weighing >30 kg with severe native coarctation at a 1:1 ratio to each treatment arm (bare versus covered), with a mean follow-up duration of 31 months. A follow-up CT aortogram would be performed 6 months post-intervention to assess for stent integrity and position, intimal hyperplasia, and also the presence of aneurysm. Patients with re-coarctation, long segment coarctation, hypoplastic transverse arch, and juxta-ductal coarctation were excluded. The mean age of the patient group was 23.6 ± 10.99 years (range 12–58), with similar baseline demographics between the two groups. Both groups of patients included severe coarctations, with a mean coarctation diameter of around 3.3 mm, as compared with that of the descending aorta of 16.7 mm at the diaphragmatic level. Patients from both arms achieved 100% procedural success, with gradient reduction from a mean of 54.6 ± 14.5 mmHg to 3.38 ± 1.61 mmHg, and coarctation dimension increased from a mean of 3.32 ± 0.65 mm to 15.94 ± 2.23 mm post-intervention. Importantly, there has been no procedural complication despite an aggressive luminal dimension improvement. There were no significant differences between the two groups in the length of hospital stay, the reduction in non-invasive blood pressure, and the reduction in the percentage of patients on antihypertensives on follow-up.

In terms of medium- to long-term safety concerns, there were no statistically significant differences in the rate of aortic wall injury on follow-up. Although more aortic pseudoaneurysms were identified in the covered stent group (two patients; 3.3% versus 0% in the bare stent group), the difference was not significant. Intriguingly, both patients presented with severe back pain that prompted an early CT aortogram (30 and 40 days post-procedure). The aneurysms were both located proximal to the implanted stent (explained possibly by prolonged and multiple attempts to negotiate the coarctation with various guidewires, potentially damaging the aortic wall), and both were managed by implanting an additional covered CP stent. There were more re-coarctations in the bare CP stent group (6.7% versus 0%), though not statistically significant, and both were managed successfully with covered CP stent.

This study has provided important insight into the applicability of bare CP stent, even in cases with severe coarctation. The acute success rate was comparable with that of covered CP stent, together with no significant increase in acute aortic wall injury. Hence, one might argue, for simple coarctation, implanting a bare CP stent would be a reasonable choice. However, one must not ignore the potential risk for delayed aortic aneurysm formation, since the per-protocol follow-up CT scans were performed at 6 months post-intervention, and not later. Theoretically, the abnormal aortic wall tissue at the previous coarctation site being treated with a bare stent would be unprotected from aortic pulsation. This would potentially increase the risk for aneurysm formation with time, especially if hypertension is unchecked. Hence, it would be interesting if a follow-up study can be performed on the patients described by Sohrabi et al. to delineate the risk of delayed aortic aneurysm formation between the groups. Due to this uncertainty of potential late aortic complications, covered CP stents are often used as first line to manage coarctation, unless there is a risk for covering important branches from the aorta—as in the patient presented here.

A final word from the expert

Timely diagnosis of coarctation of the aorta should lead to early and effective management to avoid long-term complications. These include hypertension causing cerebrovascular disease and ischaemic heart disease, as well as the formation of aneurysms and aortic dissection at the site of the coarctation. Lifelong monitoring is needed, so that treatment for residual coarctation and hypertension can be delivered before complications emerge. Whilst surgical repair is invariable in early childhood, endovascular stent implantation is becoming the modality of choice for older children and adults. Balloon dilatation tends to be reserved for re-coarctation after surgical repair in younger children or for re-dilating stents after somatic growth. Covered stents have a theoretical advantage of minimizing aneurysm formation at the coarctation site, although there is evidence that this can also occur after surgical repair, balloon dilatation, and with both uncovered and covered stent implantation. Covered stents, however, are very useful for treating aneurysms after any treatment modality, as in this case study—as long as care is taken to avoid occlusion of important head and neck vessels—and can reduce morbidity from repeat surgery.

References

1. Lock JE, Niemi T, Burke BA, Einzig S, Castaneda-Zuniga WR. Transcutaneous angioplasty of experimental aortic coarctation. *Circulation* 1982;66:1280–6.
2. Cowley CG, Orsmond GS, Feola P, McQuillan L, Shaddy RE. Long-term, randomized comparison of balloon angioplasty and surgery for native coarctation of the aorta in childhood. *Circulation* 2005;111:3453–6.
3. Fiore AC, Fischer LK, Schwartz T, et al. Comparison of angioplasty and surgery for neonatal aortic coarctation. *Ann Thorac Surg* 2005;80:1659–64; discussion 64–5.
4. Shaddy RE, Boucek MM, Sturtevant JE, et al. Comparison of angioplasty and surgery for unoperated coarctation of the aorta. *Circulation* 1993;87:793–9.
5. Walhout RJ, Lekkerkerker JC, Oron GH, Bennink GB, Meijboom EJ. Comparison of surgical repair with balloon angioplasty for native coarctation in patients from 3 months to 16 years of age. *Eur J Cardiothorac Surg* 2004;25:722–7.
6. Rao PS, Galal O, Smith PA, Wilson AD. Five- to nine-year follow-up results of balloon angioplasty of native aortic coarctation in infants and children. *J Am Coll Cardiol* 1996;27:462–70.
7. Hu ZP, Wang ZW, Dai XF, et al. Outcomes of surgical versus balloon angioplasty treatment for native coarctation of the aorta: a meta-analysis. *Ann Vasc Surg* 2014;28:394–403.
8. Harris KC, Du W, Cowley CG, Forbes TJ, Kim DW; Congenital Cardiac Intervention Study Consortium (CCISC). A prospective observational multicenter study of balloon angioplasty for the treatment of native and recurrent coarctation of the aorta. *Catheter Cardiovasc Interv* 2014;83:1116–23.

9. Forbes TJ, Kim DW, Du W, et al. Comparison of surgical, stent, and balloon angioplasty treatment of native coarctation of the aorta: an observational study by the CCISC (Congenital Cardiovascular Interventional Study Consortium). *J Am Coll Cardiol* 2011;58:2664–74.
10. Padua LM, Garcia LC, Rubira CJ, de Oliveira Carvalho PE. Stent placement versus surgery for coarctation of the thoracic aorta. *Cochrane Database Syst Rev* 2012;5:CD008204.
11. Kang SL, Tometzki A, Taliotis D, Martin R. Stent therapy for aortic coarctation in children < 30 kg: use of the low profile Valeo stent. *Pediatr Cardiol* 2017;38:1441–9.
12. Bondanza S, Calevo MG, Marasini M. Early and long-term results of stent implantation for aortic coarctation in pediatric patients compared to adolescents: a single center experience. *Cardiol Res Pract* 2016;2016:4818307.
13. Cheatham JP. Stenting of coarctation of the aorta. *Catheter Cardiovasc Interv* 2001;54:112–25.
14. Forbes TJ, Garekar S, Amin Z, et al. Procedural results and acute complications in stenting native and recurrent coarctation of the aorta in patients over 4 years of age: a multi-institutional study. *Catheter Cardiovasc Interv* 2007;70:276–85.
15. Magee AG, Brzezinska-Rajszys G, Qureshi SA, et al. Stent implantation for aortic coarctation and recoarctation. *Heart* 1999;82:600–6.
16. Mohan UR, Danon S, Levi D, Connolly D, Moore JW. Stent implantation for coarctation of the aorta in children < 30 kg. *JACC Cardiovasc Interv* 2009;2:877–83.
17. Schaeffler R, Kolax T, Hesse C, Peuster M. Implantation of stents for treatment of recurrent and native coarctation in children weighing less than 20 kilograms. *Cardiol Young* 2007;17:617–22.
18. Thanopoulos BD, Giannakoulas G, Giannopoulos A, Galdo F, Tsaoussis GS. Initial and six-year results of stent implantation for aortic coarctation in children. *Am J Cardiol* 2012;109:1499–503.
19. Feltes TF, Bacha E, Beekman RH 3rd, et al. Indications for cardiac catheterization and intervention in pediatric cardiac disease: a scientific statement from the American Heart Association. *Circulation* 2011;123:2607–52.
20. Schranz D, Zartner P, Michel-Behnke I, Akinturk H. Bioabsorbable metal stents for percutaneous treatment of critical recoarctation of the aorta in a newborn. *Catheter Cardiovasc Interv* 2006;67:671–3.
21. Ewert P, Peters B, Nagdyman N, Miera O, Kuhne T, Berger F. Early and mid-term results with the growth stent—a possible concept for transcatheter treatment of aortic coarctation from infancy to adulthood by stent implantation? *Catheter Cardiovasc Interv* 2008;71: 120–6.
22. Grohmann J, Sigler M, Siepe M, Stiller B. A new breakable stent for recoarctation in early infancy: preliminary clinical experience. *Catheter Cardiovasc Interv* 2016;87:E143–50.
23. Butera G, Chessa M, Eicken A, Thomson J, editors. *Cardiac Catheterization for Congenital Heart Disease*. Milan: Springer, 2015.
24. Seldinger SI. Catheter replacement of the needle in percutaneous arteriography; a new technique. *Acta Radiol* 1953;39:368–76.
25. AIUM practice guideline for the use of ultrasound to guide vascular access procedures. *J Ultrasound Med* 2013;32:191–215.
26. McGee DC, Gould MK. Preventing complications of central venous catheterization. *N Engl J Med* 2003;348:1123–33.
27. Stone MB, Moon C, Sutijono D, Blaivas M. Needle tip visualization during ultrasound-guided vascular access: short-axis vs long-axis approach. *Am J Emerg Med* 2010;28:343–7.
28. Rosenthal E. Coarctation of the aorta from fetus to adult: curable condition or life long disease process? *Heart* 2005;91:1495–502.
29. Harrison DA, McLaughlin PR, Lazzam C, Connelly M, Benson LN. Endovascular stents in the management of coarctation of the aorta in the adolescent and adult: one year follow up. *Heart* 2001;85:561–6.
30. Ledesma M, Alva C, Gomez FD, et al. Results of stenting for aortic coarctation. *Am J Cardiol* 2001;88:460–2.

31. Suarez de Lezo J, Pan M, Romero M, et al. Immediate and follow-up findings after stent treatment for severe coarctation of aorta. *Am J Cardiol* 1999;83:400–6.
32. Forbes TJ, Moore P, Pedra CA, et al. Intermediate follow-up following intravascular stenting for treatment of coarctation of the aorta. *Catheter Cardiovasc Interv* 2007;70:569–77.
33. Hoffman JI, Kaplan S. The incidence of congenital heart disease. *J Am Coll Cardiol* 2002;39:1890–900.
34. Morgagni J. *De Sedibus et Causis Morborum*. Venice: Remondiniana, 1760.
35. Bonnet L. Sur la lésion dite sténose congénitale de l'aorte dans la région de l'isthme. *Rev Méd (Paris)* 1903;23:108–26.
36. Edwards JE, Christensen NA, et al. Pathologic considerations of coarctation of the aorta. *Proc Staff Meet Mayo Clin* 1948;23:324–32.
37. Chen SS, Dimopoulos K, Alonso-Gonzalez R, et al. Prevalence and prognostic implication of restenosis or dilatation at the aortic coarctation repair site assessed by cardiovascular MRI in adult patients late after coarctation repair. *Int J Cardiol* 2014;173:209–15.
38. Butera G, Manica JL, Marini D, et al. From bare to covered: 15-year single center experience and follow-up in trans-catheter stent implantation for aortic coarctation. *Catheter Cardiovasc Interv* 2014;83:953–63.
39. Pedersen TA. Late morbidity after repair of aortic coarctation. *Dan Med J* 2012;59:B4436.
40. Butera G, Piazza L, Chessa M, et al. Covered stents in patients with complex aortic coarctations. *Am Heart J* 2007;154:795–800.
41. Saxena A. Recurrent coarctation: interventional techniques and results. *World J Pediatr Congenit Heart Surg* 2015;6:257–65.
42. Bocelli A, Favilli S, Pollini I, et al. Prevalence and long-term predictors of left ventricular hypertrophy, late hypertension, and hypertensive response to exercise after successful aortic coarctation repair. *Pediatr Cardiol* 2013;34:620–9.
43. Canniffe C, Ou P, Walsh K, Bonnet D, Celermajer D. Hypertension after repair of aortic coarctation: a systematic review. *Int J Cardiol* 2013;167:2456–61.
44. Choudhary P, Canniffe C, Jackson DJ, Tanous D, Walsh K, Celermajer DS. Late outcomes in adults with coarctation of the aorta. *Heart* 2015;101:1190–5.
45. Bambul Heck P, Pabst von Ohain J, Kaemmerer H, Ewert P, Hager A. Arterial Hypertension after Coarctation-Repair in Long-term Follow-up (CoAFU): predictive value of clinical variables. *Int J Cardiol* 2017;246:42–5.
46. Lee MGY, Hemmes RA, Mynard J, et al. Elevated sympathetic activity, endothelial dysfunction, and late hypertension after repair of coarctation of the aorta. *Int J Cardiol* 2017;243:185–90.
47. Ou P, Bonnet D, Auriacombe L, et al. Late systemic hypertension and aortic arch geometry after successful repair of coarctation of the aorta. *Eur Heart J* 2004;25:1853–9.
48. Foulds HJA, Giacomantonio NB, Bredin SSD, Warburton DER. A systematic review and meta-analysis of exercise and exercise hypertension in patients with aortic coarctation. *J Hum Hypertens* 2017;31:768–75.
49. O'Laughlin MP, Perry SB, Lock JE, Mullins CE. Use of endovascular stents in congenital heart disease. *Circulation* 1991;83:1923–39.
50. Holzer R, Qureshi S, Ghasemi A, et al. Stenting of aortic coarctation: acute, intermediate, and long-term results of a prospective multi-institutional registry: Congenital Cardiovascular Interventional Study Consortium (CCISC). *Catheter Cardiovasc Interv* 2010;76:553–63.
51. Sohrabi B, Jamshidi P, Yaghoubi A, et al. Comparison between covered and bare Cheatham-Platinum stents for endovascular treatment of patients with native post-ductal aortic coarctation: immediate and intermediate-term results. *JACC Cardiovasc Interv* 2014;7:416–23.
52. Ringel RE, Vincent J, Jenkins KJ, et al. Acute outcome of stent therapy for coarctation of the aorta: results of the coarctation of the aorta stent trial. *Catheter Cardiovasc Interv* 2013;82:503–10.

53. Taggart NW, Minahan M, Cabalka AK, et al. Immediate Outcomes of Covered Stent Placement for Treatment or Prevention of Aortic Wall Injury Associated With Coarctation of the Aorta (COAST II). *JACC Cardiovasc Interv* 2016;9:484–93.
54. Chang ZP, Jiang SL, Xu ZY, et al. Use of covered Cheatham-Platinum stent as the primary modality in the treatment for native coarctation of the aorta. *Chin Med J (Engl)* 2012;125:1005–9.
55. Tanous D, Collins N, Dehghani P, Benson LN, Horlick EM. Covered stents in the management of coarctation of the aorta in the adult: initial results and 1-year angiographic and hemodynamic follow-up. *Int J Cardiol* 2010;140:287–95.

12 Infective endocarditis

Salim Jivanji and Rubya Adamji

Expert commentary Michael Rigby

Case history

A 12-year-old boy with previously repaired mixed aortic valve disease presented to the emergency department at his local hospital with 2 days of fevers, general lethargy, and poor appetite.

He was born with severe aortic stenosis and, as a neonate, had undergone balloon aortic valvuloplasty, with good initial results. He subsequently developed severe aortic regurgitation with left ventricular dilatation and reducing exercise tolerance. At the age of 7 years, he underwent a Ross procedure with a right-sided pulmonary homograft. His paediatric cardiologist had followed him up on a regular basis and he was progressing well.

At his local hospital, he was described as well grown and slightly lethargic. He was tachycardic (heart rate 110 bpm) and mildly tachypnoeic (respiratory rate 24), with an axillary temperature of 37.9°C, though just prior to his arrival, the family had given him some paracetamol. He was fully saturated and had a normal blood pressure. His scars were well healed, and he had good-volume femoral pulses. His heart sounds were normal, with a grade 2/6 ejection systolic murmur in the left upper sternal edge (LUSE) and a grade 2/4 diastolic murmur in the left lower sternal edge (LLSE). His chest had good air entry bilaterally, and his abdomen was soft with no organomegaly. His ear, nose, and throat (ENT) examination was unremarkable, and there were also no stigmata to suggest subacute bacterial endocarditis. His urine dipstick was negative for nitrates and white cells.

Routine blood tests showed raised inflammatory markers (Table 12.1) and a raised white cell count (WCC). On the chest X-ray, there was a normal cardiac contour with a normal cardiothoracic ratio. There was mild calcification in the pulmonary homograft, but no focal consolidation.

There was no focus to explain his pyrexia, and the team decided to admit him for observations without starting him on antibiotics. Over the subsequent 48 hours, he had multiple spikes of temperature with a peak of 39.2°C, with concomitant tachycardia and tachypnoea. He had three further blood cultures, and his repeat bloods a day after admission had shown a rise in both his inflammatory markers and WCC (Table 12.1). Following discussion with the microbiologist, he was started on broad-spectrum antibiotics. In the absence of an obvious focus, bacterial endocarditis was high on the differential and he was discussed with the tertiary paediatric cardiology unit for review.

Table 12.1 Blood results

Blood test	On admission	Day 1 after admission
C-reactive protein (CRP)	85 mg/l	183 mg/l
Haemoglobin (Hb)	12.6 g/l	12.4 g/l
Platelet	233 g/l	320 g/l
White cell count (WCC)	18.3×10^9	24×10^9
Neutrophils	10.7×10^9	15×10^9
Lymphocytes	7.1×10^9	6.8×10^9

A more detailed history by the admitting team confirmed no recent travel or exposure to animals or pets. However, 2 months previously, he had a dental appointment for scaling and a filling under local anaesthesia in a permanent molar tooth. The procedure was not covered by antibiotics, as per the current National Institute for Health and Care Excellence (NICE) clinical guideline 64 [1].

Learning point

Patients with CHD have increased levels of dental caries [2]. More importantly, it has been reported that there are also increased levels of **untreated** dental caries in cardiac patients [3]. This could be due to a number of different factors, including oral health falling lower on the list of priorities within these families. There are reports of low levels of dental attendance in paediatric cardiology patients. De Fonseca et al. [4] found in their study that almost half of the patients with cardiac disease had never seen a dentist before. Parry and Khan [5] found that even when they do attend, only 37% of dental practitioners felt confident in providing dental treatment for children with cardiac disease.

At 50 hours, the first blood culture taken on presentation grew Gram-positive cocci. He was transferred to his local paediatric cardiology unit for further evaluation. An echocardiogram revealed a large vegetation extending from his right ventricle into his right pulmonary artery. The vegetation appeared mobile and attached, in part, to the right ventricular outflow tract (RVOT). His left ventricle had good systolic function, and there was a well-functioning mitral and neo-aortic valve. The rest of the echocardiogram was unremarkable. A computed tomography (CT) scan showed evidence of septic emboli in his distal pulmonary vasculature. He was placed on full anticoagulation with therapeutic unfractionated heparin.

Learning point Diagnosis

IE is a diagnostic and therapeutic challenge. Rapid diagnosis and initiating treatment are complicated by the strikingly diverse presentations. There remains merit in the classification of the clinical course of IE to acute and subacute—even though the lines have been blurred due to indiscriminate use of antibiotics in the community, the hospital (especially in immunosuppressed patients), and animal livestock [6, 7].

The modified Duke criteria (see Learning point: Duke criteria, p. 165) are a measure intended for research purposes and backed by AHA guidelines to evaluate patients with suspected IE; it has a lower sensitivity for patients with prosthetic valve endocarditis or cardiac device infections [8]. Definitive cardiac imaging and microbiology, together with specially conducted multidisciplinary meeting comprising a wide variety of specialists who have an interest in IE for challenging cases, are key to making the diagnosis and risk stratification. Delayed diagnosis and, as a result, hesitation in starting treatment lead to complications and poor clinical outcomes.

Learning point Duke criteria

Major criteria:

- Positive blood culture for IE:
  - Typical microorganism for IE from two separate blood cultures
  - Persistently positive blood cultures
- Evidence of endocardial involvement:
  - Oscillating intracardiac mass on valve/supporting structures or in the path of regurgitant jet in the absence of an alternative anatomical explanation
  - Abscess
  - New partial dehiscence of prosthetic valve or new valvular regurgitation.

Minor criteria:

- Predisposing heart condition or intravenous drug use
- Fever over 38°C (>100.4°F)
- Vascular phenomenon such as major arterial emboli, septic pulmonary infarcts, mycotic aneurysm, intracranial haemorrhage, conjunctival haemorrhage, Janeway lesions
- Immunological phenomenon:
  - Glomerulonephritis
  - Osler nodes
  - Roth spots
  - Rheumatoid factor
- Microbiological evidence:
  - Positive blood cultures not meeting major criteria
- Echocardiogram:
  - Consistent with IE, but not meeting major criteria.

Two major criteria, or one major and three minor criteria, or five minor criteria must be met.

There has been a recent proposal to amend the Duke criteria [9].

Clinical tip

IE is three times more common in males than in females, but there is no clear reason for this [9]. There is also no racial predilection.

The final results from his blood cultures taken locally confirmed the organism to be *Streptococcus viridans* and his antibiotics were optimized according to the sensitivities. Discussion in the multidisciplinary team (MDT) was on the conundrum of either continuing medical management or taking him for urgent surgery. In the presence of improving inflammatory markers and reducing pyrexial spikes on optimized antibiotics, it was agreed to continue on medical management.

Daily reviews with echocardiography (Figure 12.1) did not show any extension to other valves and no reduction in size of the vegetation. Concerns were raised about potentially having a large pulmonary embolism. His inflammatory markers peaked on day 3 of presentation and reached a nadir on day 5—with persistently raised C-reactive protein (CRP) at 85. The decision was to take him for urgent surgery.

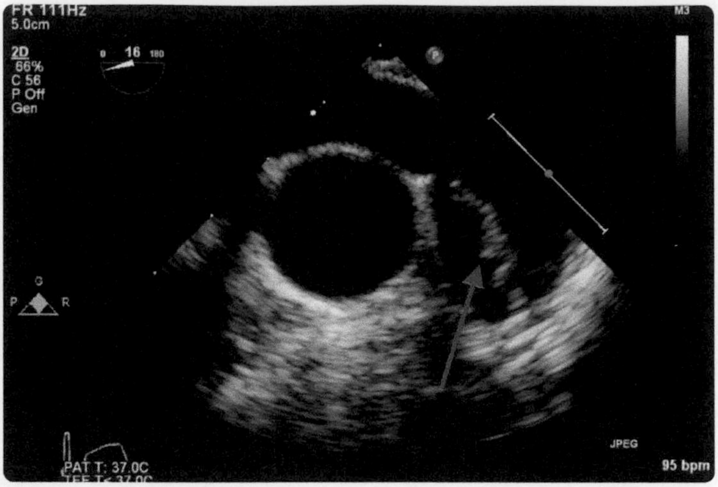

Figure 12.1 Transoesophageal echocardiogram shows a large vegetation extending from the RVOT to the pulmonary artery (red arrow).

His pulmonary homograft was excised (Figure 12.2) and a large vegetation attached to his septal leaflet was removed. The vegetation had several attachments across the RVOT and right pulmonary artery (RPA). The tricuspid valve was repaired by extension of the leaflet with CardioCel®. A new pulmonary homograft was inserted after removal of the vegetation, with reconstruction of the RPA. The surgeon reported slough-like areas in the infected area, making the procedure extremely challenging.

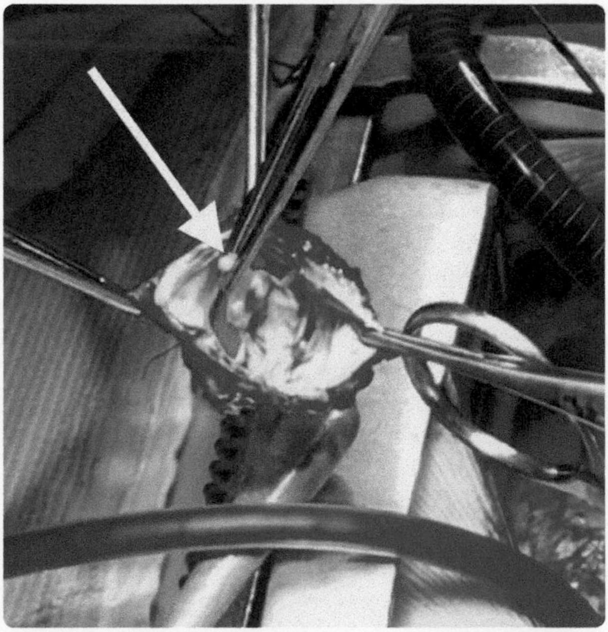

Figure 12.2 Large fleshy vegetation (white arrow) attached to the excised homograft.

Learning point

The pathophysiology of valvular bacterial endocarditis has been debated since the late 1800s. Koster [10] suggested that bacteria reached the valves by way of capillary blood vessels. This view was challenged by Dow and Harper [11] and later Harper [12] whose systematic examination of normal hearts confirmed that blood supply is present in atrioventricular valves but is limited to the first 3 mm from the line of attachment to the heart wall. In adult hearts, the distance is further reduced.

Investigating hearts infected with endocarditis, Harper and his counterparts noted that there was advancement of vessels in the valves of hearts as a result of 'previous injury'. This meant unlike normal hearts, the irregular vessels in these valves extended much more distally—along the growth of granulation tissue—which forms part of the healing process [12]. This leaves them susceptible to infection from bacterial sepsis in the bloodstream. It was also shown that, in some cases, these vessels regress.

Expert comment

For patients with a right ventricle-to-pulmonary artery (RV–PA) conduit, unexplained pyrexia is likely to be a result of endocarditis. Frequently, no vegetations are seen, but a rapid increase in the Doppler systolic gradient may be observed and can be the only finding. Conduit infection rarely responds completely to antibiotics, and the majority of patients will require surgery during the infection.

Following his surgery, he required a prolonged course of ventilation and inotropes. There were further spikes of temperature, although no further growth of organisms was recorded in repeated blood cultures. Concerns were raised as the CRP level again rose to a peak of 200. However, a CT scan to look for more evidence of septic focus in his chest and brain was unremarkable.

Three days after his surgery, there was a steady reduction in his inflammatory markers and inotropic requirements. Repeated surveillance with echocardiography demonstrated improving ventricular function with a satisfactory cardiac repair. There was mild tricuspid regurgitation, with slightly increased right-sided pressures, a well-functioning pulmonary homograft, and a good-calibre RPA.

He was weaned off his ventilation, and 2 days later, he was extubated to nasal cannula oxygen. He was transferred to the ward and remained in hospital for a total of 6 weeks to complete intravenous (IV) antibiotics and rehabilitation following his surgery.

On his last follow-up, more than 2 years after this episode, he was progressing well with good biventricular systolic function and no suggestion of active infection. He is regularly given oral hygiene and prevention advice by his dentist and the cardiology team. He has also been recommended to have antibiotic cover for future dental procedures and to avoid body piercings and tattoos.

Discussion

The issue regarding the diagnosis and management of infective endocarditis (IE) is one of endless debate. The challenge of a swift diagnosis is difficult because the presentation can be so diverse. Initiating treatment is a continual conundrum, as the alternative can have disastrous consequences. As such, numerous patients are often treated for 'suspected IE' who may have other febrile illnesses. The in-hospital mortality of 20–30% has remained unchanged for more than two decades [13–16], which explains the anxiety in managing patients who are suspected to have IE.

A recent large prospective cohort study in France covering eight centres with over 2000 patients in a 30-month period [17] showed that 11% of the population diagnosed with *Staphylococcus aureus* blood infection had infective endocarditis. This number reflected a conservative estimate as only 60% of the population had an echocardiogram. However, the percentage increased to 15.6% in those who underwent echocardiography. It also showed that injecting drug users (38%) and those with prosthetic valves (33%) were at the highest risk for developing IE. Additionally, it was noted that there was an association between the duration of bacteraemia and IE. The association may be either a cause or a consequence but emphasizes the importance of aggressive treatment of positive *S. aureus* blood cultures.

Learning point Stages of Infective Endocarditis

There are essentially three stages of IE. Initiation of treatment can take place at any stage. The first stage is usually **bacteraemia** and bacteria can enter the bloodstream via the mouth, the gastrointestinal and urinary tracts, or the skin. Additionally, any invasive procedures (medical or surgical) can lead to bacteraemia, including accessing central venous lines and dental procedures.

The likelihood of invasive procedures to produce bacteraemia varies significantly. But examples of procedures which potentially increase the risk include transoesophageal echocardiography, endoscopy, colonoscopy, and bronchoscopy.

Most cases of subacute bacterial endocarditis are thought to be secondary to bacteraemia as a result of activities of daily living (toothbrushing, bowel movements).

The second stage is **adhesion**. Although the prevalence of IE among the general population is found to be about 50% in those with no known heart disease, the endothelial lining in normal hearts is resistant to bacterial adhesion. However, in the presence of abnormal or damaged endothelial lining, bacteria (particularly Gram-positive species) are drawn via surface adhesion. With fibrin and platelet thrombus facilitating this process, these proteins mediate attachment to extracellular host matrix proteins. The thick peptidoglycan layer surrounding Gram-positive bacteria is also less sensitive to serum-induced killing and resists the bactericidal action of complement [9, 13, 14].

These bacterial adhesions (third stage) therefore give rise to **colonization**. A mature vegetation is formed as a result of cycles of bacterial proliferation, thrombosis, inflammation, and monocyte recruitment [18]. A number of the microorganisms associated with IE (including staphylococci, streptococci, and enterococci, but also less common pathogens such as *Candida* species and *Pseudomonas aeruginosa*) produce biofilms. Once established, organisms deep in the vegetation are protected by a biofilm and host immune defences. They are therefore less susceptible to bactericidal antimicrobials that interfere with bacterial cell wall synthesis [19]. Biofilm-forming capacity is now recognized as an important determinant of virulence in the development of staphylococcal device-related infections [20].

Prevention is considered to be a better strategy. The aim for prophylaxis is to eliminate bacteraemia that can cause IE in susceptible individuals. However, no randomized controlled trial has ever supported its effectiveness. We do know that oral *S. viridans* is implicated as causal organisms in IE (as has been noted in our case) and is also the leading cause in developing countries and historically in western countries. In the last decade, however, *S. aureus* has become the leading cause in Western Europe and Northern America [15–17, 21, 22], with the highest rate of morbidity and mortality [22–25].

Interventional procedures in upper and lower gastrointestinal tract, genitourinary tract, and upper and lower respiratory tract (including ear, nose, and throat) can all cause bacteraemia. However, not only does bacteraemia from the mouth occur with invasive dental procedures, but also low levels of bacteraemia can occur with daily toothbrushing and flossing. A study by Lockhart et al. [26] found bacteraemia after toothbrushing was associated with poor oral hygiene. Hence, the importance of good oral health cannot be underestimated to prevent the need for dental procedures.

Learning point

It has been recognized that patients who are at risk of developing IE often have limited understanding of the importance of prevention (including appropriate oral hygiene) and treatment (antibiotics) principles. Balmer and Bu'Lock [3] found only 64% of parents were aware of the link between the oral health of their children and IE.

Most paediatric cardiologists spend considerable time explaining the risks of body piercing and the importance of good oral health. The Child Dental Health Survey 2013—carried out every 10 years—has shown that children who are from lower-income families are more likely to have oral disease than other children of the same age [27]. This is the same population that are the most susceptible to IE.

NICE has emphasized the importance of prevention and education as the main principles in tackling IE. Routine management of all cardiac patients should include giving oral prevention advice, as recommended by the Department of Health's *Delivering Better Oral Health: an evidence-based toolkit for prevention*.

The debate of antibiotic prophylaxis, especially in dental treatment, is complex and roots back to the time when Thomas Horder in 1909 [28] recognized that the mouth was a major portal for bacterial entry. Several years later, in 1935, streptococcal bacteraemia was detected after a dental extraction [29].

The approach to dental antibiotic prophylaxis differs across the world. Since 2002, antibiotic prophylaxis has been recommended for all patients with congenital heart disease (CHD) by the Americans and Europeans (including the UK). There have been no randomized controlled trials to support its use. Additionally, the efficacy of prophylaxis is felt to be only 50% [8], although this refers to native valve endocarditis. Moreover, the development of antibiotic resistance has been gaining widespread recognition [1, 8]. Lastly, as everyday toothbrushing, flossing, and chewing cause bacteraemia, the acceptance of dental procedures as a risk factor has been questioned [30].

In 2007, the American Heart Association (AHA) suspended prophylaxis for patients with CHD who were considered to be at 'moderate risk' (previous rheumatic fever, heart murmur, or native valve disease). In 2008, NICE [1] published a new guideline which suggested 'no prophylaxis' was needed for any patients undergoing dental treatment. This was subject to much debate, and the American (AHA) and its European [European Society of Cardiology (ESC)] counterparts continued to promote the use of prophylaxis in high-risk individuals (those with a prosthetic valve, a history of IE, and cyanotic CHD).

The change in the NICE guidelines in 2008 had a profound impact in the management of patients with CHD who had dental treatment in the UK A study published in *The Lancet* [31] showed that since NICE published its guidelines, there was an almost 90% reduction in prescribing prophylactic antibiotics and a significant rise in the trend of cases of IE. Similar studies were carried out in the United States after the implementation of the AHA guidelines in 2007; however, they were shorter and of a smaller power, compared to the one published in *The Lancet*. A more recent one by Thornhill et al. [32] corroborates the findings in the United States to the UK study. The study in *The Lancet* also reviewed possible factors which could have increased the trend, including looking at implantation of prosthetic valves, the number of cardiac surgeries, insertion of permanent pacemakers (PPMs) or implantable cardioverter-defibrillators (ICDs), and the number of dental extractions during that period—all of which remained constant. The obvious increase was scaling and polishing, which had an annual increase from 12 to over 12.8 million from 2009 to 2014. However, it is not clear if this is the same population who had IE.

Was this increase as a result of increasing public awareness in dental hygiene—and, as such, greater access by CHD patients to these services—or was this as a result of avoiding dental care altogether? We do know that CHD patients do not access dental services as well as the general population [8]. The publication, however, swayed NICE to review its guidelines, resulting in a slight—albeit important— change, leaving the onus on the dentist to decide on a case-by-case basis as to the merit of dental prophylaxis [1, 33]. The recent publication of the Scottish Dental Clinical Effectiveness Programme (SDCEP) guidelines has attempted to clarify things further (Table 12.2).

Expert comment

Particularly high-risk groups are those with an RV-PA conduit in whom a percutaneous Melody® valve has been implanted and patients with a Contegra® conduit. Despite published current guidelines, cardiologists include these patients in their high-risk groups, although they are not true prosthetic valves.

Table 12.2 Timeline highlighting the key changes in antibiotic prophylaxis in the United States, Europe, and the UK

Since 2002	Antibiotic prophylaxis has been recommended for all patients with CHD by the Americans (AHA) and Europeans (ESC), including the UK; there have been no RCTs to support its use
October 2007 [34]	The AHA suspended the use of prophylaxis for patients with CHD who were considered to be at 'moderate risk' (previous rheumatic fever, heart murmur, or native valve disease)
January 2008 [35]	Revision of guidelines by the AHA to antibiotic prophylaxis recommended for: • Prosthetic cardiac valve or prosthetic material used for cardiac valve repair • Previous IE • CHD: • Unrepaired cyanotic CHD, including palliative shunts and conduits • Completely repaired CHD with prosthetic material or device, whether placed by surgery or by catheter intervention during the first 6 months after the procedure • Repaired CHD with residual defects at, or adjacent to, the site of a prosthetic patch or prosthetic device (which inhibits endothelization) • Cardiac transplantation patients who develop valvulopathy
November 2015 [36]	Support for the use of antibiotics in high-risk individuals only. Guidelines supported the AHA guidelines, except the last two points on residual defects and cardiac transplantation patients
March 2008—NICE	Guideline CG64 produced. Antibiotic prophylaxis against IE is not recommended for people undergoing dental procedures
May 2011 [37]	Population study found a 78.6% reduction in antibiotic prophylaxis prescribing. No significant increase in IE was found
March 2015 [31]	Retrospective study found the incidence of IE increased significantly in England since the introduction of the 2008 NICE guideline and almost 90% reduction in antibiotic prophylaxis prescribing
September 2015—NICE update	Insufficient evidence to warrant any change to the existing guidance and continued to recommend against antibiotic prophylaxis
July 2016—NICE amendment [1]	Antibiotic prophylaxis against IE is not recommended routinely for people undergoing dental procedures
August 2018—SDCEP [38]	Antibiotic prophylaxis to be considered if a patient is in the 'special considerations group' (children with CHD): • Contact the patient's cardiologist to determine if antibiotic prophylaxis is required for invasive dental procedures • Discuss and document the risks and benefits of antibiotic prophylaxis to ensure an informed decision is made

AHA, American Heart Association; CHD, congenital heart disease; ESC, European Society of Cardiology; RCT, randomized controlled trial.

Source data from Hughes S, Balmer R, Moffat M, Willcoxson F. The dental management of children with congenital heart disease following the publication of Paediatric Congenital Heart Disease Standards and Specifications. *Br Dent J*. 2019 Mar;226(6):447–452.

Learning point Things to consider when referring congenital heart disease patients for dental care

- In view of the **increased levels of dental caries**, compared to the general population, CHD patients often have a high treatment need [2]. This could be due to a number of factors, including the increased prevalence of enamel defects secondary to their cardiac condition; intake of sweetened medications to ensure compliance; intake of sweetened snacks due to parental indulgence; and intake of high calorific diets to promote growth [39].
- Paediatric dentists are more **aggressive in treatment planning** in view of the increased risk for IE among CHD patients. There is an emphasis in identifying and eliminating potential foci of infection,

e.g. extracting primary teeth with extensive carious lesions, rather than carrying out pulp treatments, in order to avoid future risk for infection and bacteraemia. Furthermore, treatment should be aimed to be completed in the least number of visits to keep episodes of bacteraemia to a minimum.

- Patients may have an increased **risk of bleeding** due to anticoagulant therapy or secondary to prolonged cyanosis.
- Potential increased risk of **general anaesthesia** in CHD patients. Other treatment modalities, e.g. use of nitrous oxide sedation, should be considered for anxious patients.
- Patients are known to have **increased dental anxiety**, likely secondary to their medical history [40]. Anxious children can present with more behaviour management problems [41], which can complicate their dental management.

Expert comment

Whilst advances in interventions, particularly percutaneous transcatheter valve insertion, have revolutionized how we treat patients with congenital and structural heart disease, there is a suggestion that this may also be associated with an increase in rates of IE, compared to surgically implanted valves [42–45]. Endocarditis of the aortic valve is such a serious and life-changing event that most paediatric cardiologists would insist on antibiotic prophylaxis for any patient with aortic valve disease or previous aortic valve surgery such as the Ross operation, at times of risk such as dental extraction, endoscopy, or any other operation.

Learning point What should dentists do?

The case of Montgomery vs Lanarkshire Health Board has had a great impact on the consent process and reinforces that patients have a right to be informed of all the potential risks of treatment. The Montgomery decision requires a clinician to inform a patient about 'material risks' and to find out what that specific patient would want to know [38]. This has had an impact on NICE Clinical Guideline 64.

In 2016, NICE made an amendment to its Clinical Guideline 64 (CG64):

> *'Antibiotic prophylaxis against infective endocarditis is not recommended* ***routinely*** *for people undergoing dental procedures.'*

This change in the NICE guideline places the onus on dentists to identify patients at risk for IE, to explain the risks and ways in which the risk can be reduced, and to allow patients to decide for themselves if they want antibiotic prophylaxis or not—changing the philosophy to a patient-centred decision [33].

The amendment lacked clarity and is a major challenge for dentists, as NICE did not define which individual patients should be considered for 'non-routine' management and which antibiotic regimes should be used. The SDCEP has since developed specific advice for the dental team to help implement the NICE amendment as below.

- **Routine management**—invasive dental treatment is provided without antibiotic prophylaxis, which is appropriate for the majority of cases at an increased risk of IE.
  - Ensure patients are aware of the risk of IE and provide prevention advice, including:
    - Benefits and risks of antibiotic prophylaxis and why it is not routinely recommended
    - Importance of good oral health
    - Symptoms of IE and when to seek advice
    - Risks of undergoing other invasive procedures
  - If a patient requests antibiotic prophylaxis, consider seeking advice from the cardiology team. NICE CG64 advises that 'a final decision should take into account values and preferences of patients.'
  - Ensure episodes of dental infection in patients are treated promptly.

- **Non-routine management**—invasive dental treatment for patients from a special consideration group may be considered for non-routine management. These include patients with prosthetic heart valves, previous IE, and cyanotic CHD and those patients repaired with prosthetic material.
  - Assess the patient in consultation with their cardiology team to determine whether to consider antibiotic prophylaxis for invasive dental procedures.
  - When antibiotic prophylaxis is considered, ensure the patient is aware of the risks and benefits to allow them to make an informed decision about whether prophylaxis is right for them.
  - Provide prevention advice, including:
    - Importance of good oral health
    - Symptoms of IE and when to seek advice
    - Risks of undergoing other invasive procedures
  - Ensure episodes of dental infection in patients are treated promptly.

Learning point What should paediatric cardiologists consider in the management of oral health for patients?

(See Table 12.3.)

Table 12.3 Dental standards in the Paediatric Congenital Heart Disease Standards and Service Specification (PCHDSS) 2016 [47]

	PCHDSS, Section M
1	Families will be given appropriate evidence-based preventive dental advice at the time of CHD diagnosis by the cardiologist or nurse.
2	All children and young people with planned elective cardiac surgery or intervention must have a dental assessment as part of pre-procedural planning to ensure that they are dentally fit for their planned intervention.
3	All children at increased risk for endocarditis must be referred for specialist dental assessment at 2 years of age, and have a tailored programme for specialist follow-up.
4	Each Congenital Heart Network must have a clear referral pathway for urgent dental assessments for CHD patients presenting with infective endocarditis, dental pain, acute dental infection, or dental trauma. All children and young people admitted and diagnosed with infective endocarditis must have a dental assessment within 72 hours.
5	Specialist children's surgical centres must provide access to theatre facilities and appropriate anaesthetic support for the provision of specialist-led dental treatment under general anaesthesia for children and young people with CHD.
6	Specialist children's surgical centres will refer children with CHD to a hospital dental service when local dental services will not provide care.

This document brings together the standards that emphasize the importance of prevention and the need for dentists and cardiologists to work closely together to provide holistic care for patients.
NHS England. *Paediatric Congenital Heart Disease Standards & Specification*. 2016. https://www.england.nhs.uk/wp-content/uploads/2018/08/Congenital-heart-disease-standards-and-specifications.pdf

A final word from the expert

The frequency of bacterial endocarditis is probably increasing and is a particularly dangerous condition for any patient with prosthetic material used during cardiac surgery or interventional cardiac catheterization. Although the advice regarding antibiotic prophylaxis at times of potential risk is sometimes imprecise, most cardiologists would advise such prophylaxis for patients with prosthetic valves, conduits, prosthetic shunts, and aortic valve disease. Medical reports should specifically include the advice of the attending cardiologist.

Acknowledgements

We are grateful to Dr Paul Ashley for reviewing the dental segments of the chapter. Additionally, our thanks to Mr Conal Austin for the images of the infected valve.

References

1. National Institute for Health and Care Excellence. *Prophylaxis against infective endocarditis: antimicrobial prophylaxis against infective endocarditis in adults and children undergoing interventional procedures*. Clinical guideline [CG64]. 2008. Available at: https://www.nice.org.uk/guidance/cg64
2. Stecksén-Blicks C, Rydberg A, Nyman L, Asplund S, Svanberg C. Dental caries experience in children with congenital heart disease: a case-control study. *Int J Paediatr Dent* 2004;14:94–100.
3. Balmer R, Bu'Lock FA. The experiences with oral health and dental prevention of children with congenital heart disease. *Cardiol Young* 2003;13:439–43.
4. da Fonseca MA, Evans M, Teske D, Thikkurissy S, Amini H. The impact of oral health on the quality of life of young patients with congenital cardiac disease. *Cardiol Young* 2009;19:252–6.
5. Parry JA, Khan FA. Provision of dental care for medically compromised children in the UK by general dental practitioners. *Int J Paediatr Dent* 2000;10:322–7.
6. Weinstein LW, Brusch JL. *Infective Endocarditis*. New York, NY: Oxford University Press, 1996.
7. Tang KL, Caffrey NP, Nóbrega DB, et al. Restricting the use of antibiotics in food-producing animals and its associations with antibiotic resistance in food-producing animals and human beings: a systematic review and meta-analysis. *Lancet Planet Health* 2017;1:e316–27. Erratum in: *Lancet Planet Health* 2017;1:e359.
8. Nishimura RA, Otto CM, Bonow RO, et al.; American College of Cardiology/American Heart Association Task Force on Practice Guidelines. 2014 AHA/ACC guideline for the management of patients with valvular heart disease: executive summary: a report of the American College of Cardiology/American Heart Association Task Force on Practice Guidelines. *J Am Coll Cardiol* 2014;63:2438–88.
9. Cahill TJ, Prendergast BD. Infective endocarditis. *Lancet* 2016;387:882–93.
10. Koster K. Dieembolische endocarditis. 1878; *Virchows Arch*. Bd. LXXII, S.257.
11. Harper WF. The blood supply of heart valves in relation to endocarditis. *J Anat* 1938;73(Pt 1):94–111.
12. Gross L. [Chapter 5]. In: L Gross. *The Blood Supply to the Heart in its Anatomical and Clinical Aspects*. New York, NY: Paul B Hoeber, 1921; p. 53.
13. Cahill TJ, Baddour LM, Habib G, et al. Challenges in infective endocarditis. *J Am Coll Cardiol* 2017;69:325–44.
14. Prendergast BD. The changing face of infective endocarditis. *Heart* 2006;92:879–85.
15. Tleyjeh IM, Steckelberg JM, Murad HS, et al. Temporal trends in infective endocarditis: a population-based study in Olmsted County, Minnesota. *JAMA* 2005;293:3022–8.
16. Lalani T, Chu VH, Park LP, et al. In-hospital and 1-year mortality in patients undergoing early surgery for prosthetic valve endocarditis. *JAMA Intern Med* 2013;173:1495–504.
17. Le Moing V, Alla F, Doco-Lecompte T, et al. *Staphylococcus aureus* bloodstream infection and endocarditis: a prospective cohort study. *PLoS One* 2015;10:e0127385.
18. Werdan K, Dietz S, Löffler B, et al. Mechanisms of infective endocarditis: pathogen-host interaction and risk states. *Nat Rev Cardiol* 2014;11:35–50.
19. Elgharably H, Hussain ST, Shrestha NK, Blackstone EH, Pettersson GB. Current hypotheses in cardiac surgery: biofilm in infective endocarditis. *Semin Thorac Cardiovasc Surg* Spring 2016;28:56–9.

20. Chung PY, Toh YS. Anti-biofilm agents: recent breakthrough against multi-drug resistant *Staphylococcus aureus*. *Pathog Dis* 2014;70:231–9.
21. Fowler VG Jr, Miro JM, Hoen B, et al. *Staphylococcus aureus* endocarditis: a consequence of medical progress. *JAMA* 2005;293:3012–21. Erratum: *JAMA*. 2005;294:900.
22. Selton-Suty C, Célard M, Le Moing V, et al. Preeminence of *Staphylococcus aureus* in infective endocarditis: a 1-year population-based survey. *Clin Infect Dis* 2012;54:1230–9.
23. Hoen B, Duval X. Clinical practice. Infective endocarditis. *N Engl J Med* 2013;368:1425–33. Erratum in: *N Engl J Med* 2013;368:2536.
24. Murdoch DR, Corey GR, Hoen B, et al.; International Collaboration on Endocarditis-Prospective Cohort Study (ICE-PCS) Investigators. Clinical presentation, etiology, and outcome of infective endocarditis in the 21st century: the International Collaboration on Endocarditis-Prospective Cohort Study. *Arch Intern Med* 2009;169:463–73.
25. Duval X, Alla F, Doco-Lecompte T, et al.; Association pour l'Étude et la Prévention de l'Endocardite Infectieuse (AEPEI). Diabetes mellitus and infective endocarditis: the insulin factor in patient morbidity and mortality. *Eur Heart J* 2007;28:59–64.
26. Lockhart PB, Brennan MT, Thornhill M, et al. Poor oral hygiene as a risk factor for infective endocarditis-related bacteraemia. *J Am Dent Assoc* 2009;140:1238–44.
27. NHS Digital. *Child Dental Health Survey 2013, England, Wales and Northern Ireland*. 2015. Available at: https://digital.nhs.uk/data-and-information/publications/statistical/children-s-dental-health-survey/child-dental-health-survey-2013-england-wales-and-northern-ireland
28. Horder TJ. Infective endocarditis; with an analysis of 150 cases and with special reference to the chronic form of the disease. *Q J Med* 1909;2:289–324.
29. Okell CC, Elliott SD. Bacteraemia and oral sepsis with special reference to the aetiology of subacute endocarditis. *Lancet* 1935;ii:869–72.
30. Van der Meer JT, Van Wijk W, Thompson J, et al. Efficacy of antibiotic prophylaxis for prevention of native-valve endocarditis. *Lancet* 1992;339:135–9.
31. Dayer MJ, Jones S, Prendergast B, Baddour LM, Lockhart PB, Thornhill MH. Incidence of infective endocarditis in England, 2000–13: a secular trend, interrupted time-series analysis. *Lancet* 2015;385:1219–28.
32. Thornhill MH, Gibson TB, Cutler E, et al. Antibiotic prophylaxis and incidence of endocarditis before and after the 2007 AHA Recommendations. *J Am Coll Cardiol* 2018;72:2443–54.
33. Thornhill MH, Dayer M, Lockhart PB, et al. Guidelines on prophylaxis to prevent infective endocarditis. *Br Dent J* 2016;220:51–6.
34. Wilson W, Taubert KA, Gewitz M, et al.; American Heart Association Rheumatic Fever, Endocarditis, and Kawasaki Disease Committee; American Heart Association Council on Cardiovascular Disease in the Young; American Heart Association Council on Clinical Cardiology; American Heart Association Council on Cardiovascular Surgery and Anesthesia; Quality of Care and Outcomes Research Interdisciplinary Working Group. Prevention of infective endocarditis: guidelines from the American Heart Association: a guideline from the American Heart Association Rheumatic Fever, Endocarditis, and Kawasaki Disease Committee, Council on Cardiovascular Disease in the Young, and the Council on Clinical Cardiology, Council on Cardiovascular Surgery and Anesthesia, and the Quality of Care and Outcomes Research Interdisciplinary Working Group. *Circulation* 2007;116:1736–54. Erratum in: *Circulation* 2007;116:e376–7.
35. Wilson W, Taubert KA, Gewitz M, et al.; American Heart Association. Prevention of infective endocarditis: guidelines from the American Heart Association: a guideline from the American Heart Association Rheumatic Fever, Endocarditis and Kawasaki Disease Committee, Council on Cardiovascular Disease in the Young, and the Council on Clinical Cardiology, Council on Cardiovascular Surgery and Anesthesia, and the Quality of Care and Outcomes Research Interdisciplinary Working Group. *J Am Dent Assoc* 2008;139 Suppl:3S–24S. Erratum in: *J Am Dent Assoc* 2008;139:253.

36. Habib G, Lancellotti P, Antunes MJ, et al.; ESC Scientific Document Group. 2015 ESC Guidelines for the management of infective endocarditis: The Task Force for the Management of Infective Endocarditis of the European Society of Cardiology (ESC). Endorsed by: European Association for Cardio-Thoracic Surgery (EACTS), the European Association of Nuclear Medicine (EANM). *Eur Heart J* 2015;36:3075–128.
37. Thornhill MH, Dayer MJ, Forde JM, et al. Impact of the NICE guideline recommending cessation of antibiotic prophylaxis for prevention of infective endocarditis: before and after study. *BMJ* 2011;342:d2392.
38. Scottish Dental Clinical Effectiveness Programme. *Antibiotic prophylaxis against infective endocarditis. Implementation advice*. 2018. Available at: http://www.sdcep.org.uk/wp-content/uploads/2018/08/SDCEP-Antibiotic-Prophylaxis-Implementation-Advice.pdf
39. Tasioula V, Balmer R, Parsons J. Dental health and treatment in a group of children with congenital heart disease. *Pediatr Dent* 2008;30:323–8.
40. Hollis A, Willcoxson F, Smith A, Balmer R. An investigation into dental anxiety amongst paediatric cardiology patients. *Int J Paediatr Dent* 2015;25:183–90.
41. Klaassen MA, Veerkamp JS, Hoogstraten J. Changes in children's dental fear: a longitudinal study. *Eur Arch Paediatr Dent* 2008;9(Suppl 1):29–35.
42. Amat-Santos IJ, Messika-Zeitoun D, Eltchaninoff H, et al. Infective endocarditis after transcatheter aortic valve implantation: results from a large multicenter registry. *Circulation* 2015;131:1566–74.
43. Mangner N, Woitek F, Haussig S, et al. Incidence, predictors, and outcome of patients developing infective endocarditis following transfemoral transcatheter aortic valve replacement. *J Am Coll Cardiol* 2016;67:2907–8.
44. Van Dijck I, Budts W, Cools B, et al. Infective endocarditis of a transcatheter pulmonary valve in comparison with surgical implants. *Heart* 2015;101:788–93.
45. Uebing A, Rigby ML. The problem of infective endocarditis after transcatheter pulmonary valve implantation. *Heart* 2015;101:749–51.

CASE

13 Transposition of the great arteries: to switch or not to switch?

Thomas Day

Expert commentary Michael Cheung

Case history

An infant was born via spontaneous unassisted vaginal delivery at full term, weighing 3.5 kg. He was the first child to non-consanguineous parents. His parents were both healthy and there was no known family history of congenital heart disease (CHD). At the routine 20-week anomaly scan, the sonographer had noted that although the four-chamber view appeared normal, the three-vessel view was abnormal, and a diagnosis of transposition of the great arteries (TGA) was made. A large malaligned ventricular septal defect (VSD) was also present, with posterior deviation of the outlet septum. This deviation was causing a degree of left ventricular outflow tract obstruction (subvalvar pulmonary stenosis), and the pulmonary valve also appeared small and dysplastic.

Learning point Ventricular septal defects in TGA

VSDs are the most commonly seen additional intracardiac defect in TGA, occurring in around 40% of cases [1]. The size and location of these defects are highly variable. As in hearts with normally related great arteries, VSDs can occur in any part of the ventricular septum [2]. A perimembranous defect is defined, in the setting of TGA, as fibrous continuity between the tricuspid and pulmonary valve (rather than the aortic valve), as shown in Figure 13.1. When the VSD is associated with posterior deviation of the outlet septum, it will produce obstruction of the left ventricular outflow tract (LVOT), one of the most common mechanisms of left ventricular outflow tract obstruction (LVOTO) in TGA (discussed in Learning point: Left ventricular outflow tract obstruction in TGA, p. 178).

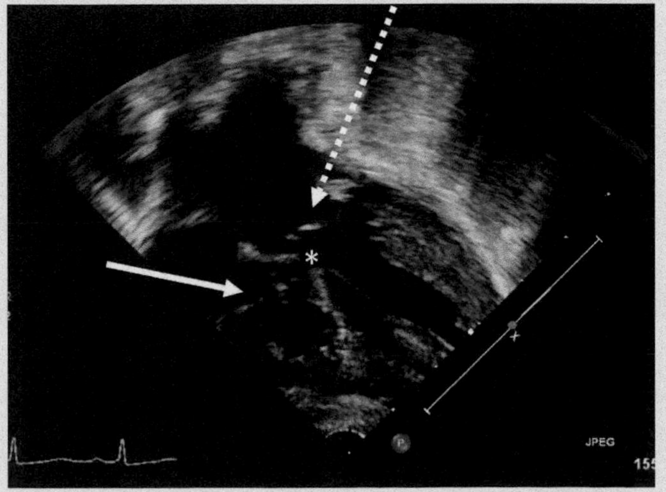

Figure 13.1 Echocardiogram (subcostal view), demonstrates the bifurcating pulmonary artery arising from the left ventricle, with a large malaligned perimembranous ventricular septal defect (asterisk). There is fibrous continuity between the pulmonary valve (dashed arrow) and the tricuspid valve (solid white arrow).

The presence of a VSD in TGA is important for several reasons. Firstly, it may alter the haemodynamics. The flow across a VSD will be mainly from the right (systemic) to the left (pulmonary) ventricle, so increasing pulmonary blood flow, with a resulting increase in oxygen saturation, and/or work of breathing. This effect will be negligible in small VSDs. Secondly, the presence of a VSD will have an impact on the surgical approach. During the arterial switch procedure, a large VSD will have to be closed to avoid later development of pulmonary over-circulation. Alternatively, if an arterial switch is not performed, then depending on its location, the VSD may be an essential component of the surgical strategy (see Learning point: Surgery for TGA with LVOTO and VSD, p. 185–186). Thirdly, the presence of a sizeable VSD may allow surgery to be delayed by maintaining the left ventricular pressure, and hence myocardial mass. There is concern, however, that the development of pulmonary vascular disease may be accelerated in patients with TGA with a VSD.

Learning point Left ventricular outflow tract obstruction in TGA

In TGA, LVOTO causes pulmonary stenosis. This reduces pulmonary blood flow, resulting in lower preoperative oxygen saturations, and may also affect the surgical strategy. As mentioned in Learning point: Ventricular septal defects (VSDs) in TGA, p. 177, a common mechanism of LVOTO is that of a malaligned VSD with posterior deviation of the outlet septum into the left ventricle. All the other usual types of outflow tract obstruction in the setting of ventriculo-arterial concordance can occur, e.g. mitral valve tissue crossing this area, ventricular tissue tags, fibromuscular ridges, annular hypoplasia, and valvar stenosis. These lesions may be surgically correctable, allowing the arterial switch to proceed [2]. If not amenable to surgical correction, an alternative to the arterial switch will be necessary.

The pregnancy progressed without complication, and the infant was delivered in good condition. In view of the antenatal cardiac diagnosis, the delivery was planned to take place in a tertiary-level maternity hospital, close to the paediatric cardiac surgical centre. No active resuscitation was required. Shortly after birth, a peripheral intravenous cannula was inserted and an infusion of prostaglandin E1 was commenced at a dose of 10 ng/kg/min (see Clinical tip: prostaglandin E1 infusions, p. 178). The infant was subsequently transferred to the cardiac surgical centre for further care.

Clinical tip Prostaglandin E1 infusions

Prostaglandin E1 (generic name: alprostadil; tradename: Prostin VR®) is a drug that is delivered by continuous infusion, in order to prevent the natural closure of the arterial duct after birth. It is used in CHD in three categories of patients: in those with a duct-dependent pulmonary circulation, those with a duct-dependent systemic circulation, and those (as in this case) who may require a patent arterial duct for adequate mixing between two parallel circulations. The usual dose range is 5–50 ng/kg/min, although higher doses can be used. Side effects are common and occur in increasing frequency as the dose increases. The most common side effects are:

- Apnoea (sometimes requiring intubation and ventilation)
- Hypotension
- Pyrexia and flushing
- Hypoglycaemia
- Irritability
- Thrombocytopenia.

If the atrial communication is small, most patients with TGA with an intact ventricular septum will have inadequate oxygenation, even in the presence of a large patent ductus arteriosus (PDA), and will therefore require an atrial septostomy. A further subset of children remain significantly desaturated, even with communication at the level of the PDA and the atrial septum. In these children, pulmonary vasodilators may be effective, but ECMO or urgent surgical repair may be required.

On arrival to the paediatric intensive care unit, the infant was well and breathing spontaneously without respiratory distress but was cyanosed, with oxygen saturations of 75% in the right hand (oxygen saturations in TGA are discussed in Clinical tip: Balloon atrial septostomy, p. 184). Auscultation revealed a 2/6 ejection systolic murmur, loudest at the left upper sternal edge and widely heard throughout the precordium. The liver edge was palpable at 1 cm below the right costal margin, and the abdomen was soft.

A transthoracic echocardiogram demonstrated normal atrial arrangement, with atrioventricular concordance and ventriculo-arterial discordance. Systemic and pulmonary venous drainage were normal. There was only a small interatrial communication, with bidirectional flow. The atrioventricular valves were normal in appearance and function. There was a moderate-sized VSD, with posterior malalignment (deviation) of the outlet septum, causing moderate subvalvar pulmonary stenosis. The pulmonary valve was significantly smaller in diameter than the aortic valve, with thickened, dysplastic leaflets (Figure 13.2). The right ventricular outflow tract was unobstructed, connected to the aorta, with a left-sided aortic arch and no coarctation. There was a large arterial duct, with low-velocity bidirectional flow. The great arteries were seen to arise from the heart in parallel, with the aortic valve anterior and to the right. The left anterior descending coronary artery was seen to arise from sinus 1 of the aortic valve (Leiden convention), along with the right coronary artery which looped anteriorly before heading to the right. The circumflex artery was seen to arise from sinus 2 (see Learning point: Leiden convention for coronary artery nomenclature in TGA, p. 180).

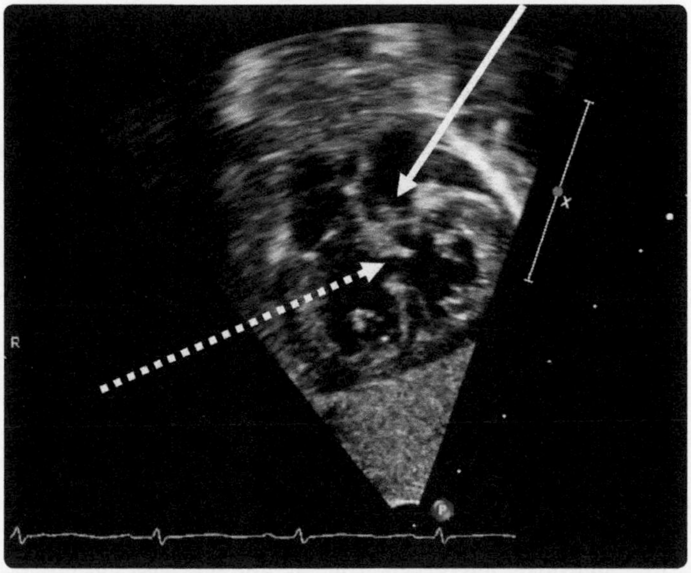

Figure 13.2 Echocardiogram, subcostal view. This demonstrates deviation of the outlet septum, causing subpulmonary obstruction (dashed arrow). In addition, the pulmonary valve is thickened and appears dysplastic, causing valvar pulmonary stenosis (solid white arrow).

Learning point Leiden convention for coronary artery nomenclature in TGA

Although certain patterns of coronary arteries are recognized in TGA, this is a highly variable area of TGA anatomy, with important clinical ramifications. As will become clear in our case, the coronary anatomy can preclude some surgical strategies, so it is vital that the various professional groups (cardiologists, echocardiographic technologists, surgeons) can communicate their findings clearly.

The so-called 'Leiden convention' (Figure 13.3) is based on the concept that the two coronary arteries almost always arise from the two aortic sinuses that are closest to the pulmonary valve (the 'facing sinuses'). The anatomically leftward coronary sinus is designated sinus 1, and the rightward sinus is designated sinus 2. From the surgeon's intraoperative viewpoint, it is possible to imagine oneself 'standing' in the non-facing sinus, with a hand in each of the two facing sinuses. Confusion may be further increased by the difference in the way that echocardiographers are viewing the aortic valve, which is essentially from the ventricular aspect, whereas the usual surgical view is from the aortic aspect. This alternative convention dictates that the sinus with the right hand in is designated sinus 1, and the one with the left hand sinus 2. It can be seen that this alternative nomenclature of the right hand-facing sinus being actually the anatomically leftward sinus, and vice versa, is confusing. Hence, we prefer to use the Leiden convention or alternatively describe the anatomical location of the coronary arteries explicitly.

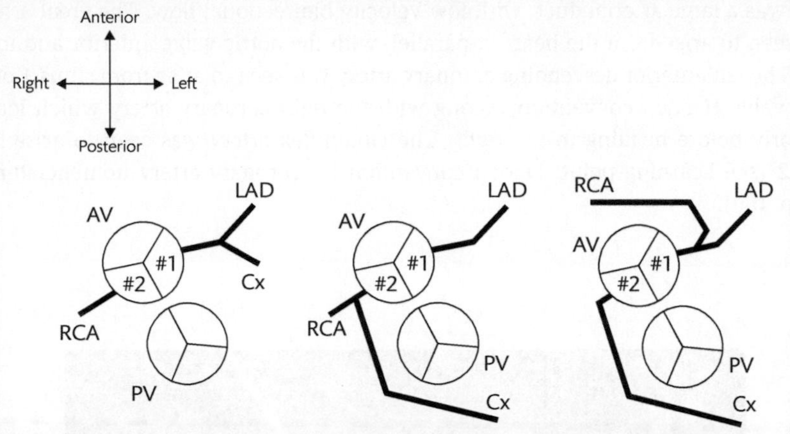

Figure 13.3 The three most common coronary arrangements seen in transposition, in descending order of frequency, from left to right. Note that these diagrams show the anatomy from an echocardiographer's perspective, i.e. from the ventricular aspect of semi-lunar valves. The arrangement on the far left accounts for >60% of cases. AV, aortic valve; PV, pulmonary valve; LAD, left anterior descending artery; Cx, circumflex artery; RCA, right coronary artery; #1, sinus number 1 (right-hand-facing sinus); #2, sinus number 2 (left-hand-facing sinus).

The most common coronary arrangement (seen in around two-thirds of TGA cases) is for the left anterior descending and circumflex arteries to arise from sinus 1, and the right coronary artery to arise from sinus 2. However, a variety of coronary artery patterns can occur [3].

Over the next few hours (whilst on prostaglandins), the oxygen saturations in the right hand (i.e. pre-ductal) fell to around 63%, despite the commencement of low-flow oxygen via nasal cannulae. In view of this, the baby was electively intubated, ventilated, and sedated, and a balloon atrial septostomy was performed via the umbilical vein. There was immediate improvement in the pre- and post-ductal oxygen saturations to 80% (see Clinical tip: Balloon atrial septostomy, p. 184).

The prostaglandin infusion was weaned and successfully stopped over the next 24 hours, with oxygen saturations remaining at around 80%. Enteral feeding was commenced without complications, and the baby was discussed in the joint cardiology and surgical conference. It was decided that he was not suitable for an arterial switch operation (ASO), because of the technical difficulties posed by the subvalvar and valvar pulmonary stenosis, including size mismatch between the aortic and pulmonary valves (see Learning point: Common contraindications to the arterial switch, p. 185). Instead, it was decided to allow the baby grow, with the aim of performing an alternative operation at a later date (see Learning point: Surgery for TGA with LVOTO and VSD, p. 185–186). The baby was discharged home after 10 days in hospital on no regular medications.

In the outpatient clinic, 2 weeks after discharge, the baby had gained a small amount of weight on breastfeeding. Examination found a 2/6 ejection systolic murmur and oxygen saturations measured in the right hand were 80%. Echocardiography confirmed an unrestrictive interatrial communication with left-to-right flow and no arterial duct. The ventricular systolic function was good, with balanced ventricular sizes. Further review was planned for 2 weeks' time.

In 2 weeks, the parents reported that the baby's feeding had become slightly more difficult. He took longer to feed and took smaller volumes of milk. Clinical examination was unchanged, except for a drop in oxygen saturations to 65%. Due to increasing cyanosis and feeding difficulties, he was admitted to the paediatric cardiology ward.

The baby remained profoundly desaturated, although there was some improvement with oxygen supplementation. There was no evidence of an intercurrent illness, and it was felt that the low saturations were a consequence of inadequate pulmonary blood flow. The surgical team felt that he was still too small to undergo definitive surgical repair, and, as such, a 3.5-mm GoreTex® tube was used to connect the brachiocephalic artery to the right pulmonary artery (right modified Blalock–Taussig shunt). It resulted in an immediate increase in oxygen saturations to 89%.

Post-operatively, low-dose aspirin was commenced (to minimize the risk for shunt thrombosis) and the infant was discharged home. He remained well, with frequent outpatient reviews to confirm good weight gain and acceptable oxygen saturations. Over the next few months, although he had adequate weight gain, his oxygen saturations slowly decreased. At 9 months, his weight was 6.7 kg and oxygen saturations were 78%. Following discussion in the multidisciplinary meeting, he was listed for elective surgical repair. Although several options were discussed, a *réparation à L'étage ventriculaire* (REV) procedure was performed (the infant's unusual coronary arrangement precluded the Nikaidoh operation, as it was felt it would put too much compression and distortion on the right coronary artery). This was carried out without complications, and the patient was discharged home after 2 weeks, with normal oxygen saturations (see Learning point: Surgery for TGA with LVOTO and VSD, p. 185–186).

Discussion

The modern management of TGA is one of the success stories of paediatric cardiology and cardiac surgery. The long-term outcome of TGA has been transformed from an almost certain death in infancy at the start of the twentieth century, through to increasing morbidity and mortality after the third to fourth decades of life following atrial switch (Mustard or Senning procedure), to excellent long-term survival with a good quality of life in the modern era of the ASO. The introduction and subsequent refinement of the operation has led to improvements in outcome over the last few decades, but as in our case, not all infants with TGA are able to undergo this procedure. This can be for a variety of anatomical reasons, and the long-term prognosis is less certain. In this chapter, we will review some of the alternative management strategies currently available.

The incidence of TGA is around 2.3–3.8 per 10,000 live births, making it one of the more common types of cyanotic CHD [4]. There is a male preponderance, and unlike other forms of cyanotic CHD, infants with TGA usually have a normal or even a higher-than-average birthweight. Simple TGA is only rarely associated with chromosomal syndromes, and extracardiac defects are uncommon [5].

The fundamental morphological feature of TGA is concordant atrioventricular connections with discordant ventriculo-arterial connections. In other words, the right ventricle, connected to the aorta, receives deoxygenated systemic venous blood from the right atrium, whilst the left ventricle gives rise to the pulmonary artery but receives oxygenated pulmonary venous blood from the left atrium. However, a wide variety of anatomical subtypes exists, especially in terms of the orientation of the great arteries, along with an array of associated cardiac anomalies. The aortic valve is usually (but not always) found anterior to, and to the right of, the pulmonary artery and is often supported by a muscular infundibulum [2]. The pulmonary valve, in contrast, is often in direct fibrous continuity with the mitral valve.

Several additional cardiac anomalies are seen commonly in patients with TGA. The presence of an interatrial communication and patency of the arterial duct are a requirement for initial survival, so these are not usually considered an anomaly as such. The two most commonly associated lesions are a VSD and LVOTO, outlined in the relevant learning points. Multiple muscular VSDs are encountered rarely.

Other lesions that may be encountered in TGA, albeit rarely, include right ventricular outflow tract obstruction, aortic coarctation/interruption, juxtaposition of the atrial appendages, and straddling tricuspid valve. These should all be investigated and excluded, as appropriate, during the initial evaluation of any infant presenting with TGA. Associated lesions can have a profound influence on the management strategy and so these must be clearly defined.

The fundamental problem in these infants is that the left and right heart circulations operate in parallel, rather than in series as in a normal heart. Clearly, if there were no communication between these two systems, this would not be compatible with life, as the systemic blood flow would become increasingly desaturated as it circulates around the body without ever reaching the lungs. Survival depends on the admixture of systemic and pulmonary venous blood through an atrial septal defect (ASD), a VSD, an arterial duct, or rarely another additional source of pulmonary blood flow, e.g. systemic pulmonary arterial collaterals.

The direction and magnitude of blood flow at these points are highly variable, dependent on the size of the communication and also on the pulmonary vascular resistance (PVR). Immediately after birth, the PVR is high, with flow through the PDA being bidirectional or even right to left. The flow of oxygenated blood from the pulmonary artery to the aorta via the PDA gives rise to the pathognomonic sign of TGA, the so-called 'reversed differential cyanosis'. In this situation, the pre-ductal oxygen saturations (usually measured in the right hand) are lower than the post-ductal oxygen saturations (usually measured in either foot). This is a very useful sign in the first few hours of life, and if seen, one can be fairly confident that the diagnosis is TGA, even before an echocardiogram is performed. It is also worth remembering that standard 'differential cyanosis' (with post-ductal saturations significantly lower than pre-ductal) cannot exist in patients with TGA. If this is seen in a baby with the diagnosis of TGA, either the measurements are wrong or the diagnosis is!

As the PVR falls after birth, the direction of flow in the PDA will change to become exclusively left to right (from the aorta to the pulmonary artery). This flow into the pulmonary arteries increases the total pulmonary blood flow, and hence increases the pulmonary venous return and the left atrial pressure. This also increases the amount of oxygenated blood flowing from the left atrium to the right atrium, through the interatrial communication, with a concomitant increase in systemic oxygen saturations. A good amount of flow at the atrial level is important for satisfactory oxygen saturations, and we will discuss how to optimize both of these (see Clinical tip: Balloon atrial septostomy, p.184).

The diagnosis of TGA is now often made prenatally, although rates of detection may vary, depending on local expertise and antenatal care systems. Antenatal diagnosis allows for delivery to be planned in a suitable centre, and prostaglandin administration to be commenced soon after birth. This has been shown to improve the preoperative condition of infants with TGA and may improve survival [6, 7]. In those not diagnosed during fetal life, cyanosis is usually the most obvious clinical feature. As explained, 'reversed differential cyanosis' is virtually diagnostic of TGA, making this a very useful clinical sign. It may only be present for the first few hours after life, however. As we have discussed, the flow of blood between the two parallel circulations is dependent on the size of the interatrial communication, PDA, and VSD (if present), as well as the PVR and systemic blood pressure. As these factors are highly variable, the degree of cyanosis and circulatory status are likewise very different between infants. The second heart sound is often single, and additional cardiac defects may give other clinical signs. A short systolic murmur of a VSD may be heard, or the ejection systolic murmur of left or right outflow tract obstruction. The intensity and character of these will be dependent upon the haemodynamics at the time of assessment. Those infants with a large VSD may show signs of pulmonary overcirculation (tachypnoea and hepatomegaly) once the PVR has dropped sufficiently.

Once the diagnosis is suspected, transthoracic echocardiography should be performed as soon as possible (see Clinical tip: Use of echocardiography in TGA, p. 183). In the modern era, no other imaging modalities are usually required prior to surgery, although magnetic resonance imaging (MRI) may be useful in particularly complex cases if the adequacy of ventricular size is uncertain. Echocardiography is generally a better imaging modality than MRI to determine the attachments of atrioventricular valves or valve function.

Expert comment Use of echocardiography in TGA

Echocardiography is now the most important preoperative imaging modality in TGA and is usually the only form of imaging that is required, both to make the diagnosis and to guide surgical strategy. Once the diagnosis of TGA is made, there are a number of additional aspects that are particularly important to define:

- The size of the interatrial communication [either patent foramen ovale (PFO) or ASD], the direction of blood flow, and the pressure gradient between the two atria
- The size and location of the VSD(s), the direction of blood flow, and the pressure gradient between the two ventricles
- The morphology, attachments, and function of the atrioventricular valves
- The outflow tracts and the presence of outflow tract obstruction, including the mechanism and severity, if present
- The size of each semi-lunar valve and the presence of any significant valvar stenosis or regurgitation
- The size of the PDA and the direction of flow
- It is important to exclude other associated lesions such as coarctation/interruption of the aorta or juxtaposition of the atrial appendages

- Coronary artery anatomy and potential intramural course. Intramural coronary arteries may be suspected by the oblique nature of the arterial origin, and depending on the surgical experience, it may be dealt with. It is important to highlight this anatomical variation to surgeons preoperatively in order to avoid injury to the coronary artery at dissection whilst mobilizing the epicardial coronary vessel.

If the interatrial communication is considered inadequate to maintain reasonable systemic saturations, then a balloon atrial septostomy should be considered if the ASO is to be delayed (see Clinical tip: Balloon atrial septostomy, p. 184). Medical management should also address any acidosis, with volume replacement to avoid hypovolaemia. Supplementary oxygen may be useful to both increase dissolved oxygen content, as well as lower the PVR. Nitric oxide may also be needed to further lower the PVR in certain patients. If all of these therapeutic manipulations fail, then an urgent arterial switch may be required, or rarely extracorporeal membrane oxygenation (ECMO).

Clinical tip Balloon atrial septostomy

First described by Rashkind and Miller in 1966, balloon atrial septostomy (BAS) revolutionized the care of infants with TGA by allowing unrestricted flow between the atria, resulting in an improvement in oxygen saturations. In many cases, the prostaglandin infusion can be safely discontinued. BAS is commonly performed with echocardiographic screening on the high dependency/intensive care unit however since the recent (2019) withdrawal of the Edwards Miller & Fogarty balloons, most centres are now performing septostomies in the cardiac catheter lab. This is because the available balloon is an over the wire system, requiring fluoroscopy.

Using the femoral or umbilical vein, a balloon-tipped catheter is advanced into the right atrium and across the interatrial communication to the left atrium. The balloon is inflated with saline and pulled sharply back into the right atrium, tearing the oval fossa and enlarging the interatrial communication (demonstrated in Figure 13.4). It is important to ensure the balloon is clear of the mitral valve and pulmonary veins before inflation.

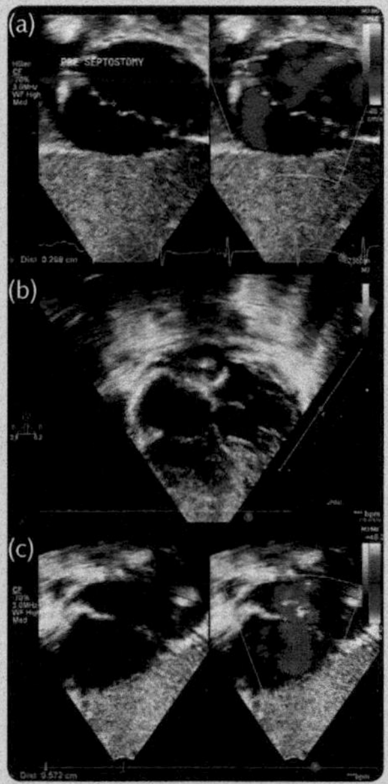

Figure 13.4 Echocardiograms, subcostal views, showing balloon atrial septostomy. (a) Small restrictive interatrial communication prior to septostomy. (b) During septostomy with the balloon in the left atrium crossing the septum. (c) Result following septostomy, with a larger interatrial communication and good left-to-right flow.

BAS is a safe procedure in experienced hands, and serious complications should be rare. However, these can include damage to the atrioventricular valves, pulmonary veins, inferior vena cava (IVC), and perforation of the heart.

Learning point Common contraindications to arterial switch

- LVOTO that cannot be rectified surgically or valvar pulmonary stenosis
- Major size discrepancy between the pulmonary and aortic valves, though rarely an isolated reason to preclude ASO
- Coronary artery anatomy that precludes coronary transfer

Expert comment Atrial switch

Surprisingly, attempts at the ASO predate atrial redirection procedures, but it was not until the first successful arterial switch in 1975 by Jatene that the procedure started to gain widespread acceptance [8]. Prior to that point, standard care involved the atrial redirection procedures (Mustard and Senning). These operations incorporated material (either autologous in the case of Senning, or synthetic in the case of Mustard) to baffle deoxygenated systemic venous blood to the left atrium, and hence to the pulmonary artery, with oxygenated pulmonary venous blood flowing to the right atrium and subsequently the aorta. This results in a physiological, but not anatomical, correction. The main drawback is that the right ventricle remains as the systemic ventricle, a task for which it is not suited in the medium term. There is a high rate of right ventricular failure, and for this reason, these procedures are now almost never performed for simple TGA [9, 10]. The Senning procedure, however, has had a renaissance as an integral part of the surgical management of 'congenitally corrected' TGA.

The ASO is the operation of choice for TGA, assuming that there is no anatomical reason that makes it unfeasible (see Learning point: Common contraindications to the arterial switch, p. 185). The main technical difficulty with this operation is the transfer of the coronary arteries from the aortic to the neo-aortic root. Mastery of this skill has allowed the ASO to become widespread. In simplistic terms, after cannulation and commencement of cardiopulmonary bypass, the aorta and main pulmonary artery are transected above the level of the sinotubular junction. The coronary arteries are then detached from the aortic root, along with rims of the aortic wall (coronary artery 'buttons'), which are then mobilized. These buttons are then attached to the pulmonary artery root (the 'neo-aortic root'). The main pulmonary artery is then brought anterior to the aorta (the Lecompte manoeuvre) and anastomosed to the aortic root, with repair of the sites of coronary artery button removal. The aorta is then anastomosed to the pulmonary root [8].

Muscular LVOTO is a well-recognized association of TGA and may preclude the arterial switch. It is usually also associated with a VSD, and the combination of TGA, VSD, and LVOTO is seen in around 4% of TGA cases [11]. In some cases, LVOTO can be surgically addressed in the same operation, thus allowing the arterial switch. However, in the majority of cases, alternative strategies are required, albeit with increased long-term morbidity and a higher rate of re-intervention. Again, as in our case, some patients with severe cyanosis may require a systemic–pulmonary artery shunt to secure adequate pulmonary blood flow prior to receiving definitive repair [1]. Learning point: Surgery for TGA with LVOTO and VSD p. 185–186 outlines the main surgical options used today.

Learning point Surgery for TGA with LVOTO and VSD

- **The Rastelli procedure** consists of using a patch to baffle the left ventricle through the VSD to the aorta. The proximal main pulmonary artery is then ligated and divided, and the right ventricle is attached to it via a conduit [12].
- **The *réparation à l'étage ventriculaire* (REV procedure)** is similar to the Rastelli procedure and also involves baffling of the left ventricle through the VSD to the aorta using a patch. It, however, avoids the use of a conduit by bringing the pulmonary arteries anteriorly (the Lecompte manoeuvre) and then anastomosing the main pulmonary artery directly to the right ventricle [13].

- **The Nikaidoh procedure** involves complete resection of the aortic root, usually with the coronary arteries still attached. The LVOTO is relieved by removal of the outlet septum and pulmonary valve annulus. The aortic root is then translocated posteriorly, sitting as much as possible over the LVOT. The VSD is closed, and the pulmonary artery is anastomosed directly to the right ventricle with the Lecompte manoeuvre [14].

The long-term outcome in patients following an ASO is excellent. One recent study of over 600 patients estimated the overall mortality to be 2.8%, with late mortality (occurring >30 days post-operatively) of only 0.9% and no deaths occurring after 5 years [15]. In addition, all survivors had excellent functional status. A separate long-term follow-up study of 1200 patients following arterial switch found a 15-year survival of 88%. Freedom from reoperation (most commonly performed due to pulmonary stenosis) was 82% at 15 years [16].

However, other studies focusing on more subtle neurodevelopmental outcomes have found significant impairment in academic achievement, memory, attention, and other aspects in adolescents, following the ASO in infancy [17]. Indeed children with TGA are recognized to have a smaller head circumference, a smaller brain volume, and also delayed brain maturation. There are also some studies showing that hypertension may occur more commonly due to the distorted shape of the aorta with more acute angulation, following the posterior translocation of the ascending aorta.

In contrast to the arterial switch, the operations described for TGA with LVOTO have a worse long-term outcome. For example, one study has estimated a 20-year survival rate of only 59% following the Rastelli procedure [18]. This may be related to the position of the right ventricle-to-pulmonary artery conduit directly behind the sternum, predisposing it to compression, and 'stealing' of some of the right ventricular volume by the intracardiac baffle from the left ventricle to the anterior aorta. Since the REV and Nikaidoh procedures are more recently developed operations, there are less data on their long-term outcome. One recent study showed only one early death and no late mortality out of 32 patients following the Nikaidoh procedure, but the median follow-up was for only 20.8 months [19]. The REV procedure may have a lower need for reoperation, according to a report of 205 patients undergoing this method of repair between 1980 and 2003. In this series, the overall survival and freedom from any reoperation at 25 years were 85% and 45%, respectively [20].

A final word from the expert

The timing of surgery in TGA varies widely, depending on the preference of individual surgical centres. An important concept is that of 'deconditioning' of the left ventricle after a prolonged period of pumping to the low-resistance pulmonary vasculature. For this reason, patients presenting late may need placement of a pulmonary artery band to train the left ventricle prior to the ASO. There are conflicting opinions regarding the timing of ASO when TGA is diagnosed before or soon after birth. Some centres prefer to delay the ASO for 1–2 weeks, allowing the baby to feed and the PVR to drop prior to cardiopulmonary bypass [21]. Others have argued that outcomes are better when the ASO is performed within 3 days [22].

Some centres will repair TGA VSD in the first couple of weeks of life, citing reduced mortality and morbidity with this approach. Our approach has been to repair these patients at 2–3 months of life, as long as the increased pulmonary blood flow is tolerated.

In cases of TGA with VSD and LVOTO, the timing of surgery is variable and depends, to a large degree, on the exact anatomy of each individual patient. In many cases, surgery can be delayed by several months, as the LVOTO will prevent deconditioning of the left ventricle, as will the VSD if it is of a significant size. Some patients, however, may require early intervention to augment pulmonary blood flow (e.g. with a modified Blalock–Taussig shunt) if the LVOTO is severe and the baby is extremely cyanosed.

References

1. Morell V, Lopez-Magallon A, Welchering N, et al. Complex transposition of the great arteries. In: da Cruz EM, editor. *Pediatric and Congenital Cardiology, Cardiac Surgery and Intensive Care*. London: Springer-Verlag, 2014; pp. 1965–81.
2. Anderson RH, Weinberg PM. The clinical anatomy of transposition. *Cardiol Young* 2005;15 Suppl 1:76–87.
3. Pasquini L, Sanders SP, Parness IA, et al. Coronary echocardiography in 406 patients with d-loop transposition of the great arteries. *J Am Coll Cardiol* 1994;24:763–8.
4. Hoffman JI., Kaplan S. The incidence of congenital heart disease. *J Am Coll Cardiol* 2002;39:1890–900.
5. Lurie IW, Kappetein AP, Loffredo CA, et al. Non-cardiac malformations in individuals with outflow tract defects of the heart: the Baltimore-Washington Infant Study (1981–1989). *Am J Med Genet* 1995;59:76–84.
6. Bonnet D, Coltri A, Butera G, et al. Detection of transposition of the great arteries in fetuses reduces neonatal morbidity and mortality. *Circulation* 1999;99:916–18.
7. Calderon J, Angeard N, Moutier S, et al. Impact of prenatal diagnosis on neurocognitive outcomes in children with transposition of the great arteries. *J Pediatr* 2012;161:94–8.e1.
8. Villafañe J, Lantin-Hermoso MR, Bhatt AB, et al. D-transposition of the great arteries: the current era of the arterial switch operation. *J Am Coll Cardiol* 2014;64:498–511.
9. Bull C, Yates R, Sarkar D, et al. Scientific, ethical, and logistical considerations in introducing a new operation: a retrospective cohort study from paediatric cardiac surgery. *BMJ* 2000;320:1168–73.
10. Hörer J, Karl E, Theodoratou G, et al. Incidence and results of reoperations following the Senning operation: 27 years of follow-up in 314 patients at a single center. *Eur J Cardiothorac Surg* 2008;33:1061–7; discussion 1067–8.
11. Williams W, McCrindle BW, Ashburn DA, et al. Outcomes of 829 neonates with complete transposition of the great arteries 12–17 years after repair. *Eur J Cardio-Thoracic Surg* 2003;24:1–10.
12. Rastelli GC, McGoon DC, Wallace RB. Anatomic correction of transposition of the great arteries with ventricular septal defect and subpulmonary stenosis. *J Thorac Cardiovasc Surg* 1969;58:545–52.
13. Lecompte Y, Neveux JY, Leca F, et al. Reconstruction of the pulmonary outflow tract without prosthetic conduit. *J Thorac Cardiovasc Surg* 1982;84:727–33.
14. Nikaidoh H. Aortic translocation and biventricular outflow tract reconstruction. A new surgical repair for transposition of the great arteries associated with ventricular septal defect and pulmonary stenosis. *J Thorac Cardiovasc Surg* 1984;88:365–72.
15. Fricke TA, d'Udekem Y, Richardson M, et al. Outcomes of the arterial switch operation for transposition of the great arteries: 25 years of experience. *Ann Thorac Surg* 2012;94:139–45.
16. Losay J, Touchot A, Serraf A, et al. Late outcome after arterial switch operation for transposition of the great arteries. *Circulation* 2001;104:121–6.
17. Bellinger DC, Wypij D, Rivkin MJ, et al. Adolescents with d-transposition of the great arteries corrected with the arterial switch procedure: neuropsychological assessment and structural brain imaging. *Circulation* 2011;124:1361–9.

18. Dearani JA, Danielson GK, Puga FJ, et al. Late results of the Rastelli operation for transposition of the great arteries. *Semin Thorac Cardiovasc Surg Pediatr Card Surg Annu* 2001;4:3–15.
19. Raju V, Myers PO, Quinonez LG, et al. Aortic root translocation (Nikaidoh procedure): intermediate follow-up and impact of conduit type. *J Thorac Cardiovasc Surg* 2015;149:1349–55.
20. Di Carlo D, Tomasco B, Cohen L, et al. Long-term results of the REV (réparation à l'étage ventriculaire) operation. *J Thorac Cardiovasc Surg* 2011;142:336–43.
21. Duncan BW, Poirier NC, Mee RB, et al. Selective timing for the arterial switch operation. *Ann Thorac Surg* 2004;77:1691–6.
22. Anderson BR, Ciarleglio AJ, Hayes DA, et al. Earlier arterial switch operation improves outcomes and reduces costs for neonates with transposition of the great arteries. *J Am Coll Cardiol* 2014;63:481–7.

CASE

14 Long QT syndrome: beyond making a diagnosis

Gabrielle Norrish

Expert commentary Juan Pablo Kaski

Case history

Following the diagnosis of long QT syndrome (LQTS) in her younger sibling, a 12-year-old girl was referred to the inherited cardiovascular disease services for cardiology assessment. The patient was clinically asymptomatic, with no history of palpitations, chest pain, syncope, or pre-syncope, and was very active. On clinical examination, she had an unremarkable cardiovascular examination, with no abnormalities detected. Her resting electrocardiogram (ECG) showed sinus rhythm with a QRS axis of +70° and a corrected QT interval of 450 ms, with abnormal T wave morphology throughout (Figure 14.1a). A transthoracic echocardiogram showed a structurally and functionally normal heart. The family were counselled that, at this time, her investigations were not diagnostic for LQTS, but suspicious in the context of her family history.

The patient was reviewed again 4 weeks later and remained clinically very well and asymptomatic from a cardiac perspective. Her screening investigations were repeated; however, her resting ECG on this occasion was clearly abnormal with a corrected QT interval of 550 ms and widespread T wave morphology abnormalities (Figure 14.1b). A treadmill test was undertaken at this time. Characteristically, at peak exercise, the QTc was further prolonged and notching of her T waves was seen (Figure 14.1c). Based upon the ECG abnormalities and family history, a diagnosis of LQTS was made.

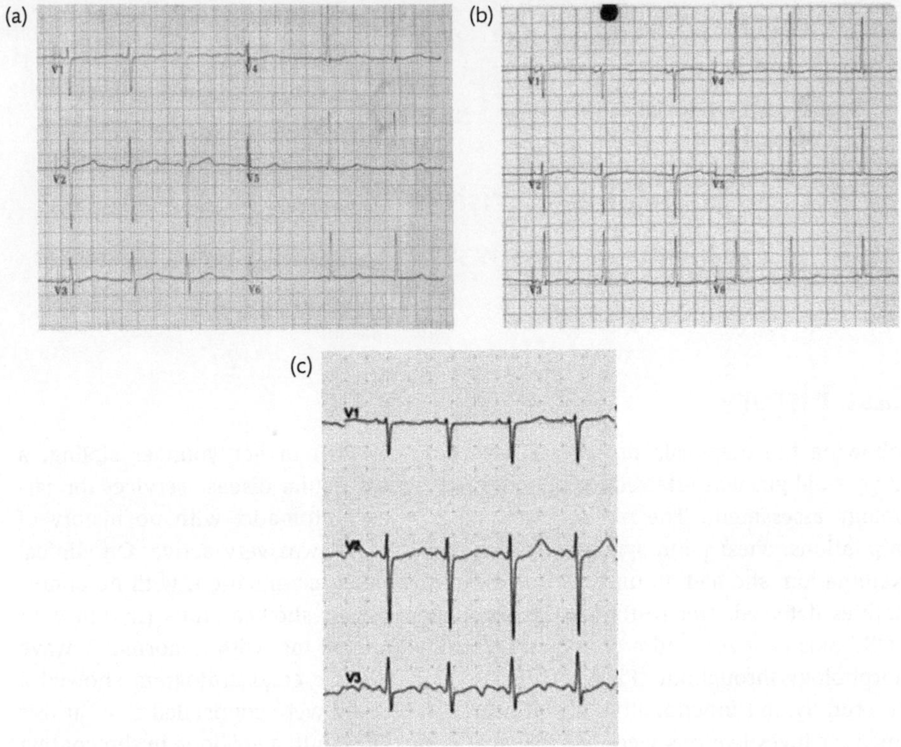

Figure 14.1 (a) Resting ECG at presentation—corrected QT interval 450 ms, flat and broad T waves. (b) Resting ECG 4 weeks later—corrected QT interval 550 ms, flat and broad T waves. (c) ECG 4 minutes into recovery of exercise test—QTc 543 ms, T waves notched.

Clinical tip ECG findings in LQTS

Patients with LQTS often have abnormalities on a resting ECG.

QT prolongation

The QT interval should be corrected for heart rate, and the longest calculated value taken. This is most commonly done using the Bazett's formula [1] in leads II, V4, or V5. However, it is worth noting that this formula is less accurate at higher heart rates (above 100 bpm) and that other formulae, such as Fridericia's, can be used. Further guidance relating to measuring the QT interval in specific circumstances can be found in recent reviews [2].

$$QTc = \frac{QT}{\sqrt{RR}}$$

Different normative values have been proposed for QTc in childhood. It is generally accepted that normal values for QTc are <450 ms for boys and <460 ms for girls.

T wave morphology

Patients with LQTS may have a wide range of abnormal T wave morphology. Different characteristic repolarization patterns have been described in the three major LQTS genotypes (Figure 14.2) [3]:

- Late-onset peaked/biphasic
- Bifid T waves
- Broad-based T waves.

Expert comment

It is important to realise than ECG abnormalities may be dynamic and transient as the QT interval and repolarisation are affected by a number of variables including serum electrolyte concentrations, parasympathetic and sympathetic drive and underlying myocardial disease. A 'normal' resting ECG therefore does not exclude a diagnosis of LQTS.

Learning point How do you diagnose LQTS?

When patients present with syncope and are found to have marked QTc prolongation, the diagnosis of LQTS is quite straightforward. However, in asymptomatic patients or those in whom the resting QTc is within normal limits/borderline, the diagnosis is more challenging. For such circumstances, a clinical scoring system (Schwartz criteria see Table 14.1) has been proposed which accounts for clinical characteristics other than the QTc interval such as abnormal T wave morphology (Figure 14.2) [4]. However, more recently, it has been shown that whilst this criterion has a high specificity for identifying mutation carriers, it has a low sensitivity [5].

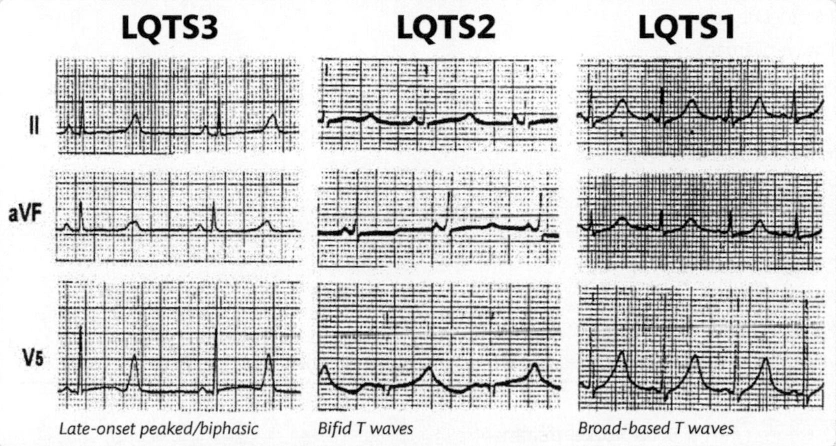

Figure 14.2 Characteristic T wave morphology according to LQTS genotype.
Reproduced from Moss, A., Zareba, W., Benhorin, J., et al, ECG T-Wave Patterns in Genetically Distinct Forms of the Hereditary Long QT Syndrome, *Circulation*. 1995;92:2929–2934, (1995) with permission from Wolters Kluwer.

The most recent European Society of Cardiology guidelines [6] recommends that:

1. LQTS diagnosis is made:
   a. In the presence of an LQTS risk score of >3.5 in the absence of a secondary cause for prolongation **and/or**
   b. In the presence of an unequivocally pathogenic mutation in the QTS genes **or**
   c. In the presence of a corrected QT interval for heart rate using Bazett's formula (QTc) ≥500ms in repeated 12-lead ECGs and in the absence of a secondary cause for QT prolongation
2. LQTS can be diagnosed in the presence of QTc interval of between 480 and 499 ms in repeated 12-lead ECGs in a patient with unexplained syncope in the absence of a secondary cause for QT prolongation and in the absence of a pathogenic mutation.

Following the diagnosis of LQTS, the patient was counselled to avoid medications that cause secondary prolongation of QTc and was started on a low-dose beta-blocker (bisoprolol).

After starting treatment with a beta-blocker, the patient was seen regularly for clinical review. Exercise tests and 24-hour tapes were performed at regular intervals to assess the adequacy of beta-blockade and to detect subclinical ventricular arrhythmias. At times, the patient complained of side effects of the beta-blocker, which included feeling tired and lethargic.

Clinical tip Avoiding secondary QTc prolongation

As part of patient counselling, patients should be advised to avoid medications known to cause QTc prolongation (https://www.crediblemeds.org).

Expert comment How do you assess the adequacy of beta-blockade?

No specific guidelines exist as to how to assess the adequacy of beta-blockade.

However, in clinical practice, clinicians monitor the resting heart rate on 24-hour ECG Holter, targeting a relative bradycardia and also the peak heart rate during exercise testing. This is interpreted in light of the patient's age and balanced against the side effects of both sinus bradycardia and beta-blockers themselves.

Table 14.1 Diagnosing LQTS

Finding	Score
Electrocardiographic	
Corrected QT interval (ms):	
≥480	3
460–470	2
450 (in males)	1
QTc fourth minute of recovery from exercise stress test ≥480 ms	1
Torsades de pointes	2
T wave alternans	1
Notched T waves in three leads	1
Low heart rate for age	0.5
Clinical history	
Syncope:	
With stress	2
Without stress	1
Congenital deafness	0.5
Family history	
Family members with definite LQTS	1
Unexplained sudden cardiac death in immediate family members aged <30 years	0.5

Learning point Beta-blocker treatment

Patients with LQTS are at risk for sudden cardiac death secondary to ventricular arrhythmias, with a 13% incidence of cardiac arrest or sudden cardiac death in untreated patients before the age of 40 years (Figure 14.3) [7].

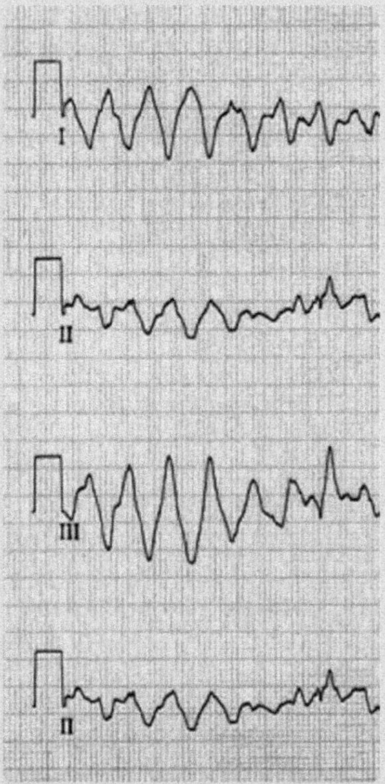

Figure 14.3 Cardiac monitor showing torsades de pointes (polymorphic ventricular tachycardia).

Beta-blockers have been shown to reduce the risk for an adverse arrhythmic event in LQTS [8]. The specific mechanisms by which beta-blockers reduce mortality remain unclear. A recent study reported a heart rate-dependent effect of beta-blockade on QT and QTc intervals in LQT1 patients, with shortening of these intervals at higher heart rates, thus providing a potential mechanism of risk reduction for this group of patients [9].

In clinical practice today, there are an increasing number of patients diagnosed with LQTS through genetic screening who are genotype-positive but phenotype-negative (i.e. positive for a pathogenic mutation, but clinically asymptomatic with normal resting ECG). However, despite being asymptomatic, this group of patients are at an increased risk for adverse cardiac events, compared to unaffected family members, and may therefore benefit from beta-blocker therapy [10].

Prospective studies comparing the efficacy of different beta-blockers in patients with LQTS have not been performed, and we therefore rely on information obtained from observational retrospective studies. Previous studies have shown that both non-selective (e.g. propranolol) and β1-selective beta-blockers (e.g. nadolol and metoprolol) are equally effective at preventing adverse cardiac events [11, 12]. However, a more recent retrospective registry reported an increased efficacy of cardio-selective beta-blockers (metoprolol), compared to propranolol, in symptomatic patients [13, 14]. Prospective studies are required to further elucidate the role of different beta-blockers in the management of LQTS patients.

Current guidelines [6] report:

1. Beta-blockers **are recommended** in patients with a diagnosis of LQTS who are:
   a. Asymptomatic with QTc ≥470 ms and/or
   b. Symptomatic with syncope or documented ventricular tachycardia/ventricular fibrillation (VT/VF)
2. Beta blockers **can be useful** in patients with a diagnosis of LQTS who are asymptomatic with QTc ≤470 ms.

Following the diagnosis of LQTS in the two sisters, clinical cascade screening for other family members was recommended. During family screening, the patient's mother was also found to have an abnormal ECG, diagnostic for LQTS with QTc prolongation and similar abnormal T wave morphology. Genotype testing in the mother identified a pathogenic mutation associated with LQTS type 1 (*KCNQ1*), which was subsequently confirmed to be present in both her daughters. The identification of a pathogenic mutation allowed for further genetic cascade screening in the extended family.

Learning point Genetics of LQTS

LQTS is an inherited ion channelopathy which predisposes individuals to torsades de pointes and sudden arrhythmic death. It is usually inherited in an autosomal dominant fashion. However, it exhibits incomplete penetrance and variable expression among affected family members. Currently, 75% of patients with a diagnosis of LQTS possess a known pathogenic mutation. Of these, approximately 20–25% have a normal corrected QT interval [7, 10]. Yet these patients remain at an increased risk for ventricular arrhythmias [10].

There are currently 16 different types of LQTS recognized, although types 1, 2, and 3 account for over 90% of genotyped cases. Gene-specific differences in phenotype are now well recognized. Schwartz et al. compared triggers for arrhythmic events in LQTS patients and found that, whilst exercise was a common trigger for arrhythmia in LQTS1, auditory stimuli, such as an alarm clock, were more prevalent in LQTS2 and arrhythmias during sleep were a feature of LQTS3 (Table 14.2) [13].

Genotype analysis is now an important part of the management of LQTS patients and is performed routinely. For patients in whom a pathogenic mutation is identified, genetic screening of first-degree relatives is recommended to identify asymptomatic carriers [6]. For patients in whom no known causative mutation is identified, first-degree relatives should be clinically screened at regular intervals with a resting ECG. Research has shown that families are more likely to accept screening if the proband is genotype-positive. However, the yield of family screening is the same for both genotype-positive and negative patients [15].

Table 14.2 Genetics of LQTS

LQTS variant	Chromosome locus	Gene	Affected current	Arrythmia trigger
LQTS1	11p15.5	*KCNQ1*	↓ I_{Ks} (slowly activated delayed rectifier potassium current)	Exercise (particularly swimming)
LQTS2	7q35-36	*KCNH2*	↓ I_{Kr} (rapidly activated delayed rectifier potassium current)	Emotional stress or auditory stimuli
LQTS3	3p21-24	*SCN5A*	↑ I_{Na} (cardiac voltage-gated sodium channel gene)	During sleep

Four years after her initial diagnosis, our patient complained of recurrent episodes of painful palpitations which were associated with pre-syncopal feelings of dizziness, although she had not fainted or collapsed with any of these episodes. She had presented to accident and emergency on several of these occasions when a resting ECG showed no arrhythmia or change from her baseline abnormalities. As these episodes were occurring frequently, a further 24-hour ECG Holter was fitted, which surprisingly captured an episode of non-sustained monomorphic ventricular tachycardia occurring whilst she was asleep.

Learning point Risk stratification for sudden cardiac death in LQTS

Untreated LQTS patients have a 13% incidence of cardiac arrest or sudden cardiac death before the age of 40 years [7]. However, the risk is not equal for all patients and identifying those patients at highest risk can be challenging.

Priori et al. [7] reported genotype-specific differences in the natural history of untreated LQTS, with LQTS 1 patients having significantly higher cardiac event-free survival, compared to those with LQTS2 or 3 (Figure 14.4). A progressive increase in the corrected QT interval was an independent predictor of an adverse cardiac event in the entire LQTS population (QTc >500 ms accepted as high risk), whereas gender was not significantly associated. However, on subgroup analysis, important genotype differences were demonstrated. For example, although gender was not a predictor of adverse risk in the whole cohort, male LQTS3 patients were found to be at a significantly higher risk, compared to their female counterparts, whilst female LQTS2 patients were at a significantly higher risk, compared to male LQTS2 patients; the reason for this gender variability is not currently known. In addition, whilst an increased QTc duration was predictive of the risk in LQTS1 and 2 patients, it was not associated with risk in LQTS3 patients where gender appears to be more important for risk stratification (Figure 14.5). Age at first presentation has also been shown to be important with patients presenting before the age of 7 years with syncope or aborted cardiac arrest (ACA) being at high risk for further events.

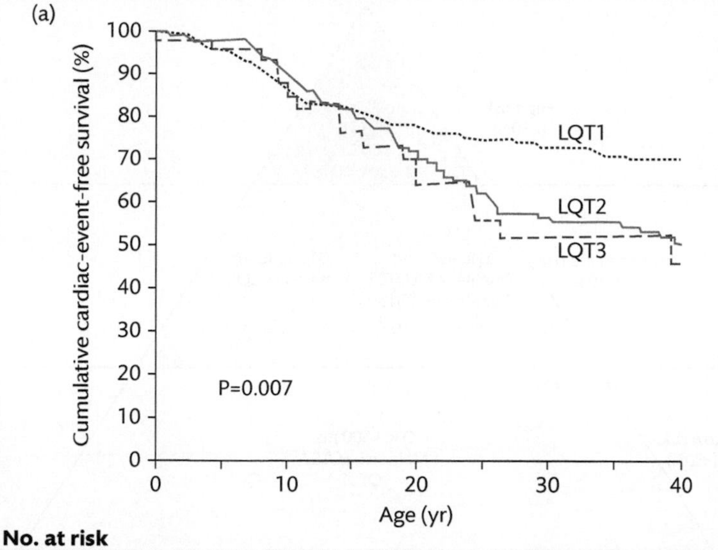

No. at risk

LQT1	355	249	192	146	100
LQT2	176	130	187	57	34
LQT3	49	30	20	9	7

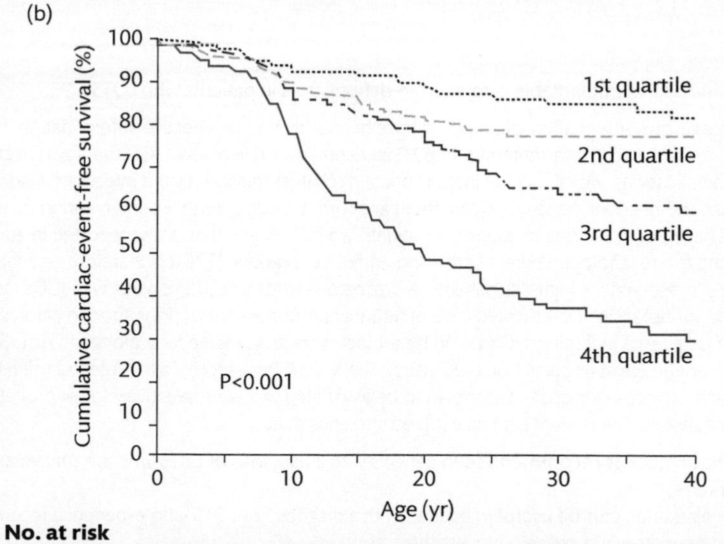

No. at risk

1st quartile	148	112	96	76	45
2nd quartile	150	104	80	62	45
3rd quartile	140	103	78	49	33
4th quartile	142	92	45	28	18

Figure 14.4 Kaplan–Meier estimates of cumulative survival free of cardiac events in long QT syndrome patients according to: (a) genetic locus of mutation; (b) quartile of corrected QT interval.

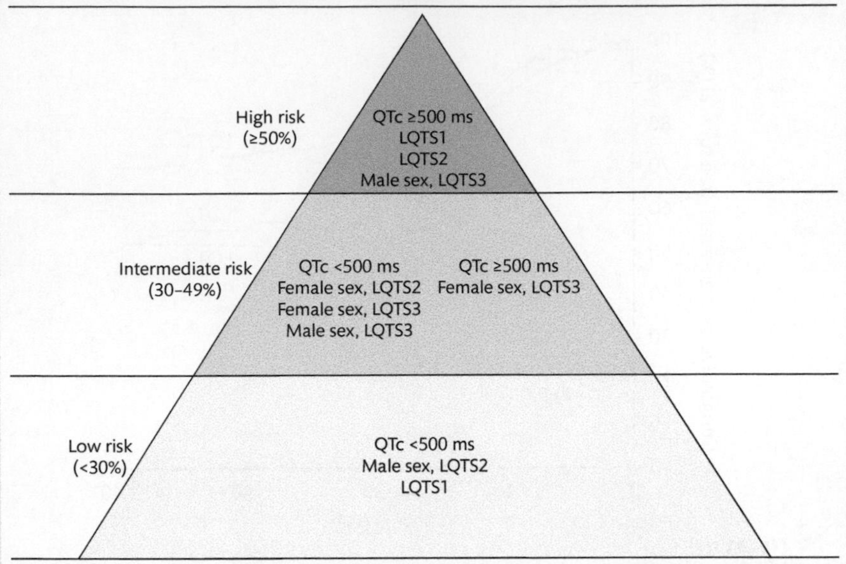

Figure 14.5 Proposed scheme for risk stratification of patients with LQTS according to genotype and sex.

Reproduced from Priori S, Schwartz P, Napolitano C, et al, Risk stratification in the Long-QT syndrome, *N Engl J Med* 2003;348:1866–74. Copyright © 2003 Massachusetts Medical Society.

Learning point Implantable cardioverter-defibrillators in patients with LQTS

Implantable cardioverter-defibrillators (ICDs) have been shown to be effective at terminating potentially lethal ventricular arrhythmias in LQTS patients [16, 17]. However, ICD therapy is not without complications, which include inappropriate discharges, device-related infections, lead fracture, and the need for device replacement in line with somatic growth. Re-intervention rates of up to 48% have been reported in paediatric patients, which is higher than those reported in adult patients, and the psychological effect of this should not be forgotten [17]. It is therefore essential that this therapy is reserved for high-risk patients. A prospective study of LQTS patients with ICDs identified four clinical variables significantly predictive of future appropriate shocks: prior aborted cardiac arrest; cardiac events, including syncope on beta-blocker therapy; markedly prolonged QTc (>500 ms); and younger age at implantation (<20 years). The M-FACT risk score was developed using these variables and an increasing score was shown to be associated with a progressively lower probability of appropriate shocks. The current guidance [6] recommends that:

1. ICD implantation **is recommended** in patients with a diagnosis of LQTS who are survivors of a cardiac arrest
2. ICD implantation **can be useful** in patients with a diagnosis of LQTS who experience recurrent syncopal events whilst on beta-blocker therapy
3. ICD implantation **is not indicated** in asymptomatic LQTS patients who have not been tried on beta-blocker therapy (except under exceptional circumstances).

An urgent clinic review was subsequently arranged, during which primary prevention in the form of an ICD was recommended to the family. Following psychological preparation, the family accepted this recommendation and a transvenous ICD was implanted shortly after.

Learning point Beyond beta-blockers

Although beta-blockers are effective at reducing the risk for ventricular arrhythmias, there are subsets of patients in whom they are contraindicated (e.g. brittle asthmatics) or not tolerated.

The role of the left stellate ganglion and the sympathetic nervous system in triggering ventricular arrhythmias was first reported in 1966 by Yanowitz et al. [18]. This led to interest in the therapeutic effect of modifying sympathetic innervation by left cardiac sympathetic denervation (LCSD), which could be particularly useful for LQTS where arrhythmic events are closely linked to situations with high sympathetic activity such as exercise or emotional stress. Schwartz et al. [19] reported a significant reduction in mean yearly cardiac events (syncope, ACA) following LCSD in high-risk patients, which was associated with a shortening of the calculated QT interval. Although ICD implantation is now recommended in high-risk individuals, there is a theoretical concern that an appropriate ICD shock with a secondary sympathetic surge could trigger an electrical storm. LCSD itself does not treat any ventricular arrhythmias but does reduce the likelihood of them occurring.

Current guidance [6] recommends:

1. LCSD **is recommended** in high-risk patients with a diagnosis of LQTS in whom:
   a. ICD therapy is contraindicated or refused and/or
   b. Beta-blockers are either not effective in preventing syncope/arrhythmias, not tolerated, not accepted, or contraindicated
2. LCSD **can be useful** in patients with a diagnosis of LQTS who experience breakthrough events whilst on therapy with beta-blockers/ICD.

Expert comment

ICD therapy is not without complications, which include inappropriate discharges, device-related infections, lead fracture, and the need for device replacement in line with somatic growth. Re-intervention rates of up to 48% have been reported in paediatric patients, which is higher than that reported in adult patients and the psychological effect of this should not be forgotten [17]. It is therefore essential that this therapy is reserved for high-risk patients.

A final word from the expert Future directions: should we screen for LQTS?

In common with other inherited conditions which affect young people, there is an interest in the feasibility of population-based screening for the condition. This is an area of controversy among experts in the field. Screening for inherited channelopathy could be performed in different situations, including in those with a family history of sudden cardiac death, athletes who could theoretically be at higher risk for exercise-induced arrhythmias, or the general population.

Sudden arrhythmic death (SAD) is defined as a sudden unexpected cardiac death that remains unexplained, occurring with a rate of approximately 1.38 per 100,000 population in the United Kingdom. Despite no recognizable cause identified in the proband, evidence supports the clinical screening of first-degree paediatric relatives of SAD victims. Kaski et al. reported a positive diagnosis of an inherited channelopathy [20] [Brugada syndrome, LQTS, catecholaminergic polymorphic ventricular tachycardia (CPVT)] in 13.5% of first-degree paediatric relatives screened. Similar results have been reported in other series [21]. This likely reflects the variable penetrance and expression of autosomal dominant channelopathy mutations among members of the same family. Screening in this situation is now recommended [6].

A more difficult question is whether all young people should be screened and, if so, when the most ideal time is. There is disagreement among experts as to whether neonatal screening is feasible and cost-effective [22, 23]. To avoid the large physiological variation of QTc in the first week of life, it has been recommended that this would need to take place at 3–4 weeks of life prior to the age at which sudden infant death syndrome (SIDS) is often seen (2–6 months). Whilst recent cost-effective analyses [24] have shown this approach to be cost-effective, others have raised concerns regarding the sensitivity of an ECG and the possibility of inappropriate treatment of young infants [23].

References

1. Bazett HC. An analysis of the time-relations of electrocardiograms. *Heart* 1920;7:353–70.
2. Rautaharju PM, Surawicz B, Gettes LS, et al.; American Heart Association Electrocardiography and Arrhythmias Committee, Council on Clinical Cardiology;

American College of Cardiology Foundation; Heart Rhythm Society. AHA/ACCF/HRS Recommendations for the Standardization and Interpretation of the Electrocardiogram. Part IV: The ST Segment, T and U Waves, and the QT Interval: A Scientific Statement From the American Heart Association Electrocardiography and Arrhythmias Committee, Council on Clinical Cardiology; the American College of Cardiology Foundation; and the Heart Rhythm Society: Endorsed by the International Society for Computerized Electrocardiology. *J Am Coll Cardiol* 2009;53:982–91.

3. Moss AJ, Zareba W, Benhorin J, et al. ECG T wave patterns in genetically distinct forms of the hereditary long QT syndrome. *Circulation* 1995;92:2929–34.
4. Schwartz PJ, Moss AJ, Vincent GM, Crampton RS. Diagnostic criteria for the long QT syndrome: an update. *Circulation* 1993;88:782–4.
5. Hofman N, Wilde AA, Kääb S, et al. Diagnostic criteria for congenital long QT syndrome in the era of molecular genetics: do we need a scoring system? *Eur Heart J* 2007;28:575–80.
6. Priori SG, Wilde AA, Horie M, et al. Executive summary: HRS/EHRA/APHRS expert consensus statement on the diagnosis and management of patients with inherited primary arrhythmia syndromes. *Europace* 2013;15:1389–406.
7. Priori S, Schwartz P, Napolitano C, et al. Risk stratification in the long-QT syndrome. *N Engl J Med* 2003;348:1866–74.
8. Oss A, Zareba W, Hall J, et al. Effectiveness and limitations of beta-blocker therapy in congenital long QT syndrome. *Circulation* 2000;101:616–23.
9. Bennett M, Gula L, Klein G, et al. Effect of beta-clockers on QT dynamics in the long QT syndrome: measuring the benefit. *Europace* 2014;16:1847–51.
10. Goldenberg I, Horr S, Moss AJ, et al. Risk for life-threatening cardiac events in patients with genotype-confirmed long-QT syndrome and normal-range corrected QT intervals. *J Am Coll Cardiol* 2011;57:51–9.
11. Chockalingam P, Crotti L, Giardengo G, et al. Not all beta-blockers are equal in the management of long QT syndrome types 1 and 2: higher recurrence of events under metoprolol. *J Am Coll Cardiol* 2012;60:2092–9.
12. Wilde A, Ackerman M. Beta-blockers in the treatment of congenital Long QT syndrome—is one beta-blocker superior to another? *J Am Coll Cardiol* 2014;64:1359–61.
13. Schwartz PJ, Priori SG, Spazzolini C, et al. Genotype–phenotype correlation in the long QT syndrome: gene-specific triggers for life-threatening arrhythmias. *Circulation* 2001;103:89–95.
14. Abu-Zeitone A, Peterson DR, Polonsky B, McNitt S, Moss AJ. Efficacy of different beta-blockers in the treatment of long QT syndrome. *J Am Coll Cardiol* 2014;64:1352–8.
15. Hanninen M, Klein G, Laksman Z, et al. Reduced uptake of family screening in genotype-negative versus genotype-positive long QTS syndrome. *J Genet Couns* 2015;24:558–64.
16. Schwartz PJ, Spazzolini C, Priori SG, et al. Who are the long QT syndrome patients who receive an implantable cardioverter–defibrillator and what happens to them? Data from the European Long QT Syndrome implantable Cardioverter–Defibrillator (LQTS ICD) Registry. *Circulation* 2010;122:1272–82.
17. Etheridge SP, Sanatani S, Cohen MI, Albaro CA, Saarel EV, Bradley DJ. Long QT syndrome in children in the era of implantable defibrillators. *J Am Coll Cardiol* 2007;50:1335–440.
18. Yanowitz J, Preston J, Abildskov J. Functional distribution of right and left stellate innervation to the ventricles. Production of neurogenic electrocardiographic changes by unilateral alteration of sympathetic tone. *Circ Res* 1966;18:416–28.
19. Nordkamp O, Driessen A, Odero A, Koolbergen D, Schwartz P, Wilde A. Left cardiac sympathetic denervation in the Netherlands for the treatment of inherited arrhythmia syndromes. *Neth Heart J* 2014;22:160–6.
20. Giudici V, Spanaki A, Hendry J, et al. Sudden arrhythmic death syndrome: diagnostic yield of comprehensive clinical evaluation of pediatric first-degree relatives. *Pacing Clin Electrophysiol* 2014;37:1681–5.

21. Wong L, Roses-Noguer F, Till J, Behr E. Cardiac evaluation of pediatric relatives in sudden arrythmic death syndrome. A 2 center experience. *Circ Arrhythm Electrophysiol* 2014;7:800–6.
22. Saul J, Schwartz P, Ackerman M, Triedman J. Rationale nd objectives for ECG screening in infancy. *Heart Rhythm* 2014;11:2316–21.
23. Van Hare G, Perry J, Berul C, Triedman J. Cost effectiveness of neonatal ECG screening for the long QT syndrome: letter to the editor. *Eur Heart J* 2007;28:137–41.
24. Quaglini S, Rognoni C, Spazzolini C, Priori SG, Mannarino S, Schwartz PJ. Cost effectiveness of neonatal ECG screening for the long QT syndrome. *Eur Heart J* 2006;27:1824–32.

CASE

15 Fetal management of hypoplastic left heart syndrome

Michael Harris

Expert commentary Gurleen Sharland

Case history

A 25-year-old primiparous woman was referred to a tertiary fetal cardiology service at 21 weeks' gestation, following her routine anomaly scan. The local unit was concerned that there were abnormal views of the fetal heart suggestive of congenital heart disease. Her early trimester screening showed a normal nuchal translucency measurement and her adjusted risk for aneuploidy was low.

There was no significant family history of congenital heart disease, and the woman herself was medically fit, taking no medications, apart from the usual pregnancy vitamins. Detailed fetal echocardiography confirmed normal atrial arrangement, with a hypoplastic, echogenic, globular, and poorly functioning left ventricle. The mitral valve was patent, with a small amount of forward flow and a minor degree of mitral regurgitation. There was no forward flow across the aortic valve, and the ascending aorta was severely hypoplastic. There was evidence of retrograde flow from the duct into the aorta. There was a small left-to-right shunt across the atrial septum. The pulmonary veins appeared dilated. A diagnosis of hypoplastic left heart syndrome (HLHS) was made (Figures 15.1 and 15.2). A fetal cardiologist and a clinical nurse specialist counselled the couple, before an appointment was made for them to see a fetal medicine specialist for a detailed fetal assessment.

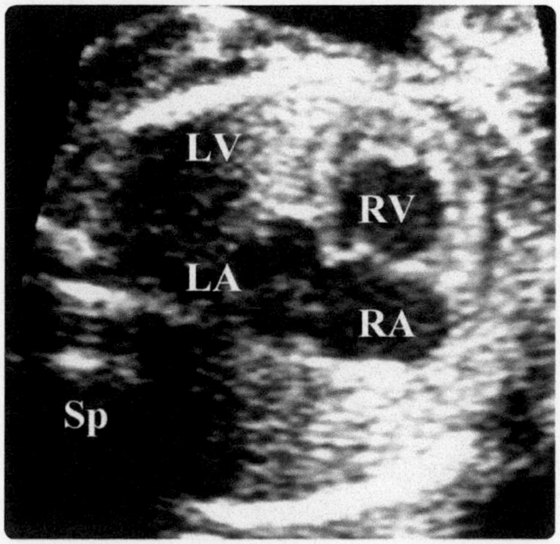

Figure 15.1 Four-chamber wiew showing slit-like left ventricle in fetal hypoplastic left heart syndrome. LA, left atrium; LV, left ventricle; RA, right atrium; RV, right ventricle; Sp, spine.

Expert comment

The significance of noting the nuchal translucency measurement is that an increased value, particularly when above the 99th centile (3.5 mm), is associated with major heart defects, including left heart obstructive lesions such as hypoplastic left heart syndrome.

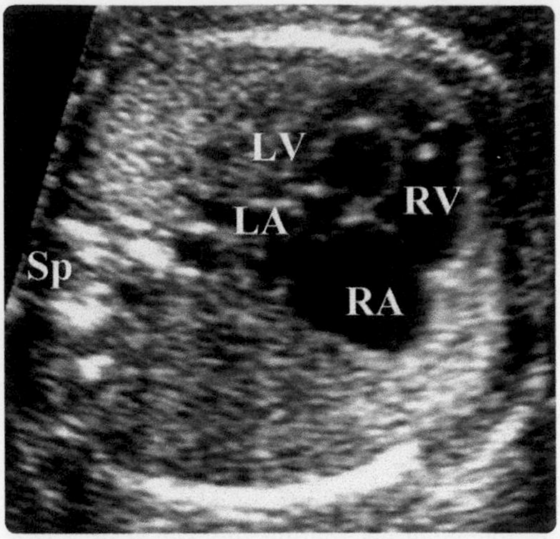

Figure 15.2 Four-chamber view showing globular, echogenic left ventricle in fetal hypoplastic left heart syndrome. LA, left atrium; LV, left ventricle; RA, right atrium; RV, right ventricle; Sp, spine.

Learning point What is hypoplastic left heart syndrome?

Hypoplastic left heart syndrome consists of aortic and mitral valve hypoplasia or atresia, with a small left ventricle and varying degrees of aortic arch obstruction. The aortic valve is usually atretic. The mitral valve may be atretic or patent. The ascending aorta and aortic arch are usually severely hypoplastic. In cases with a patent mitral valve, there may be mitral regurgitation. The hypoplastic left ventricle can be: (1) slit-like and almost impossible to discern; or (2) larger and more globular, in which case it is poorly contractile and echogenic.

In true HLHS, the left atrium is also small. In comparison to the normal situation in fetal life where the umbilical venous return is directed from right to left across the atrial septum, in HLHS, there is a left-to-right shunt at the atrial level, except in cases of an intact atrial septum. In the rare cases where the atrial septum is intact or restrictive to flow, then the pulmonary veins are often dilated, unless there is a decompressing vein from the left atrium. Pulmonary venous Doppler studies may be helpful in assessing the degree of restriction. Some series report up to 67% risk of mortality after birth and surgery in fetuses with an intact or restrictive atrial septum, placing them in a much higher-risk category [1].

Expert comment

Less commonly, the severe end of the spectrum of cases with coarctation of the aorta or critical aortic stenosis with severe left heart hypoplasia may fall into the spectrum of HLHS.

Expert comment

A left-to-right shunt at the atrial level in the fetus is a marker of severe left heart obstruction.

Learning point How is HLHS detected in fetal life?

HLHS is readily detectable during obstetric anomaly scans. One study from Australia showed that nearly 85% of cases of HLHS were detected antenatally [2]. In Wales, between 2002 and 2008, 50 of 55 cases of HLHS were antenatally detected [3]. Antenatal detection rates for congenital heart disease per se have increased in the United Kingdom over the last decade, but specific data for HLHS are difficult to come by. HLHS is one of the lesions that can be readily detected in the standard fetal cardiac views in any fetal screening programme.

Expert comment

There are different forms of HLHS, and the echocardiographic appearances will vary, depending on the anatomical variant. In cases with aortic atresia and a patent mitral valve, the left ventricle will appear echogenic and globular, as well as being hypoplastic and poorly functioning. The echogenicity correlates with endocardial fibroelastosis and is a feature of cases where there is inflow into the chamber but no outflow. In cases with mitral and aortic atresia, the left ventricle is slit-like and barely discernible.

Learning point What about the right ventricle and tricuspid valve?

The right ventricle is usually normal in structure, although it may be mildly dilated. Function is usually preserved, although not always. An assessment of the tricuspid valve is important. The presence of moderate or worse degrees of tricuspid regurgitation is a worrying feature, as the tricuspid valve becomes the systemic valve in postnatal life in single-ventricle palliation. Significant tricuspid regurgitation impacts on the efficacy of the single-ventricle Fontan circulation. Severe tricuspid regurgitation detected in the fetal period is usually a bad prognostic indicator, and parents should be counselled accordingly.

The fetal cardiologist was careful to fully explain the diagnosis to the couple and proceeded to give them more information about what to expect, should they continue with the pregnancy. The various postnatal treatment options were explained to them.

Clinical tip How does the baby with HLHS present after birth and how is it managed?

Whilst HLHS is a serious and severe form of congenital heart disease, *in utero*, the fetuses are normally stable. Following delivery, however, the systemic circulation is dependent on ductal flow, with blood pumped by the right ventricle, whilst the left ventricle is incapable of supporting the systemic circulation. In cases where the duct closes or is allowed to close after delivery, the baby deteriorates acutely and will not survive without medical and surgical intervention. Clearly, if the diagnosis has been made antenatally, then such babies can have intravenous prostaglandin initiated electively after birth to maintain ductal patency. In cases where the diagnosis becomes apparent postnatally, such babies often present with collapse acutely in the first 48–72 hours after birth and require resuscitation. The category of fetuses with an intact or restrictive atrial septum, in addition, may have the serious additional problem of acute left atrial hypertension with concomitant pulmonary venous obstruction. This is a very precarious state, with profound hypoxaemia and poor cardiac output. Unless emergent atrial septoplasty is undertaken, the baby will die.

Learning point What treatment options are available for HLHS?

Treatment of this condition requires initial stabilization of the circulation after birth prior to a palliative procedure. There are several surgical options available for this, including the classical Norwood operation in which the native aorta is anastomosed to the pulmonary artery to form the neo-aorta. This usually requires a homograft patch for augmentation. Pulmonary blood flow is via an arterio-pulmonary shunt. The Norwood operation with the Sano modification has become more utilized in the last 15 or so years. In this procedure, in addition to the creation of the neo-aorta, a conduit is placed directly between the right ventricle and the left or right pulmonary artery, rather than using an arterio-pulmonary shunt [4]. The hybrid procedure is used in some centres particularly for high-risk patients and has been used in some countries outside the UK as a bridge to transplantation. In the UK, the hybrid procedure is used for those neonates thought to be at risk due to low birthweight, prematurity, and other extracardiac factors. In addition, those with an intact or restrictive interatrial septum would fall into this group, as would those with poor ventricular function or severe aortic atresia or isthmus obstruction [5]. In this procedure, ductal patency is assured via the percutaneous placement of a stent, although some centres maintain ductal patency with long-term prostaglandin infusion. Furthermore, the application of bilateral pulmonary artery bands helps to limit pulmonary blood flow and balance the systemic and pulmonary circulations. The final step is ensuring patency of the atrial septum and this is usually achieved via a balloon atrial septostomy. Which of these options are chosen depends upon the surgical centre and the patient risk factors. Survival is variable [6].

Expert comment

Counselling following prenatal diagnosis of HLHS includes a detailed explanation of the problem with the aid of diagrams and discussion of the treatment strategies, the risk for associated lesions, and all the management options, including termination of pregnancy. Written information should be provided, as well as contact details for parent support groups. The parents should also be given the opportunity to meet with a paediatric cardiac surgeon.

As is common in such situations, the couple were keen to know whether there was anything that they had done that had caused the heart problem. They asked whether or not there were other problems with the baby, apart from the heart.

Expert comment

HLHS is one of the most common lesions seen in fetal series as it is associated with an abnormal four-chamber view and is easily detectable during obstetric screening.

Learning point How common is hypoplastic left heart syndrome?

This lesion accounts for <0.1% of live births but is a relatively common form of congenital heart disease, accounting for 8% of all congenital heart defects [7]. This equates to about 200 diagnoses per year in the UK and Ireland. Recurrence rates for congenital heart disease in another pregnancy are in the order of 2–5%.

It is more common in males than females but, if untreated, is responsible for 25–40% of all neonatal cardiac deaths [8]. Outcomes for HLHS remain challenging. Rates of survival following initial palliation for HLHS are variable, with some quoting rates of 90%, although figures of 73–80% [9] are more commonly cited. In those with higher-risk anatomical substrates, the mortality rate can by approximately 50%, with rates improving from 43% survival to 53% survival for those with HLHS and an intact or restrictive septum [10]. Survival through all palliation stages up to Fontan is in the order of 60–65% [11], although recently published Australian and New Zealand data for Fontan after HLHS suggests 10-year freedom from Fontan failure of 79% where Fontan failure is defined as death, heart transplant, Fontan conversion or takedown, protein-losing enteropathy, plastic bronchitis, or New York Heart Association functional class III or IV [12].

Termination rates are quite variable, and in the UK, this seems to depend, to a degree, on the geographical region. The reasons for this are not clear and are likely multi-factorial, resulting from cultural, educational, and religious considerations. One study from a large tertiary centre in the West Midlands showed their termination rate to be around 25%, which had fallen from 43.7% over a 5-year period [13], whereas others in London have had rates of 45% in more recent years [11]. The reason for the drop in termination rates is not completely clear but may be to do with improved outcomes for Norwood surgery, compared to the previous era.

Expert comment

Reported termination rates for HLHS vary considerably between regions and between countries. However, in the last two decades, there has been a very notable fall in termination rates for this condition.

Learning point Associations with HLHS

HLHS is not generally associated with chromosomal abnormalities. Of course, cases have been described with trisomies 13 and 18, Turner's syndrome (XO), and other genetic translocations or deletions, but these are not the rule. In a large series from a single tertiary fetal cardiology centre, only 4% of cases of HLHS had associated chromosomal anomalies [11]. Additionally, a small percentage (4% in the same series) will have associated extracardiac anomalies.

Expert comment

Cases of HLHS with aortic atresia and a patent mitral valve are very rarely associated with either chromosomal or other extracardiac abnormalities. However, those who have associated mitral atresia are at an increased risk for associated abnormalities, though this risk is <5% for chromosomal abnormalities.

The couple had further questions regarding their options during the pregnancy and what they might expect after the delivery should they continue with the pregnancy.

Learning point The role of fetal cardiology in HLHS

Fetal cardiology has an important and growing role in this condition. Firstly, HLHS is one of the more commonly detected cardiac conditions in antenatal life. The detection of this cardiac lesion is an end in itself, but as it can occasionally be a marker of extracardiac anomalies, this facilitates a fuller prenatal examination of the fetus and opportunities for invasive karyotyping. Clearly, important discussions about prognosis can be had and all options for continuing or interrupting the pregnancy can be put to the prospective parents.

A key contribution is to allow appropriate preparation to optimize postnatal outcome. Fetal diagnosis provides an opportunity for planning of delivery and ensuring that appropriate measures are taken to stabilize the baby in the immediate neonatal period. There is evidence that babies with HLHS born following antenatal diagnosis are in a better condition preoperatively in terms of need for intubation, key acid–base markers, and renal function [14]. The effect on mortality is less certain but may be more to do with the fact that neonatal HLHS surgery is some of the riskiest surgeries performed, and there are multiple peri- and intraoperative factors that contribute to the relatively high mortality of this procedure [14–16].

Expert comment

It is important to remember, when comparing outcomes of those babies with a prenatal diagnosis to those in whom the diagnosis was made after birth, that those with a postnatal diagnosis will only take into account those babies that have reached the cardiac centre for diagnosis and treatment. Those with prenatal diagnosis include babies that may have had an intrauterine death or have died in the early neonatal period without treatment, as well as high-risk groups such as those with a restricted atrial septum who may not have survived long enough to reach the cardiac centre if a prenatal diagnosis has not been made.

Clinical tip The interatrial septum in HLHS

The interatrial septum is one of the key determinants of risk and mortality in HLHS. Assessing the interatrial septum in fetal life can be difficult. The foramen ovale is often sited in an unusual position, being high and more posterior [17]. The smallness of the left atrium can make assessing the actual size of the aperture and obtaining trans-septal flow velocity Dopplers difficult. Moreover, these features do not necessarily correlate well with postnatal anatomy and haemodynamics [18]. However, pulmonary venous Doppler traces are much more readily and reliably obtainable and there is good evidence that these can be used to assess left atrial hypertension and foramen ovale flow restriction. This may help to indicate the need for possible emergent atrial septoplasty [17, 19]. The septum is patent in most cases of HLHS, but in up to 22%, it is restrictive and intact in 6% [18].

Restriction at the atrial septum is thought to contribute to left atrial hypertension. Pulmonary venous flow in the fetus accounts for up to 25% of cardiac output as pregnancy progresses [18] and increases further after delivery. In the context of a stenotic or atretic left atrioventricular valve and a restrictive foramen that limits left-to-right flow, the pulmonary venous return has restricted flow pathways. This is thought to contribute to pulmonary venous disease with arterialization of the pulmonary veins. Pulmonary arterial hypertension results, and in both the short and long term, this leads to a poor outcome for the child. In the short term after delivery, there is an acute rise in the pulmonary venous pressure, with pulmonary venous congestion and pulmonary oedema. Such babies are profoundly hypoxaemic and acidotic and require emergent surgical atrial septectomy or balloon septoplasty or stent placement. In the long term, lung vascular changes as a result of pulmonary venous hypertension have important implications for survival and morbidity in the Fontan circulation.

Learning point Prenatal assessment of atrial septal restriction and the need for emergent atrial septoplasty

The normal pulmonary venous waveform consists of S, D, and A waves. The S wave corresponds to forward flow in systole through the lungs into the pulmonary venous system and into the left atrium and as mitral valve opens. The D wave consists of forward flow in diastole and corresponds with the E wave of passive mitral inflow that occurs in early diastole. The A wave corresponds to atrial contraction, and active forward flow from the left atrium into the left ventricle. The A wave in the pulmonary venous Doppler indicates the nadir of pulmonary venous flow [17] and is identified as reduced or absent forward flow (Figure 15.3). Occasionally, there is even some brief retrograde flow.

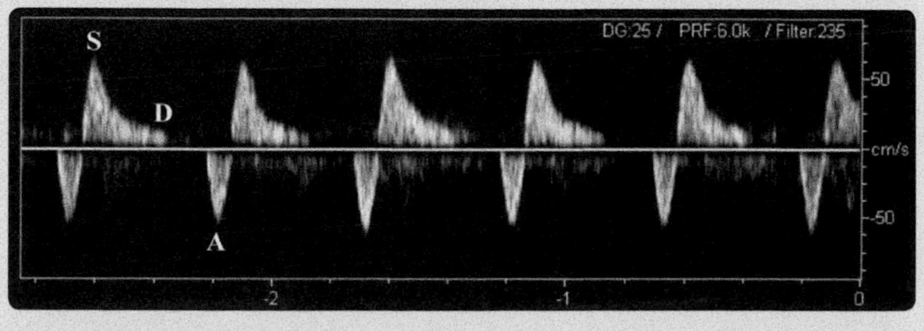

Figure 15.3 Pulmonary venous Doppler trace in restrictive interatrial septum. A, A wave; D, D wave; S, S wave.

Many fetal cardiologists use varying S, D, and A parameters as a marker of atrial restriction. The absolute value of the S wave has been shown to be raised in HLHS, but even more so in those with a restrictive or intact atrial septum [17, 19]. In those with a mean gestational age of 25.6 weeks, the normal S wave velocity was 21.4 cm/s versus 27.7 cm/s in HLHS with an unrestrictive septum and 33.7 cm/s in HLHS with a restrictive septum [17]. The difference in S wave velocity between those with a restrictive or those with an open foramen ovale is not as marked as the difference between those with a normal heart and those with HLHS. The D wave velocity shows a reduction, which is logical, considering that this normally corresponds to the passive filling of the atrium in diastole due to flow across the open mitral valve. In cases of mitral atresia or hypoplasia, this is clearly not possible, with the blood instead flowing across the open foramen ovale. Others have looked at the A wave velocity (which is reversed) and noted that this velocity increases, up to 35 cm/s, in those subsequently requiring emergent atrial septostomy [19]. However, none of these absolute values in and of themselves are absolutely predictive of foramen restriction. Consequently, some groups have looked at other parameters, including A wave duration, A wave velocity time integral (VTI), the S wave-to-D wave ratio, forward and reverse flow VTIs, and the ratio of the former to the latter and the A-wave/D-wave ratio. They have concluded that a forward/reverse flow VTI ratio of <3 is the strongest predictor of the need for emergent atrial septostomy in the neonatal period (Table 15.1) [19].

Table 15.1 Pulmonary venous Doppler parameters associated with a need for emergent balloon atrial septostomy [19]

A wave duration	>77 ms
S/D velocity ratio	>2.5
A/D velocity ratio	>1.35
A wave VTI	>1.4 cm
Forward/reverse VTI ratio	<5

Source data from Michelfelder, E. et al., 2005. Predictive Value of Fetal Pulmonary Venous Flow Patterns in Identifying the Need for Atrial Septoplasty in the Newborn With Hypoplastic Left Ventricle. *Circulation*, Volume 112, pp. 2974–2979.

Expert comment

In practice, cases with Doppler traces at the extremes are easy to identify, but there remains a grey area in the middle ground with overlap between cases with a restrictive atrial septum that will run into difficulty after birth and those that will not.

Predicting atrial septal restriction is not an exact science and is more a question of probabilities. Some of the reasons for this may include the fact that little is known about the structure and characteristics of the left atrium itself, particularly left atrial compliance. Furthermore, it is possible that the right ventricle, which is poorly understood in HLHS, has some bearing on flow at the level of the atrial septum.

Clinical tip What is the value of being able to predict possible atrial septal restriction?

The value of being able to predict atrial restriction in fetal life is twofold. Firstly, it is crucial in being able to counsel appropriately prospective parents that their baby presents an especially high risk in terms of mortality. This may alter what they choose to do with the pregnancy. Secondly, it allows planning of delivery, which, in these circumstances, may require emergent procedures to ensure patency of the atrial septum. This may be via emergency balloon septoplasty, stent placement, or surgical atrial septectomy.

Learning point An emerging role for fetal MRI in risk stratification in HLHS?

Pulmonary lymphangiectasia is a rarely occurring condition. It is characterized by the dilatation of the pulmonary lymphatic vessels. It can occur either as a primary pulmonary problem, secondary to pulmonary venous obstruction due to pulmonary venous or cardiac anatomical abnormalities, or can be part of a generalized lymphatic problem [20]. HLHS with an intact or restrictive septum clearly is an anatomical substrate for pulmonary venous obstruction and consequent pulmonary lymphangiectasia. Victoria and Andronikou [21] coined the term 'nutmeg lung' on the basis of findings on fetal magnetic resonance imaging (MRI) scans of eight patients, only one of whom had HLHS. The appearances are similar to those seen on computed tomography (CT) of a congested liver and consist of fluid-filled tubular channels that extend from the hila to the surface of the lungs. Subsequently, the same group from Philadelphia identified 44 MRI scans in fetuses with HLHS [22]. Four of these were found to have 'nutmeg lung'. Three of these had restrictive lesions on echocardiography and subsequently died. The fourth died at 5 months of age, secondary to refractory respiratory distress. Of the 40 without 'nutmeg lung', five had restrictive lesions on echocardiography. Three of these died. Mortality in the remaining 35 was 35%. This indicates firstly that not all of those with HLHS develop 'nutmeg lung', which is self-evident. Secondly, not all of those with restrictive lesions develop 'nutmeg lung'. However, in those with restrictive lesions and 'nutmeg lung', mortality is 100%, compared to those without nutmeg lung or restriction (Table 15.2). Consequently, this finding may be of great benefit as a prognostic indicator and counselling tool, not just in cases of suspected atrial restriction, but also in HLHS more generally.

Table 15.2 'Nutmeg' lung, restrictive atrial septum, and mortality [22]

Total HLHS + MRI (n = 44)	Restrictive lesions on echo	Mortality (%)
Nutmeg lung, 4	3	100
No nutmeg lung, 40	5	60
	No restrictive lesion, 35	35

Source data from Saul, D. et al., 2016. Hypoplastic left heart syndrome and nutmeg lung pattern *in utero*: a cause and effect relationship or prognostic indicator?. *Pediatr Radiol*, Volume 46, pp. 483–489.

Expert comment

Studies have described pulmonary abnormalities, including 'arterialization' of the pulmonary veins and lymphatic dilatation, in cases of HLHS associated with a restricted or an intact atrial septum. This has been attributed to left atrial hypertension. In this setting, it can be very helpful to use fetal MRI to look for evidence of lung lymphangiectasia.

Learning point Fetal intervention in atrial septal restriction

The restrictive or intact atrial septum is a tempting therapeutic target to try to reduce the mortality risk for this group of fetuses with HLHS. The advantages would be not only to alter the unfavourable haemodynamics of such a situation, but also to alter the pulmonary vascular abnormalities that are seen in association with chronic pulmonary venous hypertension. The former is crucial for the initial stabilization and preoperative status of the baby, whilst the latter also has important ramifications for the single-ventricle Fontan circulation in which having a low-resistance pulmonary circuit is so crucial for success.

Kalish and co-workers [23] from Boston described their initial experience of actual or attempted in utero atrial stent placement in nine fetuses with HLHS and an intact atrial septum. Previous work on balloon septostomy [24–26] with either static balloon dilatation or use of cutting balloons has shown the lack of efficacy of reliably generating a patent atrial septum in this condition. Hence, the rationale for stenting of the atrial septum was firstly that it had been shown to be technically possible, and secondly, and most importantly, that it may provide a means of producing a persistent atrial septal defect.

Of the nine fetuses, five had successful placement of an atrial septal stent, with four of these showing flow through the stent. In one of these five, whilst the stent was placed in a transseptal position, flow could not be demonstrated through it. The remaining four of the nine fetuses did not have successful atrial septal stent placement, however in three of these four, there was acute decompression of the left atrium due to dilatation of the atrial septum. One of the nine fetuses died *in utero*, and eight survived to delivery, of which four died in the neonatal period. Two of these four had had atrial septal stent placement. Four of the surviving fetuses past the neonatal period; one survived to biventricular repair, and two survived to bidirectional Glenn, one of which died after the operation. There was one fetus which was stable at birth which had no data at the time of publication. There were no maternal complications [23].

Time and further experience after the learning curve will demonstrate whether this is a viable therapeutic option for that group of HLHS patients that are at higher risk of mortality.

A final word from the expert

Studies have shown that fetal intervention for a restrictive or an intact septum is technically possible in the fetus. It is less clear how beneficial this intervention may be in the longer term and further studies are required. It may be that damage to the lungs has already occurred before the intervention takes place, and case selection is therefore paramount.

References

1. Rychik J, Rome JJ, Collins MH, DeCampli WM, Spray TL. The hypoplastic left heart syndrome with intact atrial septum: atrial morphology, pulmonary vascular histopathology and outcome. *J Am Coll Cardiol* 1999;34:554–60.
2. Chew C, Halliday J, Riley M, Penny D. Population-based study of antenatal detection of congenital heart disease by ultrasound examination. *Ultrasound Obstet Gynecol* 2007;29:619–24.
3. Sinha A, Gopalakrishnan P, Tucker D, Uzun O. Outcome after prenatal diagnosis of hypoplastic left heart syndrome (HLHS) in south wales over a 7 year period. *Arch Dis Child Fetal Neonatal Ed* 2011;96:Fa67.
4. Barron DJ, Kilby MD, Davies B, Wright JG, Jones TJ, Brawn WJ. Hypoplastic left heart syndrome. *Lancet* 2009;374:551–64.
5. Honjo O, Caldarone C. Hybrid palliation for neonates with hypoplastic left heart syndrome: current strategies and outcomes. *Korean Circ J* 2010;40:103–11.
6. Chen Q, Parry AJ. The current role of hybrid procedures in the stage 1 palliation of patients with hypoplastic left heart syndrome. *Eur J Cardiothorac Surg* 2009;36:77–83.
7. Andrews R, Cook A, Yates R. Concordance for hypoplastic left heart syndrome in a monochorionic twin pregnancy. *Heart* 2003;89:e13.
8. Shenoy R, Parness I. Hypoplastic left heart syndrome—looking back, looking forward. *J Am Coll Cardiol* 2014;64:2036–8.
9. McGuirk S, Griselli M, Stumper OF, et al. Staged surgical management of hypoplastic left heart syndrome: a single institution 12 year experience. *Heart* 2006;92:364–70.
10. Vlahos A, Lock J, McElhinney D, van der Velde M. Hypoplastic left heart syndrome with intact or highly restrictive atrial septum: outcome after neonatal transcatheter atrial septostomy. *Circulation* 2004;109:2326–30.
11. Sharland G. *Fetal Cardiology Simplified*, first edition. London: tfm Publishing Ltd, 2013.
12. d'Udekem Y, Iyengar AJ, Galati JC, et al. Redefining expectations of long-term survival after the Fontan procedure. Twenty-five years of follow-up from the entire population of Australia and New Zealand. *Circulation* 2014;130(11 Suppl 1):S32–8.
13. Rasiah SV, Ewer AK, Miller P, et al. Antenatal perspective of hypoplastic left heart syndrome: 5 years on. *Arch Dis Child Fetal Neonatal Ed* 2008;93:F192–7.
14. Sivarajan V, Penny DJ, Filan P, Brizard C, Shekerdemian LS. The impact of antenatal diagnosis of hypoplastic left heart syndrome on the clinical presentation and surgical outcomes: the Australian experience. *J Paediatr Child Health* 2009;45:112–17.
15. Peake LK, Draper ES, Budd JL, Field D. Outcomes when congenital heart disease is diagnosed antenatally versus postnatally in the UK: a retrospective population-based study. *BMC Pediatr* 2015;15:58.
16. Andrews R, Tulloh R, Sharland G, et al. Outcome of staged reconstructive surgery for hypoplastic left heart syndrome following antenatal diagnosis. *Arch Dis Child* 2001;85:474–7.
17. Better D, Apfel H, Zidere V, Allan L. Pattern of pulmonary venous blood flow in the hypoplastic left heart syndrome in the fetus. *Heart* 1999;81:646–9.
18. Manning N, Archer N. Fetal pulmonary venous Doppler flow patterns in hypoplastic left heart syndrome. *Heart* 2008;94:1374–5.

19. Michelfelder E, Gomez C, Border W, Gottliebson W, Franklin C. Predictive value of fetal pulmonary venous flow patterns in identifying the need for atrial septoplasty in the newborn with hypoplastic left ventricle. *Circulation* 2005;112:2974–9.
20. Seed M, Bradley T, Bourgeois J, Jaeggi E, Yoo SJ. Antenatal MR imaging of pulmonary lymphangiectasia secondary to hypoplastic left heart syndrome. *Pediatr Radiol* 2009;39:747–9.
21. Victoria T, Andronikou S. The fetal MR appearance of 'nutmeg lung': findings in 8 cases linked to pulmonary lymphangiectasia. *Pediatr Radiol* 2014;44:1237–42.
22. Saul D, Degenhardt K, Iyoob SD, et al. Hypoplastic left heart syndrome and nutmeg lung pattern in utero: a cause and effect relationship or prognostic indicator? *Pediatr Radiol* 2016;46:483–9.
23. Kalish B, Tworetzky W, Benson CB, et al. Technical challenges of atrial septal stent placement in fetuses with hypoplastic left heart syndrome and intact atrial septum. *Catheter Cardiovasc Interv* 2014;84:77–85.
24. Bar-Cohen Y, Perry SB, Keane JF, Lock JE. Use of stents to maintain atrial defects and fontan fenestrations in congenital heart disease. *J Interv Cardiol* 2005;18:111–18.
25. Marshall AC, van der Velde ME, Tworetzky W, et al. Creation of an atrial septal defect *in utero* for fetuses with hypoplastic left heart syndrome and intact or highly restrictive atrial septum. *Circulation* 2004;110:253–8.
26. Marshall AC, Levine J, Morash D, et al. Results of *in utero* atrial septoplasty in fetuses with hypoplastic left heart syndrome. *Prenat Diagn* 2008;28:1023–8.

CASE

16 Near syncope is not always benign

Paraskevi Theocharis

Expert commentary Roberta Bini

Case history

A six-and-a-half-year-old girl presented to the local accident and emergency (A & E) after an episode of a 'racing heart'. She was found lying on the floor by her mother, complaining of chest pain and dizziness, and was noted to be sweaty, pale, and lethargic. Prior to that, she had an episode of vomiting, following her evening meal. On arrival to A & E, she was diagnosed with supraventricular tachycardia (SVT), requiring adenosine to revert her to sinus rhythm.

Examination revealed a clear chest on auscultation, with a respiratory rate of 25 breaths/minute and saturations of 98% on room air. The first heart sound was normal, with an accentuated pulmonary component of the second heart sound and a 2/6 systolic murmur at the left lower sternal border. She had a 3-cm liver that was palpable below the costal margin. She had no oedema, with good-volume peripheral pulses, and the jugular venous pressure was only mildly elevated.

Echocardiography revealed a structurally normal heart with signs of severe pulmonary hypertension (PH), including a dilated, hypertrophied right ventricle with reduced longitudinal and radial systolic function. The right atrium was also dilated, and there was moderate tricuspid regurgitation with a maximum velocity of 5 m/s across it. The main and branch pulmonary arteries were dilated and there was mild pulmonary insufficiency, (See Figure 16.1 and Table 16.1). She was referred to the national centre of PH for assessment.

In retrospect, the mother felt that the patient has had a gradual decline in effort tolerance over the previous 12 months. At the time of presentation, the patient had been crawling up the stairs and was only able to walk for 10 minutes on the flat. The family felt that the symptoms were due to excessive tiredness secondary to increased school activities and her usual indolence and, as such, did not seek medical advice. Clinically, she fulfilled World Health Organization (WHO) functional class IV.

Over the previous year, she had two episodes of loss of consciousness. The first episode was on the way to school when she experienced leg pain and started shivering before collapsing to the floor and losing consciousness for 2 minutes. It was considered as a first episode of 'afebrile seizure'. She had a second episode a few months later under similar circumstances. Otherwise she had an unremarkable past medical history and was on no regular medications. A paediatrician reviewed her, and an electrocardiogram (ECG) and cardiac and neurological examinations were felt to be normal.

Clinical tip

SVT is not uncommon in the paediatric age. It may be the underlying cause of symptoms such as palpitations, fainting spell, chest pain, decreasing exercise tolerance, and congestive heart failure, especially in younger children and infants. When screening for SVT, an echocardiogram should always be performed to rule out structural cardiac anomalies and to assess ventricular function. In this patient, it revealed an unexpected finding of PH, which, in children, is rare [1].

Learning point Echocardiographic assessment of PH

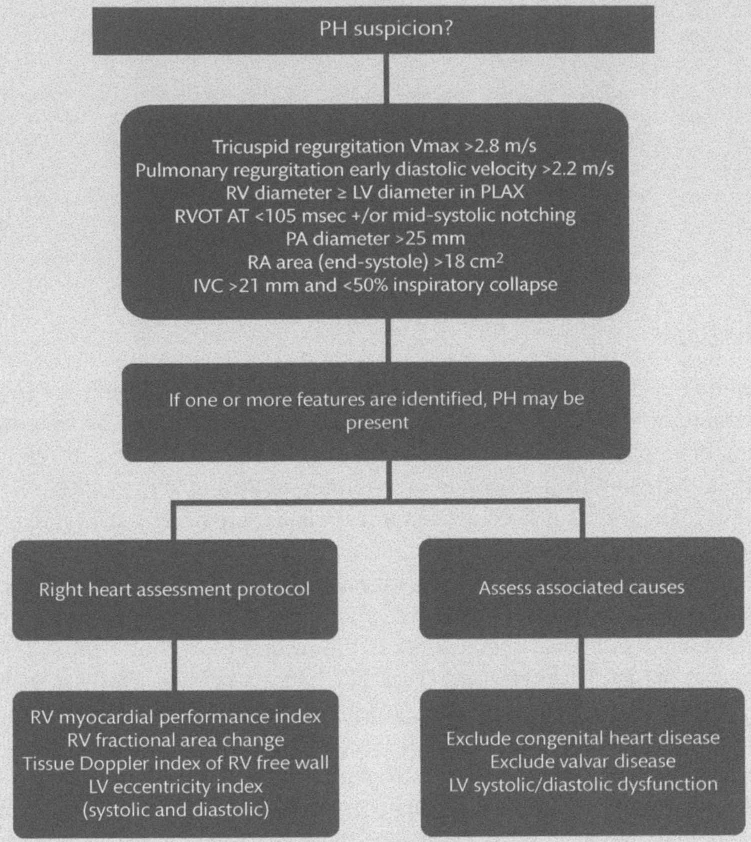

Figure 16.1 Diagnostic algorithm for pulmonary hypertension following echocardiographic assessment in patients with a structurally normal heart.

Table 16.1 Echocardiographic probability of pulmonary hypertension in symptomatic patients with a suspicion of pulmonary hypertension [2]

Peak tricuspid regurgitation velocity (m/s)	Presence of other echocardiographic pulmonary hypertension signs	Echocardiographic probability of pulmonary hypertension
≤2.8	No	Low
≤2.8	Yes	Intermediate
2.9–3.4	No	
2.9–3.4	Yes	High
>3.4	Not required	

Source data from Galie N, Humbert M, Vachiery JL, et al, 2015 ESC/ERS Guidelines for the diagnosis and treatment of pulmonary hypertension: The Joint Task Force for the Diagnosis and Treatment of Pulmonary Hypertension of the European Society of Cardiology (ESC) and the European Respiratory Society (ERS): Endorsed by: Association for European Paediatric and Congenital Cardiology (AEPC), International Society for Heart and Lung Transplantation (ISHLT). *Eur Heart J*, 2015;37(1):67–119.

Clinical tip

At the time of initial diagnosis of PH, the patient should be urgently referred to a specialist centre for evaluation and further management, as there is evidence that early treatment initiation improves long-term outcome. A comprehensive history and physical examination are important, which, combined with diagnostic testing for the assessment of PH pathogenesis/classification and formal assessment of cardiac function, should be performed before the initiation of therapy, including extensive blood tests to exclude autoimmune disease, vasculitis, and prothrombotic conditions (Table 16.2).

Table 16.2 Diagnostic testing and severity assessment in pulmonary hypertension

Diagnostic tests	Associated lesions
Chest X-ray	Large right atrium and ventricle Dilated central pulmonary arteries Variable peripheral lung fields, depending on the amount of pulmonary blood flow (loss of peripheral vascularity) Skeletal abnormalities
Electrocardiogram	Signs of right atrial enlargement Right axis deviation Right ventricular hypertrophy with secondary T wave changes
Computed tomography/ pulmonary angiography	Assess enlargement of pulmonary arteries Central filling defects and webs in pulmonary arteries Presence of parenchymal lung disease
Abdominal ultrasound	Exclude arteriovenous malformation Exclude portal hypertension Exclude portocaval shunt
Lung function tests	20–50% of patients have mild restrictive lung defect and the majority of patients have a reduction in the diffusion capacity
Ventilation/perfusion scan	Ventilation–perfusion mismatch is seen in chronic thromboembolic disease
Cardiopulmonary exercise test	Children with pulmonary hypertension often have significant impairment in aerobic capacity, with a peak oxygen consumption of 20.7 ± 6.9 versus 35.5 ± 7.4 ml/kg/min when compared to healthy controls
Blood tests	ANA, dsDNA, ENA, anti-cardiolipin antibodies LFTs, AST, U&Es, bone profile CRP, pro-BNP, C3, C4, clotting screen ESR, lupus anticoagulant Rheumatoid factor, T3, T4, TSH FBC, IgA/IgM/IgG, NT-pro-BNP

ANA, anti-nuclear antibodies; AST, aspartate aminotransferase; BNP, b-type natriuretic peptide; CRP, C-reactive protein; dsDNA, double-stranded deoxyribonucleic acid; ENA, extractable nuclear antibodies; ESR, erythrocyte sedimentation rate; FBC, full blood count; IgA, immunoglobulin A; IgG, immunoglobulin G; IgM, immunoglobulin M; LFTs, liver function tests; TSH, thyroid-stimulating hormone; U&Es, urea and electrolytes.

Learning point

Idiopathic pulmonary arterial hypertension (IPAH) is a debilitating progressive disease characterized by increased pulmonary vascular resistance (PVR), right ventricular failure, and death. Median survival in untreated children is <1 year. The incidence of IPAH in children is 0.48 per million children per year. Presenting symptoms include dyspnoea (most common presenting feature), syncope (more common in the paediatric population than in adults), and absence of oedema in young children. The majority of patients present in WHO functional classes III and IV (moderate to severe limitation) [3] (Table 16.3).

Clinical tip

Dyspnoea, fatigue and failure to thrive are common PRESENTING symptoms; syncope is more common in children, but overt RV failure is a late event and the child may die of sudden death before the occurrence of RV failure.

Table 16.3 World Health Organization classification of functional status of patients with pulmonary hypertension [4]

Functional class	Description
I	Patients with pulmonary hypertension in whom there is no limitation of usual physical activity; ordinary physical activity does not cause increased dyspnoea, fatigue, chest pain, or pre-syncope
II	Patients with pulmonary hypertension who have mild limitation of physical activity. There is no discomfort at rest, but normal physical activity causes increased dyspnoea, fatigue, chest pain, or pre-syncope
III	Patients with pulmonary hypertension who have a marked limitation of physical activity. There is no discomfort at rest, but less-than-ordinary activity causes increased dyspnoea, fatigue, chest pain, or pre-syncope
IV	Patients with pulmonary hypertension who are unable to perform any physical activity at rest and who may have signs of right ventricular failure. Dyspnoea and/or fatigue may be present at rest and symptoms are increased by almost any physical activity

Reproduced from Barst RJ, McGoon M, Torbicki A, Sitbon O, Krowka MJ, Olschewski H, Gaine S. Diagnosis and differential assessment of pulmonary arterial hypertension. *J Am Coll Cardiol*, 2004;43(12 Suppl S):40S-47S with permission from Elsevier.

Learning point

IPAH is a pulmonary vasculopathy that remains a diagnosis of exclusion, specifically indicating the absence of diseases of the left side of the heart or valves, lung parenchyma, thromboembolism, or other miscellaneous causes.

Pulmonary arterial hypertension (PAH) is defined as mean pulmonary artery pressure (mPAP) ≥25 mmHg with pulmonary arterial wedge pressure (PAWP) <15 mmHg and pulmonary vascular resistance indexed (PVRI) >2 WU.m^2. IPAH or isolated PAH is PAH with no underlying disease that is known to be associated with the condition [5].

A mutation in the bone morphogenetic protein receptor 2 (*BMPR2)* gene can be identified in approximately 10–40% of IPAH cases and in approximately 70% of hereditary pulmonary arterial hypertension (HPAH) cases [6, 7]. Familial cases of PAH have been long recognized and are usually inherited in an autosomal dominant fashion [8]. HPAH accounts for 6% of all cases and shows genetic anticipation, with presentation occurring at a younger age in successive generations [9, 10]. Germline mutations associated with HPAH currently include those detected in the *BMPR2* gene, the activin receptor-like kinase type-1 (*ALK-1*) gene, and the endoglin gene encoding different receptors for bone morphogenetic proteins, which belong to the transforming growth factor-β superfamily and are involved in the control of vascular cell proliferation [2, 6].

Expert comment

The European Society of Cardiology (ESC), the European Respiratory Society (ERS), and the American Heart Association (AHA) have recently published guidelines for the diagnosis and treatment of PH in adult and paediatric populations. IPAH is classified in category 1 with other causative conditions, as listed in Box 16.1 [2, 5]. The rationale for inclusion of all these conditions in one category is the characteristic histology and endothelial cell abnormalities of category 1 PAH diseases are indistinguishable from one another. The plexiform lesion is the epitome of severe disease in all category 1 diseases (Figure 16.2). Lung biopsy is rarely justified in children with PH. The exceptions are when there is suspicion of pulmonary vascular occlusive disease (PVOD) or pulmonary capillary haemangiomatosis (PCH), of alveolar hypoplasia/dysplasia in persistent pulmonary hypertension of the newborn (PPHN), and very rarely in children with complex congenital heart disease in whom it might still be possible to operate (e.g. left ventricular obstructive lesions) [11].

Box 16.1 Condensed clinical classification of pulmonary hypertension (updated from Simonneau et al. [12])

1. Pulmonary arterial hypertension (PAH)
1.1 Idiopathic
1.2 Heritable
  1.2.1 *BMPR2* mutation
  1.2.2 Other mutations
1.3 Drug and toxin induced
1.4 Associated with:
  1.4.1 Connective tissue disease
  1.4.2 HIV infection
  1.4.3 Portal hypertension
  1.4.4 Congenital heart disease
  1.4.5 Schistosomiasis

1′ Pulmonary veno-occlusive disease and/or pulmonary capillary haemangiomatosis

1′′ Persistent pulmonary hypertension of the newborn

2. Pulmonary hypertension due to left heart disease
2.1 Left ventricular systolic dysfunction
2.2 Left ventricular diastolic dysfunction
2.3 Valvar disease
2.4 Congenital/acquired left heart inflow/outflow tract obstruction and congenital cardiomyopathies
2.5 Other

3. Pulmonary hypertension due to lung diseases and/or hypoxia
3.1 Chronic obstructive pulmonary disease
3.2 Interstitial lung disease
3.3 Other pulmonary diseases with mixed restrictive and obstructive pattern
3.4 Sleep-disordered breathing
3.5 Alveolar hypoventilation disorders
3.6 Chronic exposure to high altitude
3.7 Developmental lung diseases

4. Chronic thromboembolic pulmonary hypertension and other pulmonary artery obstructions
4.1 Chronic thromboembolic pulmonary hypertension
4.2 Other pulmonary artery obstructions

5. Pulmonary hypertension with unclear and/or multi-factorial mechanisms
5.1 Haematological disorders
5.2 Systemic disorders
5.3 Metabolic disorders
5.4 Others

Source data from Simonneau G, Gatzoulis MA, Adatia I, Celermajer D, Denton C, Ghofrani A, Gomez Sanchez MA, Krishna Kumar R, Landzberg M, Machado RF, Olschewski H, Robbins IM, Souza R. Updated clinical classification of pulmonary hypertension. *J Am Coll Cardiol*, 2013;62(25 Suppl):D34-41.

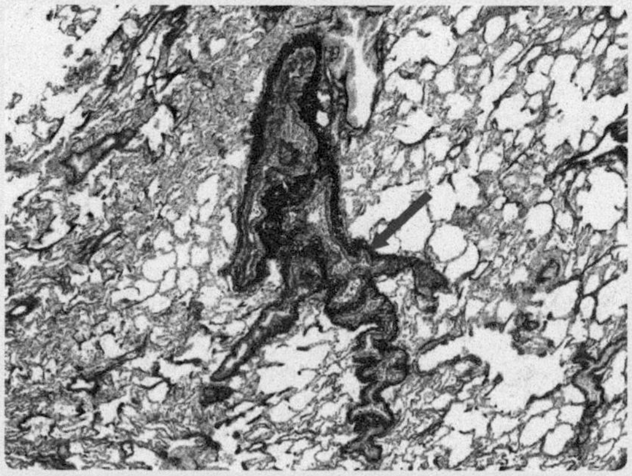

Figure 16.2 Plexiform lesions (arrow) are complex vascular formations originating from the remodelling of small pulmonary arteries and arterioles, with varying degrees of endothelial cell proliferation, muscular hypertrophy, and intimal fibrosis, ultimately leading to an obliteration of precapillary vessels.

On arrival at the national centre for PH, the patient's chest X-ray revealed central pulmonary arterial dilatation, with loss of peripheral blood vessels and signs of right atrial and right ventricular enlargement (Figure 16.3). The ECG showed RV-dominant force with right axis deviation and RV hypertrophy by voltage criteria.

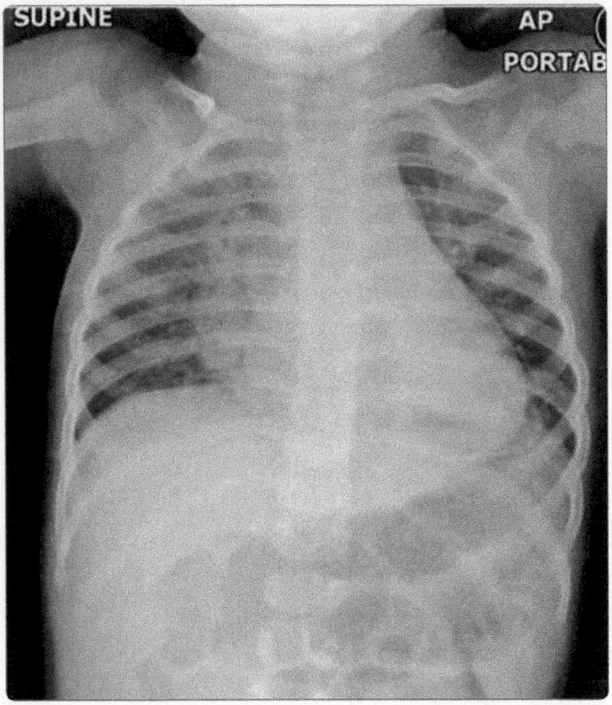

Figure 16.3 Chest X-ray with prominent right atrial and right ventricular enlargement, main pulmonary artery dilatation, and loss of peripheral lung blood vessels.

Clinical tip

RV pressure and volume overload can lead to an abnormal shape and function of the interventricular septum, resulting in septal flattening altering the LV geometry.

Left Ventricular Eccentricity Index in systole or diastole is the ratio of the LV anteroposterior to septolateral diameters measured in the short axis parasternal views at the level of the papillary muscles. [LV-EI(D)>1 suggests RV volume overload whilst LV-EI(S)>1 suggests RV pressure overload].

Left Ventricular Eccentricity index in systole or diastole is the ratio of the LV Anteroposterior to Septolateral diameters measured in the short axis partasternal view at the level of the papillary muscles. [LV- EI(D)]>1 means RV volume overload, [LV- EI(S)]>1 means RV pressure overload [13].

Echocardiography confirmed a normal cardiac anatomy but showed a severely dilated and hypertrophied right ventricle with reduced longitudinal and radial function. The tricuspid regurgitation (TR) jet gave rise to a velocity of 4.4 m/s, and there was moderate pulmonary regurgitation (PR), with an end-diastolic velocity of 2.2 m/s. There was moderate to severe flattening of the interventricular septum. The left ventricular eccentricity index in diastole [LV-EI(D)] was 1.22, and the left ventricular eccentricity index in systole [LV-EI(S)] 1.3, with preserved left ventricular systolic function and no evidence of left heart or valvar disease. The mechanism of adaptation of the right ventricle to high pressure is to increase wall thickness by accumulating muscle mass and to assume a more rounded shape, which pushes the interventricular septum to the left, thus altering the left ventricular geometry (Figures 16.4, 16.5, and 16.6).

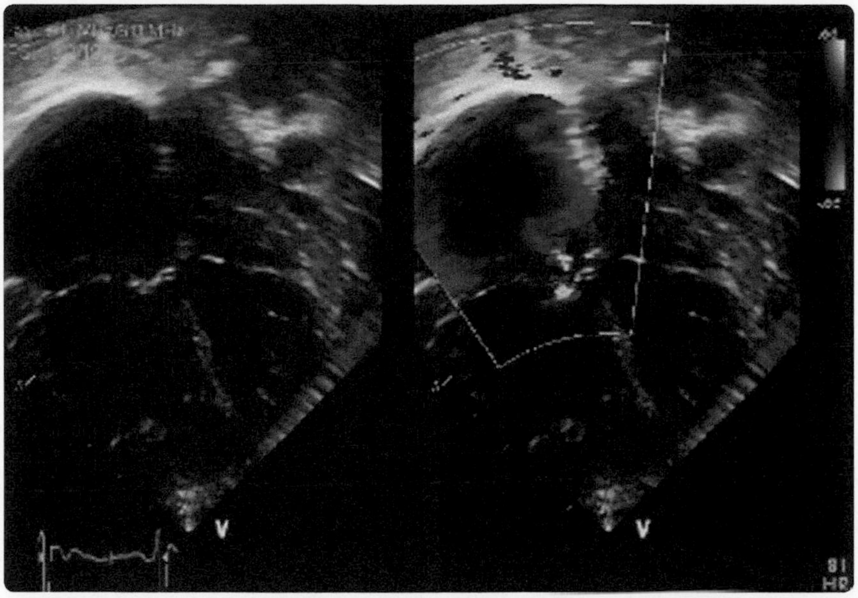

Figure 16.4 Four-chamber view revealing a markedly dilated right atrium and right ventricle with significant right ventricular hypertrophy. There is a broad tricuspid regurgitation jet demonstrated on colour Doppler.

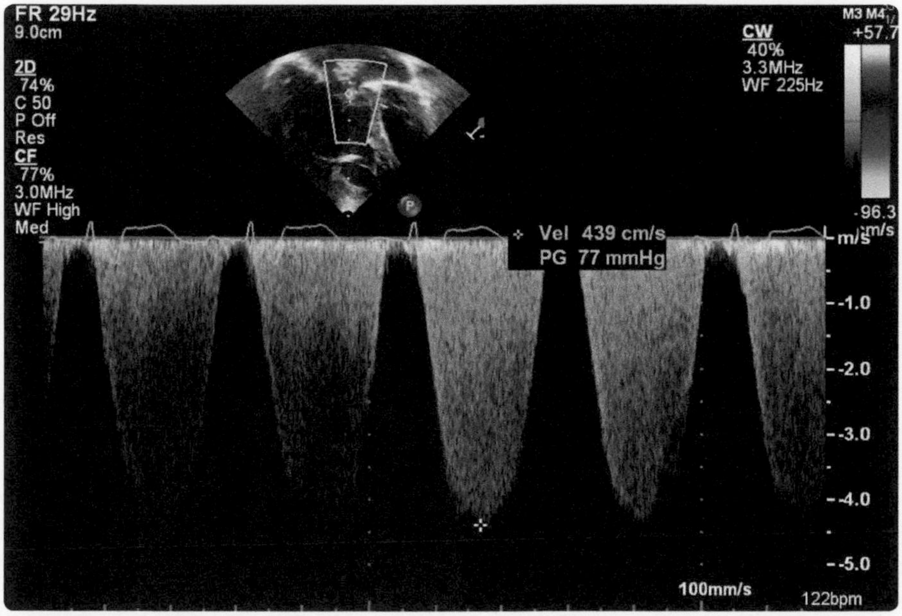

Figure 16.5 Continuous-wave (CW) Doppler indicating a high pressure drop from the right ventricle to the right atrium.

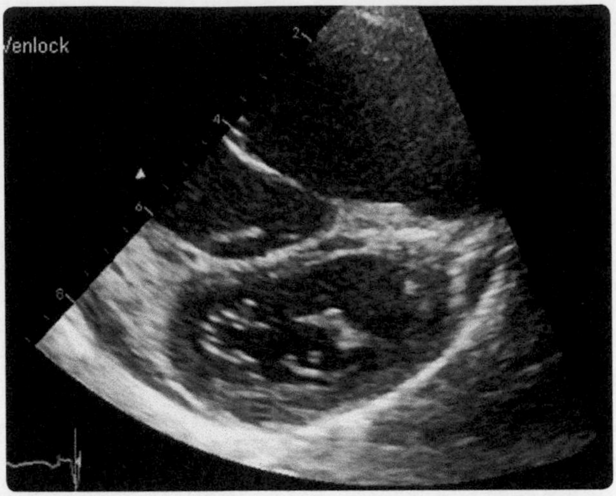

Figure 16.6 Short axis parasternal view with severe septal flattening, reflecting severe pressure loading of the right ventricle.

Computed tomography pulmonary angiography (CTPA) of the chest revealed marked pulmonary arterial dilatation with an abnormal arborization pattern, in keeping with established pulmonary vascular disease and no PVOD changes or thromboembolic disease Figure 16.7.

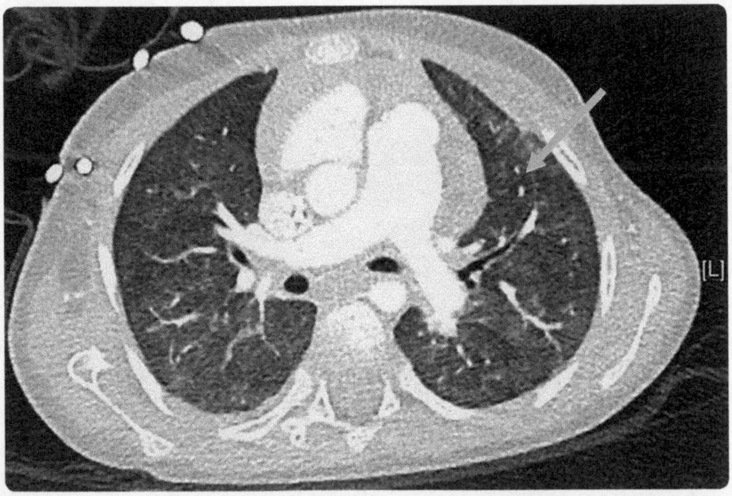

Figure 16.7 Thoracic CT demonstrating significant dilatation of the branch pulmonary arteries, in comparison to the aorta, and irregular arborization in keeping with established pulmonary vascular disease. Plexiform lesions (arrow) with areas of mosaic attenuation and ground-glass appearance are visible within the lung parenchyma.

Abdominal ultrasound showed no signs of portal hypertension, arteriovenous malformation, or portosystemic shunt.

Extensive blood investigations for connective tissue disease and vasculitis, thyroid function tests, liver, bone, and kidney biochemistry, electrolytes, HIV antibodies, inflammatory markers, full blood count (FBC), erythrocyte sedimentation rate (ESR), and coagulation markers were performed and did not show any abnormal values. On admission, N-terminal pro-b-type natriuretic peptide (NT-pro-BNP) was elevated significantly at 9996 pg/l (normal values 29–206).

Clinical tip

An initial comprehensive **echocardiographic** evaluation should be performed, with repeat evaluations in the setting of changes in therapy or clinical condition. Imaging to exclude pulmonary thromboembolic disease, peripheral pulmonary artery stenosis, pulmonary vein stenosis, PVOD, and parenchymal lung disease should be performed during the initial investigations. Ventilation-perfusion lung scanning is indicated in patients in whom IPAH is suspected to exclude chronic thromboembolic disease as a cause of the elevated pulmonary artery pressure, which may be amenable to surgery. In chronic thromboembolic PH, the lung scan usually demonstrates one major ventilation–perfusion mismatch [14, 15].

NT-pro-BNP should be measured at diagnosis and during follow-up to supplement clinical decisions. It is a useful biomarker of disease progression.

Cardiac magnetic resonance imaging (MRI) remains the gold standard for evaluating the right ventricle. The most common use for MRI in paediatric PH patients is to assess RV size, mass, and function in the initial evaluation and during follow-up. Cardiac MRI is also used to quantify biventricular volumes and pulmonary blood flow, to assess cardiopulmonary anatomy, and to determine pulmonary artery mechanical properties. Septal curvature metrics are used to estimate RV afterload and track acute changes in pulmonary haemodynamics during vasodilator testing. This suggests that septal curvature configuration could be used for routine continuing assessment of load in a non-invasive way in PH to estimate the mPAP [16].

Given the severity of the presentation, the patient was commenced on oral sildenafil (a phosphodiesterase type 5 inhibitor) and intravenous (IV) epoprostenol (a natural vasodilator). Combined cardiac catheterization and MRI study was performed on the above treatment at an epoprostenol dose of 17 ng/kg/min, the results of which are summarized in Table 16.4.

Table 16.4 Drop in the PVRI indicates an acute vasodilator responder status

	mPAP (mmHg)	iQp (l/min/m^2)	PVRI (WU.m^2)
Baseline FiO_2 (0.21)	35	3.5	8
Vasodilation (FiO_2 1 + iNO 20 ppm)	18	3.5	2.4

iQp: indexed pulmonary flow.

Hickman line was inserted under the same anaesthesia to secure continuous central epoprostenol administration. As the cardiac catheter demonstrated a good response to the medical treatment, the epoprostenol dose was not increased further and a calcium channel blocker (CCB) was commenced. Repeat awake (non-general anaesthesia) MRIs were performed during the admission, which showed progressive reduction of the RV diastolic volume and improvement of the RV ejection fraction. The patient was discharged home 3 weeks later with a diagnosis of IPAH, as no other cause of the raised pressures and PVRI were identified. Biomarkers like NT-pro-BNP were monitored and showed significant reduction (752 pg/l at discharge).

Learning point

Cardiac catheterization is recommended before initiation of PAH-targeted therapy, unless the patient is critically ill and requires immediate empirical therapy. The procedure should include acute vasodilation testing (AVT), unless there is a specific contraindication (severe ventricular dysfunction on the echocardiogram or severe cardiac failure). AVT may be performed with inhaled nitric oxide (NO) (20–80 ppm), 100% oxygen, inhaled or IV prostaglandin 2 (PGI2) analogues, or IV adenosine or sildenafil [17–20]. In children with IPAH, the response to vasodilator testing is used to define the prognosis and the likelihood of response to long-term treatment with CCB therapy.

The patient is considered as a responder if there is:

1. A decrease in mPAP of at least 10 mmHg to <40 mmHg, with a normal or increased cardiac output (CO) [21, 22]
2. A decrease in mPAP of ≥20%, an increase or no change in cardiac index, and a decrease or no change in PVR/systemic vascular resistance (SVR) ratio [23]
3. If PVRI during AVT returns to normal levels [3]

Repeat cardiac catheterization is recommended within 3–12 months after the initiation of therapy to assess response or when required for decision-making in regards to escalation of medical therapy.

Clinical tip

The **6-minute walking distance (6MWD) test** should be used to follow exercise tolerance in paediatric PH patients of school age onwards. There are no robust standardized normal values and no data to support the use of 6MWT to predict survival in children with PH. Most clinicians use changes in serial 6MWTs for longitudinal follow-up.

Cardiopulmonary exercise testing (CPET) is frequently used to evaluate and follow up patients with PH. Paediatric CPET using the bicycle ergometer is used in cooperative children who are >7 years of age. Heart rate and rhythm, oxygen saturation, and blood pressure are recorded in all subjects. In the assessment of asymptomatic paediatric PH patients with CPET, the following variables are useful: maximal oxygen consumption, carbon dioxide elimination, maximal cardiac output, and anaerobic threshold. Children with PH often have significant impairment in aerobic capacity, with a peak oxygen consumption of 20.7 ± 6.9 versus 35.5 ± 7.4 ml/kg/min, when compared to healthy controls (p <0.0001) [24].

NT-pro-BNP should be measured at diagnosis and during follow-up to supplement clinical decisions. NT-pro-BNP, the more stable by-product of BNP, is released from the atria and ventricles in response to stretch from volume overload. BNP and NT-pro-BNP are not specific markers for mechanisms of pulmonary vascular or RV remodelling but are markers that increase with atrial dilatation or failure of either ventricle. BNP and NT-pro-BNP values are used in the paediatric population to monitor response to therapy, and levels decrease as RV function improves with therapy [25–28].

Expert comment

Survival of children aged >1 year without RV failure who were found to be AVT responders and were treated with CCBs was 97% and 81% at 1 and 10 years, respectively, and sustained treatment success was 84% and 47%, respectively [29]. CCBs may possess a potential negative inotropic effect in patients with low CO [30]. Long-term CCB therapies recommended for use in acute responders include nifedipine, diltiazem, and amlodipine.

In patients with a negative acute response to vasodilation and lower-risk characteristics, initiation of oral monotherapy is recommended and should include either a phosphodiesterase type 5 (PDE5) inhibitor or an endothelin (ET) receptor antagonist (ERA) [5].

Sildenafil, an oral active, potent selective inhibitor of PDE5 used in randomized controlled trials in PAH, has shown favourable results on exercise capacity, symptoms, and/or haemodynamics in adults [31], with similar effects in children with PAH [18, 32].

Tadalafil, a once-daily selective PDE5 inhibitor, has shown favourable results on exercise capacity, symptoms, haemodynamics, and time to clinical worsening at high doses [33] and has improved the clinical condition in children with PAH as well [34, 35].

Bosentan, an oral ERA, improves exercise endurance, haemodynamics, and functional class over the short term in children with IPAH [36]. Similarly, ambrisentan, another ERA, has been shown to improve symptoms, exercise capacity, haemodynamics, and time to clinical worsening in patients with IPAH [37–39].

Patients who deteriorate despite therapy with either ERAs or PDE5 inhibitors may benefit from consideration of early combination therapy (add-on or upfront) [40]. Galie et al. in a recent study revealed that the combination of ambrisentan and tadalafil in patients with PAH who had not received previous treatment resulted in a significantly lower risk for clinical failure events with single-medication therapy [41].

IV (epoprostenol) and subcutaneous (treprostinil) PGI2 or its analogues should be initiated without delay in patients with higher-risk PAH [5]. Continuous IV epoprostenol infusion improves symptoms, exercise capacity, and haemodynamics in patients with IPAH and is the only treatment shown to reduce mortality in IPAH [2]. Transition from parenteral to oral or inhaled therapy may be considered in asymptomatic children with PAH who have demonstrated sustained near-normal pulmonary haemodynamics and require close monitoring in an experienced paediatric PH centre.

A month following hospital discharge, the patient was reviewed and it was noted that her effort tolerance continued to improve. She was now able to ride her bicycle and run up the stairs without becoming breathless or tired (WHO functional class I). On examination, she had normal heart sounds and no hepatomegaly. The echocardiogram continued to show a dilated right atrium and right ventricle, with mildly impaired longitudinal and radial function. There was trivial TR with Vmax of 2.4 m/s and trivial PR. Two months later, the cardiac MRI demonstrated normal RV volumes and normal biventricular function. Epoprostenol was weaned slowly and discontinued, with a view to repeat cardiac catheterization combined with an MRI study to reassess her haemodynamics.

Four months later, a combined cardiac catheterization–MRI study was performed on treatment (sildenafil and a CCB), demonstrating an mPAP of 25 mmHg and a PVRI of 6.5 WU.m^2 at baseline, coming down to 1.0 WU.m^2 on the vasodilation stage.

Discussion

Natural course of the disease

The prognosis of untreated PAH is poor. Median survival in untreated children is < 1 year. The clinical and haemodynamic features at presentation which can be predictive of reduced transplant-free survival period include reduced WHO functional class, an elevated PVRI at baseline, and an elevated PVRI and PAP during AVT [3]. The main determinant of treatment is the response to vasodilator testing with NO during cardiac catheterization. In those with a positive response, the PAP and PVR must fall to a near-normal level, with no fall in CO, and this applies to > 10% of those with IPAH. Children who improve and are stable on a CCB need repeat cardiac catheterization after 1 year or less, as they can become resistant to the drug and may need escalation of therapy before they deteriorate. Treatment with CCBs is only effective in responders, and responder status is associated with increased survival period [42, 43]. The majority of negative responders present with WHO functional classes III–IV and frequently need to be started on IV epoprostenol therapy immediately [11].

Lung biopsy is rarely used as part of the routine work-up, given the relatively high risk of the procedure in children with PH. Lung biopsy would be indicated if there was a suspicion of PVOD or PCH, which would require alternative management. PAH histologically follows a specific pattern of advanced remodelling of all layers of the pulmonary arterial wall. In particular, the small 'resistance' pulmonary arteries are affected. Remodelling involves proliferation of endothelial and smooth muscle cells, adventitial thickening, fibrosis, thrombosis, inflammation, and ultimately the development of complex plexiform lesions [44–46].

Palliative procedures

Syncopal children require urgent creation of an interatrial communication (e.g. blade septectomy, radiofrequency-assisted trans-septal puncture, and static balloon dilatation of the atrial septum or insertion of an atrial flow regulator), thus decompressing the right heart chambers and increasing left ventricular pre-load and CO [47, 48]. This improves systemic oxygen transport despite arterial oxygen desaturation and decreases sympathetic hyperactivity.

In patients with severe right heart failure and markedly elevated PVR, atrial septectomy can be fatal due to insufficient pulmonary blood flow and subsequent severe hypoxaemia The current WHO exclusion criteria for atrial septectomy are right atrial pressure of > 20 mmHg, systemic arterial oxygen saturation of < 90%, predicted 1-year survival of < 40%, and PVR of > 55 units.m^2. The Potts shunt is a novel alternative technique for decompressing the right ventricle without significant upper body cyanosis. It is a surgical technique in which a side-to-side anastomosis is created from the left pulmonary artery to the descending aorta, resulting in a right-to-left shunt. It is theoretically advantageous in that it decompresses the failing right ventricle without increasing upper body cyanosis. The Potts shunt may be considered as an alternative option—palliative treatment and bridge to transplantation in patients with idiopathic PH and severe right heart failure refractory to medical management. It allows prolonged survival and dramatic long-lasting improvement in functional capacities in these patients. The same concept applies to a transcatheter technique consisting of retrograde radiofrequency perforation of the descending aorta at the side of apposition to the left pulmonary artery [49].

Patients in WHO functional class III or IV on maximally optimized medical treatment or patients with rapidly progressive disease should be referred to lung transplantation centres for suitability assessment. The current predicted 50% survival for lung transplant in children is 4.3 years, with 75% survival at 1 year, and there are only few donors [50].

Novel treatment perspectives

Despite improvements in the treatment of IPAH, it remains a debilitating disease with a poor prognosis. Therefore, additional therapeutic strategies targeted at diverse pathobiological changes are being explored. New drugs which are being studied include NO-dependent stimulators and activators of cyclic guanosine monophosphate (cGMP), vasoactive intestinal peptide, non-prostanoid prostacyclin agonists, growth factor inhibitors, and serotonin antagonists [51].

Another novel therapeutic strategy involves regeneration of the pulmonary vasculature via increased incorporation of endothelial progenitor cells (EPCs), which are bone marrow-derived cells that can differentiate into endothelial cells and are injected into the injured vascular endothelium, resulting in re-endothelialization and neovascularization [52–54].

A final word from the expert

Children with IPAH should be evaluated and treated at specialized paediatric pulmonary hypertension centres. They should also have regular follow-up at 3- to 6-monthly intervals, with more frequent visits for patients with advanced disease or after initiation of, or changes in, therapy. Preventive measures including respiratory syncytial virus prophylaxis (if eligible), influenza and pneumococcal vaccinations, rigorous monitoring of growth parameters, and prompt recognition and treatment of infectious respiratory illnesses are recommended. Patients undergoing surgery or other invasive intervention requiring a general anaesthetic need careful planning, consultation with experienced cardiac anaesthetists, and clear plans for appropriate post-procedural care.

Patients with pulmonary hypertension on medical treatment belong to the vulnerable group of patients that are in increased risk of becoming unwell with respiratory infections, including COVID-19, and should therefore be particularly strict in following the social distancing measures outlined by the respective Government guidelines: this would exclude attendance of such individuals at nurseries, school, college or universities. Avoidance of situations such as socialising with family, going to restaurants and children's parties would also apply in the same way as the advice for high risk groups. Until there is a suitable robust vaccination programme, some/or all of these measures will need to remain.

IPAH is associated with significant maternal and fetal mortality during pregnancy; it is recommended that female adolescents with PH are provided age-appropriate counselling about pregnancy risks and options for contraception.

Patients with IPAH should have a thorough evaluation, including CPET. Treatment should be initiated before engaging in physical (symptom-limited) activities because of the risk for syncope or sudden death with exertion. However, paediatric patients with severe or a recent history of syncope should not participate in competitive sports.

Paediatric patients with PH should engage in light to moderate aerobic activity, avoid strenuous and isometric exertion, remain well hydrated, and be allowed to self-limit as required. Additionally, during airplane travel, supplemental oxygen use is reasonable in paediatric patients with PH.

Lastly, paediatric PAH carries a significant burden on the entire family, so caregivers and siblings should be assessed for psychosocial stress and be readily provided with support as needed.

References

1. Page RL, Joglar JA, Caldwell MA, et al. 2015 ACC/AHA/HRS Guideline for the management of adult patients with supraventricular tachycardia: A Report of the American College of Cardiology/American Heart Association Task Force on Clinical Practice Guidelines and the Heart Rhythm Society. *J Am Coll Cardiol* 2016;67:e27–115.
2. Galie N, Humbert M, Vachiery JL, et al. 2015 ESC/ERS Guidelines for the diagnosis and treatment of pulmonary hypertension: The Joint Task Force for the Diagnosis and Treatment of Pulmonary Hypertension of the European Society of Cardiology (ESC) and the European Respiratory Society (ERS): Endorsed by: Association for European Paediatric and Congenital Cardiology (AEPC), International Society for Heart and Lung Transplantation (ISHLT). *Eur Heart J* 2015;37:67–119.
3. Moledina S, Hislop AA, Foster H, Schulze-Neick I, Haworth SG. Childhood idiopathic pulmonary arterial hypertension: a national cohort study. *Heart* 2010;96:1401–6.
4. Barst RJ, McGoon M, Torbicki A, et al. Diagnosis and differential assessment of pulmonary arterial hypertension. *J Am Coll Cardiol* 2004;43(12 Suppl S):40S–7S.

5. Abman SH, Hansmann G, Archer SL, et al. Pediatric pulmonary hypertension: Guidelines From the American Heart Association and American Thoracic Society. *Circulation* 2015;132:2037–99.
6. Aldred MA, Vijayakrishnan J, James V, et al. *BMPR2* gene rearrangements account for a significant proportion of mutations in familial and idiopathic pulmonary arterial hypertension. *Hum Mutat* 2006;27:212–13.
7. Cogan JD, Vnencak-Jones CL, Phillips JA, 3rd, et al. Gross *BMPR2* gene rearrangements constitute a new cause for primary pulmonary hypertension. *Genet Med* 2005;7:169–74.
8. Dresdale DT, Michtom RJ, Schultz M. Recent studies in primary pulmonary hypertension, including pharmacodynamic observations on pulmonary vascular resistance. *Bull N Y Acad Med* 1954;30:195–207.
9. Lane KB, Machado RD, Pauciulo MW, et al. Heterozygous germline mutations in BMPR2, encoding a TGF-beta receptor, cause familial primary pulmonary hypertension. *Nat Genet* 2000;26:81–4.
10. Loyd JE, Butler MG, Foroud TM, Conneally PM, Phillips JA, 3rd, Newman JH. Genetic anticipation and abnormal gender ratio at birth in familial primary pulmonary hypertension. *Am J Respir Crit Care Med* 1995;152:93–7.
11. Haworth SG. The management of pulmonary hypertension in children. *Arch Dis Child* 2008;93:620–5.
12. Simonneau G, Gatzoulis MA, Adatia I, et al. Updated clinical classification of pulmonary hypertension. *J Am Coll Cardiol* 2013;62(25 Suppl):D34–41.
13. Augustine DX, Coates-Bradshaw LD, Willis J, Harkness A, Ring L, Grapsa J, Coghlan G, Kaye N, Oxborough D, Robinson S, Sandoval J, Rana BS, Siva A, Nihoyannopoulos P, Howard LS, Fox K, Bhattacharyya S, Sharma V, Steeds RP, Mathew T. Echocardiographic assessment of pulmonary hypertension: a guideline protocol from the British Society of Echocardiography. *Echo Res Pract*. 2018 Sep; 5(3):G11–G24. doi: 1010.1530/ERP-17-0071.71.0
14. Moser KM, Page GT, Ashburn WL, Fedullo PF. Perfusion lung scans provide a guide to which patients with apparent primary pulmonary hypertension merit angiography. *West J Med* 1988;148:167–70.
15. Fedullo PF, Auger WR, Kerr KM, Rubin LJ. Chronic thromboembolic pulmonary hypertension. *N Engl J Med* 2001;345:1465–72.
16. Pandya B, Quail MA, Steeden JA, et al. Real-time magnetic resonance assessment of septal curvature accurately tracks acute hemodynamic changes in pediatric pulmonary hypertension. *Circ Cardiovasc Imaging* 2014;7:706–13.
17. Atz AM, Adatia I, Lock JE, Wessel DL. Combined effects of nitric oxide and oxygen during acute pulmonary vasodilator testing. *J Am Coll Cardiol* 1999;33:813–19.
18. Singh R, Choudhury M, Saxena A, Kapoor PM, Juneja R, Kiran U. Inhaled nitroglycerin versus inhaled milrinone in children with congenital heart disease suffering from pulmonary artery hypertension. *J Cardiothorac Vasc Anesth* 2010;24:797–801.
19. Apitz C, Reyes JT, Holtby H, Humpl T, Redington AN. Pharmacokinetic and hemodynamic responses to oral sildenafil during invasive testing in children with pulmonary hypertension. *J Am Coll Cardiol* 2010;55:1456–62.
20. Schulze-Neick I, Hartenstein P, Li J, et al. Intravenous sildenafil is a potent pulmonary vasodilator in children with congenital heart disease. *Circulation* 2003;108 Suppl 1:II167–73.
21. Robbins IM, Moore TM, Blaisdell CJ, Abman SH. National Heart, Lung, and Blood Institute Workshop: improving outcomes for pulmonary vascular disease. *Circulation* 2012;125:2165–70.
22. Barst RJ, Ertel SI, Beghetti M, Ivy DD. Pulmonary arterial hypertension: a comparison between children and adults. *Eur Respir J* 2011;37:665–77.
23. Barst RJ, McGoon MD, Elliott CG, Foreman AJ, Miller DP, Ivy DD. Survival in childhood pulmonary arterial hypertension: insights from the registry to evaluate early and long-term pulmonary arterial hypertension disease management. *Circulation* 2012;125:113–22.

24. Yetman AT, Taylor AL, Doran A, Ivy DD. Utility of cardiopulmonary stress testing in assessing disease severity in children with pulmonary arterial hypertension. *Am J Cardiol* 2005;95:697–9.
25. Fijalkowska A, Kurzyna M, Torbicki A, et al. Serum N-terminal brain natriuretic peptide as a prognostic parameter in patients with pulmonary hypertension. *Chest* 2006;129:1313–21.
26. Nagaya N, Nishikimi T, Uematsu M, et al. Plasma brain natriuretic peptide as a prognostic indicator in patients with primary pulmonary hypertension. *Circulation* 2000;102:865–70.
27. Lowenthal A, Camacho BV, Lowenthal S, et al. Usefulness of B-type natriuretic peptide and N-terminal pro-B-type natriuretic peptide as biomarkers for heart failure in young children with single ventricle congenital heart disease. *Am J Cardiol* 2012;109:866–72.
28. Tobias JD. B-type natriuretic peptide: diagnostic and therapeutic applications in infants and children. *J Intensive Care Med* 2011;26:183–95.
29. Yung D, Widlitz AC, Rosenzweig EB, Kerstein D, Maislin G, Barst RJ. Outcomes in children with idiopathic pulmonary arterial hypertension. *Circulation* 2004;110:660–5.
30. Beghetti M. Congenital heart disease and pulmonary hypertension. *Rev Port Cardiol* 2004;23:273–81.
31. Galie N, Ghofrani HA, Torbicki A, et al. Sildenafil citrate therapy for pulmonary arterial hypertension. *N Engl J Med* 2005;353:2148–57.
32. Barst RJ, Ivy DD, Gaitan G, et al. A randomized, double-blind, placebo-controlled, dose-ranging study of oral sildenafil citrate in treatment-naive children with pulmonary arterial hypertension. *Circulation* 2012;125:324–34.
33. Galie N, Brundage BH, Ghofrani HA, et al. Tadalafil therapy for pulmonary arterial hypertension. *Circulation* 2009;119:2894–903.
34. Rosenzweig EB. Tadalafil for the treatment of pulmonary arterial hypertension. *Expert Opin Pharmacother* 2010;11:127–32.
35. Takatsuki S, Calderbank M, Ivy DD. Initial experience with tadalafil in pediatric pulmonary arterial hypertension. *Pediatr Cardiol* 2012;33:683–8.
36. McLaughlin VV, Sitbon O, Badesch DB, et al. Survival with first-line bosentan in patients with primary pulmonary hypertension. *Eur Respir J* 2005;25:244–9.
37. Galie N, Badesch D, Oudiz R, et al. Ambrisentan therapy for pulmonary arterial hypertension. *J Am Coll Cardiol* 2005;46:529–35.
38. Galie N, Olschewski H, Oudiz RJ, et al. Ambrisentan for the treatment of pulmonary arterial hypertension: results of the ambrisentan in pulmonary arterial hypertension, randomized, double-blind, placebo-controlled, multicenter, efficacy (ARIES) study 1 and 2. *Circulation* 2008;117:3010–19.
39. Takatsuki S, Rosenzweig EB, Zuckerman W, Brady D, Calderbank M, Ivy DD. Clinical safety, pharmacokinetics, and efficacy of ambrisentan therapy in children with pulmonary arterial hypertension. *Pediatr Pulmonol* 2013;48:27–34.
40. Ivy DD, Abman SH, Barst RJ, et al. Pediatric pulmonary hypertension. *J Am Coll Cardiol* 2013;62(25 Suppl):D117–26.
41. Galie N, Barbera JA, Frost AE, et al. Initial use of ambrisentan plus tadalafil in pulmonary arterial hypertension. *N Engl J Med* 2015;373:834–44.
42. Sitbon O, Humbert M, Jais X, et al. Long-term response to calcium channel blockers in idiopathic pulmonary arterial hypertension. *Circulation* 2005;111:3105–11.
43. Barst RJ, Maislin G, Fishman AP. Vasodilator therapy for primary pulmonary hypertension in children. *Circulation* 1999;99:1197–208.
44. Humbert M, Morrell NW, Archer SL, et al. Cellular and molecular pathobiology of pulmonary arterial hypertension. *J Am Coll Cardiol* 2004;43(12 Suppl S):13S–24S.
45. Jeffery TK, Morrell NW. Molecular and cellular basis of pulmonary vascular remodeling in pulmonary hypertension. *Prog Cardiovasc Dis* 2002;45:173–202.
46. Pietra GG, Capron F, Stewart S, et al. Pathologic assessment of vasculopathies in pulmonary hypertension. *J Am Coll Cardiol* 2004;43(12 Suppl S):25S–32S.

47. Sandoval J, Gaspar J, Pulido T, et al. Graded balloon dilation atrial septostomy in severe primary pulmonary hypertension. A therapeutic alternative for patients nonresponsive to vasodilator treatment. *J Am Coll Cardiol* 1998;32:297–304.
48. Kurzyna M, Dabrowski M, Bielecki D, et al. Atrial septostomy in treatment of end-stage right heart failure in patients with pulmonary hypertension. *Chest* 2007;131:977–83.
49. Baruteau AE, Belli E, Boudjemline Y, et al. Palliative Potts shunt for the treatment of children with drug-refractory pulmonary arterial hypertension: updated data from the first 24 patients. *Eur J Cardiothorac Surg* 2015;47:e105–10.
50. Haworth SG, Hislop AA. Treatment and survival in children with pulmonary arterial hypertension: the UK Pulmonary Hypertension Service for Children 2001–2006. *Heart* 2009;95:312–17.
51. Rabinovitch M. Molecular pathogenesis of pulmonary arterial hypertension. *J Clin Invest* 2008;118:2372–9.
52. Ghofrani HA, Barst RJ, Benza RL, et al. Future perspectives for the treatment of pulmonary arterial hypertension. *J Am Coll Cardiol* 2009;54(1 Suppl):S108–17.
53. Westenbrink BD, Lipsic E, van der Meer P, et al. Erythropoietin improves cardiac function through endothelial progenitor cell and vascular endothelial growth factor mediated neovascularization. *Eur Heart J* 2007;28:2018–27.
54. van Albada ME, du Marchie Sarvaas GJ, Koster J, Houwertjes MC, Berger RM, Schoemaker RG. Effects of erythropoietin on advanced pulmonary vascular remodelling. *Eur Respir J* 2008;31:126–34.

CASE

17 The preterm patent ductus arteriosus: the controversy of closure

Mohammad Ryan Abumehdi

Expert commentary Lindsey Hunter

Case history

A male infant was born at 26 + 0 weeks' gestation via an emergency Caesarean section due to maternal pre-eclampsia, weighing 770 g. Antenatal scans prior to delivery demonstrated reversed end-diastolic blood flow in the umbilical artery.

In an effort to control maternal hypertension, the infant's mother was treated with both labetalol and nifedipine. In addition, betamethasone was administered prior to delivery to promote lung maturation. Following delivery, the infant was noted to have a poor respiratory effort, with an Apgar score of 4 at 1 minute and of 8 at 5 minutes, requiring subsequent intubation and surfactant therapy.

The infant was transferred to the neonatal intensive care unit (NICU) for treatment. Intensive care monitoring included near infrared spectroscopy (NIRS) of both cerebral and abdomen oxygen saturations. Shortly after birth, the infant deteriorated, requiring inotropic support and dexamethasone therapy to maintain an adequate systemic blood pressure.

Expert comment Developing techniques

Near infrared spectroscopy

NIRS is employed to non-invasively monitor tissue oxygenation of end-organs, both cerebral and somatic, where traditional cardiovascular monitoring may not detect hypoperfusion. A significant reduction in NIRS has been observed in preterm infants with a PDA and this evidence of hypoperfusion may represent a haemodynamically significant PDA.

A study by Dix et al. studied the relationship between echocardiographic parameters, cerebral oxygenation, and haemodynamically significant PDAs in 380 preterm infants. In infants born <32 weeks' gestation, there was a statistically significant increase in echocardiographic ductal diameter and reduction in cerebral oxygenation [1]. Although not statistically significant, a higher left atrial: aortic root (LA:Ao) and lower cerebral oxygenation was observed in infants with a haemodynamically significant PDA. In addition, lower cerebral oxygen saturations were observed in those who underwent surgical management of their PDA.

Brain natriuretic peptide

Serum brain natriuretic peptide (BNP) levels have been reported to be elevated in infants with a clinically significant PDA. However, published evidence is limited to a few studies correlating an elevation in BNP levels with increased mortality and the incidence of severe intraventricular haemorrhage (IVH) [2].

Routine examination on day 3 of life detected a systolic murmur suggestive of a PDA. Echocardiography demonstrated normal atrioventricular and ventricular arterial connections, but evidence of a large PDA (diameter 1.9 mm), with pulsatile left-to-right flow. The PDA had a conical morphology, corresponding to type A of the angiographic Krichenko criteria. The left atrium and ventricle were dilated and there was no evidence of ventricular hypertrophy.

The next day, following a failed extubation, the infant deteriorated requiring reintubation and a period of high-frequency oscillatory ventilation (HFOV). In an attempt to medically close his PDA, oral ibuprofen was administered. This was unsuccessful, and in keeping with the departmental policy, a course of paracetamol was commenced.

Expert comment Risk factors for PDA

The most significant risk factor for a haemodynamically significant PDA is gestational age, with the risk of increased morbidity and mortality being inversely proportional to gestational age [3]. In infants below 30 weeks' gestation, approximately 65% will have a PDA identified by day 4 of life [4]. Other risk factors include respiratory distress syndrome, low birthweight, and failure to receive antenatal steroids.

Clinical tip Features of PDA

Clinical signs of a haemodynamically significant duct present a few days after birth as the pulmonary vascular resistance falls:

- Murmur—auscultated loudest at the left upper sternal edge and in the left infraclavicular region. The classical continuous murmur of a duct is not heard until the aortic pressures are greater than systolic and diastolic pulmonary pressures
- Left ventricular heave
- Bounding pulses
- Wide pulse pressure
- Tachypnoea
- Apnoea
- Carbon dioxide retention
- Ventilator dependence
- High oxygenation index.

Learning point Echocardiography

Transthoracic echocardiography remains the gold standard for PDA assessment. Several echocardiographic findings are commonly utilized to determine the significance of a PDA:

- **PDA dimension**—a transductal diameter of >1.5 mm [5] is associated with a haemodynamically significant shunt. Several studies have not demonstrated a correlation between ductal size and gestational age [6].
- **PDA:left pulmonary artery (LPA) ratio**—large >1, moderate 0.5–1, small <1. This ratio, coupled with a low gestational age or low birthweight, increases the sensitivity and specificity of predicting a symptomatic duct [7].

Learning point

Indomethacin

- Historically first-line treatment for medical management of a persistent duct.
- As the infant grows older, the influence of prostaglandins on the patency of the duct is reduced; therefore, the efficacy of indomethacin also decreases.
- Vasoconstrictive effects are not limited to the PDA, and side effects may include necrotizing enterocolitis (NEC), platelet dysfunction, intestinal perforation, and renal injury.

Ibuprofen

- Promotes vasoconstriction of the PDA but reported to cause less systemic vasoconstriction.
- Side effects may include acute kidney injury, pulmonary hypertension, and hyperbilirubinaemia.

A Cochrane review comparing indomethacin, ibuprofen, and a placebo in preterm and low-birthweight infants found ibuprofen to be as effective as indomethacin for PDA closure [8]. Ibuprofen demonstrated a lower incidence of complications—NEC, duration of ventilatory support, and transient renal insufficiency. There was no difference in the efficacy of oral and IV ibuprofen preparations. The half-life of enteral ibuprofen is longer, and enteral ibuprofen is superior to IV ibuprofen in reducing the incidence of NEC. However, the optimal dosing regimen at each gestational age remains unclear.

Paracetamol

- Paracetamol (acetaminophen) is a viable alternative to ibuprofen and indomethacin.
- Uncertainty surrounding possible hepatotoxicity and effect on the neurodevelopment of preterm infants in higher than recommended doses.

A Cochrane review of two randomized controlled trials compared the efficacy and safety of paracetamol to prostaglandin inhibitors [9].

In summary:

- No significant difference was reported in the rate of closure between oral ibuprofen and paracetamol.

Clinical tip Echocardiographic features of PDA

Signs of pulmonary over-circulation

- Increased LA:Ao ratio
- Increased flow in the LPA in diastole
- Increased mean PA flow
- Reversed mitral E/A ratio

Signs of systemic hypoperfusion

- Retrograde flow in the descending aorta/mesenteric arteries
- Left ventricular output:superior vena cava flow ratio >4.0

- The duration for the need for supplemental oxygen and hyperbilirubinaemia level was found to be lower in those who received paracetamol.
- Complications such as renal and liver dysfunction and gastrointestinal complications were lower in infants treated with paracetamol.
- Evidence is limited, and further longer-term follow-up is required [9].

Clinical tip Contraindications to ibuprofen and indomethacin

- Suspected/confirmed NEC
- Active bleeding
- Suspected/confirmed sepsis
- Significant renal impairment
- Coagulation defects and thrombocytopenia
- Duct-dependent congenital heart defects

Oxygenation proved difficult, with the infant requiring relatively high-pressure ventilation to maintain adequate tidal volumes, with a moderately high oxygen requirement (30–55%). The baby was treated for sepsis and required multiple transfusions to optimize haemoglobin levels and maintain adequate oxygen saturations.

Despite ongoing intensive therapy and a period of relative stability, on day 21 of life, the infant developed signs of congestive cardiac failure. On examination, there was a gallop rhythm, tachycardia, bounding femoral pulses, and 3 cm hepatomegaly. The clinical status was compounded by evidence of bilateral lung opacities on chest X-ray, suggesting the development of chronic lung disease (CLD) (Figure 17.1). The infant had periods of spontaneous desaturations and was commenced on diuretic therapy to alleviate the symptoms of increased pulmonary blood flow.

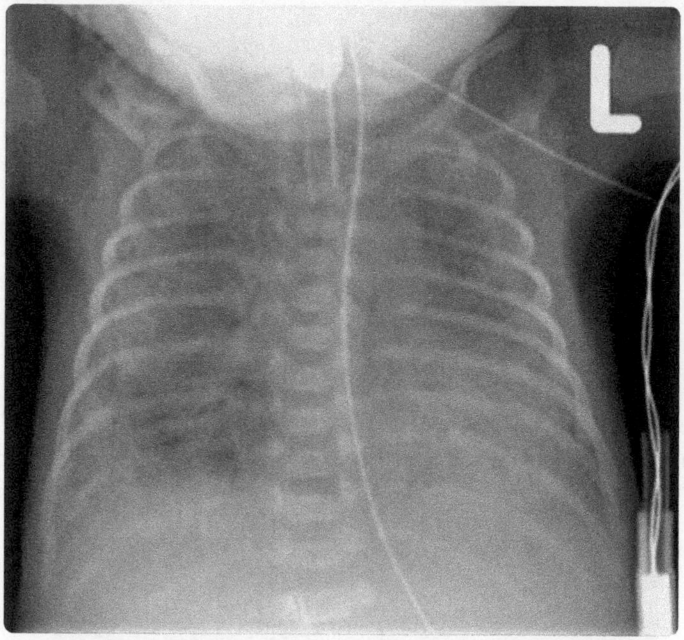

Figure 17.1 Anteroposterior chest X-ray demonstrating features of congestive cardiac failure: bilateral pleural effusions, cardiomegaly, Kerley B lines, interstitial oedema, and pulmonary venous congestion.

Clinical tip Conservative medical management

There is institutional variation, but management may include:

- **Antenatal steroids.** Clear evidence that antenatal steroids, in addition to postnatal surfactant, promote and improve lung maturation. In addition, their influence on the pathophysiology and incidence of preterm PDA is thought to be beneficial [10].
- **Fluid restriction.** Although widely used, evidence is limited. Most institutions do not exceed fluid volumes of 130 ml/kg/day.

- **Diuretics.** The use of furosemide may stimulate the synthesis of prostaglandin, which maintains the ductus arteriosus in the first 2 weeks of life. Furosemide may be useful in infants with evidence of pulmonary over-circulation. However, balancing diuretics and fluid restriction can be challenging in preterm infants, leading to potential electrolyte imbalance and renal dysfunction.
- **Optimal temperature control, oxygenation, and permissive hypercapnia.** Aim to reduce the demands of cardiac output. The use of positive end-expiratory pressure improves gas exchange and the likelihood of successful extubation. Permissive hypercapnia promotes a reduction in tidal volumes and prevents barotrauma. Relative pulmonary vasoconstriction may decrease the shunt into the pulmonary circulation.
- **Optimal haemoglobin and haematocrit levels.** Limited evidence, optimal oxygen-carrying capacity, and oxygen uptake by tissues may be beneficial.

Echocardiography confirmed a persistent PDA which had increased in diameter to 2.7 mm, an LA:Ao ratio of 2.5:1, and low-velocity left-to-right flow. There was bidirectional flow across a small patent foramen ovale, and the left heart appeared dilated but with preserved systolic contraction (Figures 17.2 and 17.3).

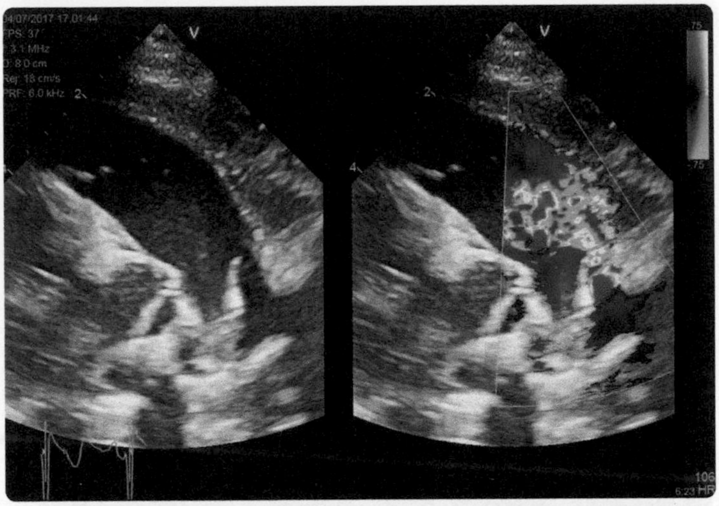

Figure 17.2 Parasternal short axis 'ductal view' demonstrating pulmonary artery flow, with ductal flow returning into the pulmonary artery.

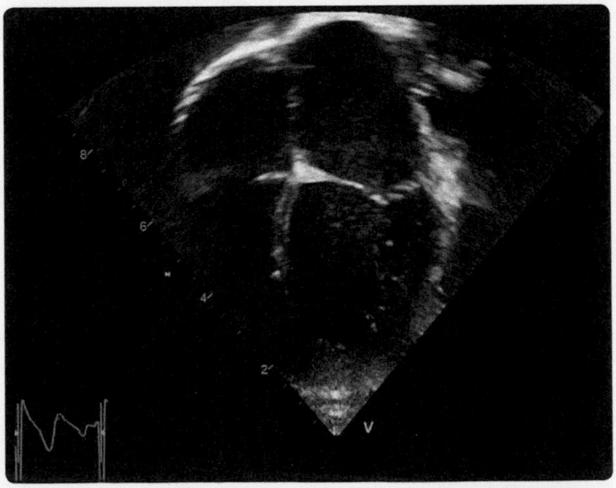

Figure 17.3 Apical four-chamber view demonstrating dilated left atrium and ventricle.

Learning point Flow patterns within the duct

There is a high correlation with transductal diameter, the widest in type 1 and the narrowest in type 4 [9, 11] (Figure 17.4):

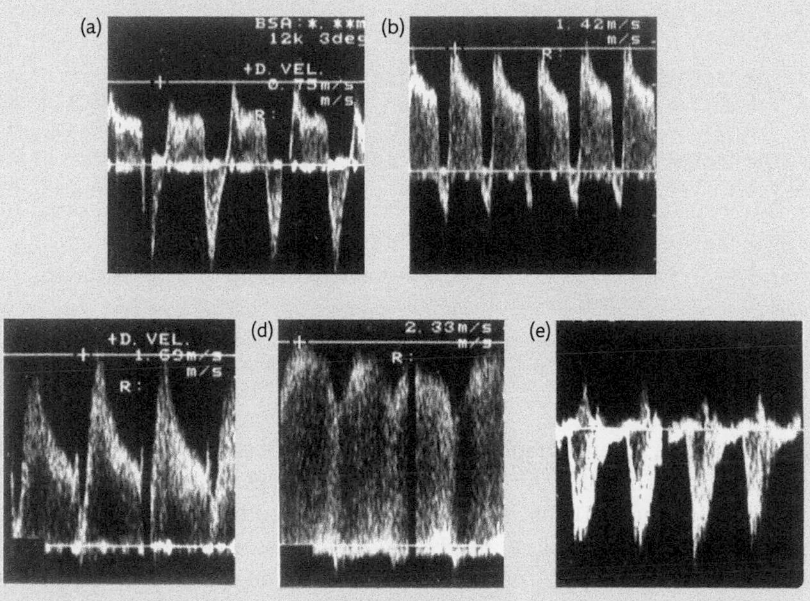

Figure 17.4 (a) Type 1 (pulmonary hypertension pattern): bidirectional shunt from right to left in early systole, followed by a small left to right shunt in diastole. (b) Type 2 (growing pattern): shunting is bidirectional; a decreasing right to left shunt and an increasing left to right shunt in systole, representing falling pulmonary vascular resistance. (c) Type 3 (pulsatile pattern): pulsatile left to right flow; no right to left shunting. (d) Type 4 (closing pattern)—continuous left to right flow; no rhythmical pulsatile change in left to right flow. (e) Type 5 (closed pattern)—closed pattern similar to pulmonary artery flow pattern.

Reproduced from Echocardiographic assessment of patent ductus arteriosus flow pattern in premature infants. Su B, Watandbe T, Shimizu M, *et al*, *Archives of Disease in Childhood* 1997;77:F36–F40 with permission from BMJ Publishing Group Ltd.

At 4 weeks of age, 31+^{0} weeks corrected gestational age (CGA), the local unit felt that, in view of the high oxygen requirements and symptoms of cardiac failure, the infant should be transferred to the regional cardiac centre for cardiology review and consideration of surgical PDA closure. The cardiac multidisciplinary team (MDT) concluded surgical PDA ligation was preferable to percutaneous device closure due to the infant's weight of 1.07 kg. Percutaneous duct closure in small babies has been implemented in some centres. However, after reviewing the data in this specific case, the MDT felt surgical ligation would be superior.

Learning point Percutaneous PDA occlusion

Although it is a well-established technique in term infants, use in premature infants is dependent on institutional experience, and data regarding outcomes in very preterm infants (<32 weeks' gestation) are varied and limited [12]. There is no pre-defined lower weight limit for the safe closure of a PDA. However, most device manufacturers suggest a lower limit of 6 kg, although this is a relative contraindication.

Percutaneous occlusion has been demonstrated to be a generally safe and successful option in very preterm infants below 4 kg, reducing the need for mechanical ventilation [12]. A recent UK national study looking at device closure in infants under 6 kg showed favourable outcomes nationally, with 92% undergoing successful implantation and 95% having complete occlusion at their last follow-up [13]. Relative adverse events were more apparent in the smallest of infants, with acute arterial injury being the most common complication. Some centres have demonstrated that venous-only access avoids this complication, with no increase in rates of device embolization or malposition.

There has been marked variability in the criteria for referral and optimal timing for device closure, compared to surgical alternatives.

It seems that premature infants under 1500 g can undergo percutaneous transvenous PDA closure with relative safety, and the technique is likely to be used more frequently.

Preoperative echocardiography demonstrated left heart dilatation with good systolic contraction. The left ventricle measured 18 mm (Z = +2.68) in diastole, and the left atrial diameter 11 mm (Z = +1.0) and the aortic root 6 mm (Z = −2.14), demonstrating an LA:Ao ratio of nearly 2:1. A patent foramen ovale showed bidirectional flow. Ductal flow in diastole was low velocity, and the PDA measured 3 mm in diameter.

At 4 weeks of age, CGA 31^{+3}, and weighing 1070 g, the infant remained ventilator-dependent and underwent surgical ligation, off bypass, via a lateral thoracotomy using a double clip. The procedure required repeated breaks from lung retraction due to frequent desaturations. In the presence of a significant PDA and recurrent desaturations, the decision was made to clip, rather than ligate, the duct with a suture. The additional benefit of a small residual PDA would allow offloading in the presence of CLD—this was felt to be of clinical benefit and could be closed with a percutaneous device at later stage.

Learning point Post-ligation cardiac syndrome

Following PDA ligation, there is an abrupt change in physiology and haemodynamics, predisposing infants to post-ligation cardiac syndrome. The sudden increase in left ventricular afterload and reduction in pre-load may lead to a rapid drop in cardiac output, with reduction in systolic and diastolic function. In other patients, post-ligation cardiac syndrome may present with severe hypertension.

Risk factors include:

- <28 days of age
- Weight <1000 g [14].

Post-operative administration of prophylactic intravenous (IV) milrinone, a phosphodiesterase type 3 inhibitor, may prevent significant haemodynamic instability post-PDA ligation and may counteract the effects of post-ligation cardiac syndrome [14, 15].

Expert comment Surgical management

A more conservative surgical management approach has been taken in recent years, resulting in surgical ligation of PDAs being reserved when medical management fails. However, a primary role for surgical ligation may exist in select cases of extremely low-weight preterm infants (<800 g) or in those in whom prostaglandin inhibitors are contraindicated [16, 17].

The success rates of surgical closure are, as expected, much higher, although malposition/dislodgement of the ductal clip do rarely occur.

Procedural-related risks include:

- Pneumothorax
- Hypothermia
- Bleeding
- Phrenic and vocal nerve palsy
- Wound infection
- Thoracic scoliosis.

A Cochrane review found no statistically significant difference between surgical ligation and closure using indomethacin [risk ratio (RR) 0.67; 95% confidence interval (CI) 0.34 to 1.31; risk difference (RD) −0.07; 95% CI −0.20 to 0.05) [18]. There was no difference in the rates of CLD, IVH, and NEC and in creatinine levels. However, surgical ligation was associated with a statistically significant increase in the incidence of pneumothorax and retinopathy of prematurity (ROP) [18].

Following the procedure, the infant's diastolic blood pressure improved from 30 mmHg to 40 mmHg. Post-procedural echocardiography demonstrated no residual PDA flow (Figure 17.5). The left ventricle, although dilated, had preserved systolic contraction. The left atrial size decreased to 9 mm (Z = −0.42), and the left ventricle in diastole 16 mm (Z = +1.51).

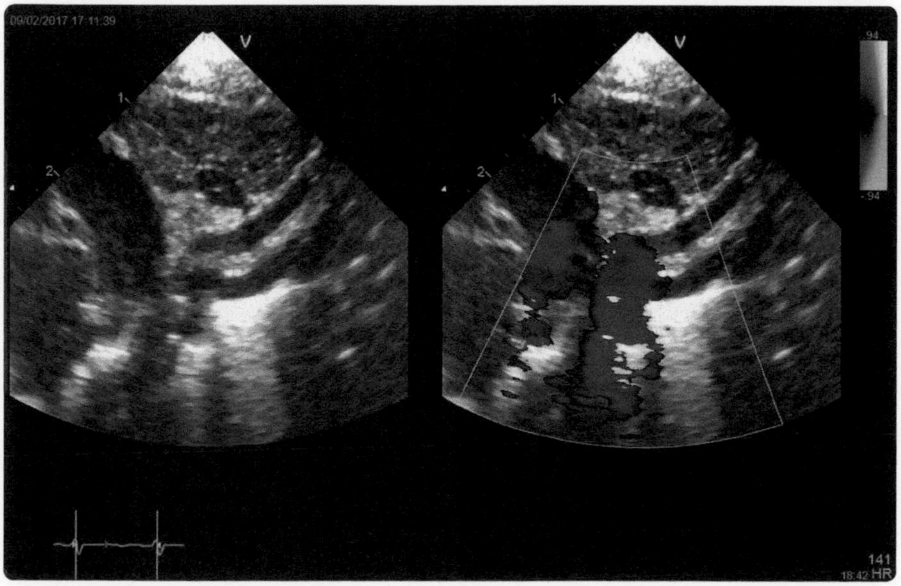

Figure 17.5 Parasternal short axis view, following surgical ligation, demonstrating no residual flow.

Even after PDA ligation, the infant maintained a significant oxygen requirement and so was recommenced on dexamethasone and was eventually extubated onto biphasic positive airway pressure on day 36 of life (CGA 32 weeks), 6 days after ligation. Dexamethasone was gradually weaned and stopped on day 47 (CGA 32^{+4} weeks).

Expert comment Long-term prognosis

If left untreated, preterm infants born with a haemodynamically significant PDA are reported to have mortality levels four times those of similar aged infants without a PDA. Infants who respond positively to medical management with ductal closure return to comparable mortality levels.

Currently, no clinical trials or meta-analyses have demonstrated that PDA closure improves medium- and long-term outcomes such as the incidence of pulmonary haemorrhage, CLD, and NEC [19].

Throughout the course of the infant's hospital admission, serial cranial ultrasound scans detected prominent periventricular flare with a simplified gyral pattern, typical of prematurity, and a small bilateral subependymal haemorrhage. The infant received regular monitoring of head growth and neurodevelopmental follow-up. ROP was treated by the ophthalmology team. Despite two episodes of presumed sepsis, the infant progressed to non-invasive respiratory support on day 72 (CGA 36^{+2}) and was subsequently discharged home (CGA 45 weeks) on nasal cannula oxygen and beclomethasone therapy for CLD.

A final word from the expert

In neonatal medicine, no single topic divides opinion more than the management of the PDA in preterm infants. Throughout its history, the 'en vogue' management has ranged from prophylactic medical closure, symptomatic medical closure, and surgical ligation to a conservative approach. Despite multiple studies and reviews, no international management consensus has been reached. Trials often have selection bias with multiple variables, including gestational age, birthweight, gender, use of antenatal steroids, and timing of treatment or interventions [14].

The pathophysiology of a PDA and its associated comorbidities requires a greater level of understanding. Therefore, defining a haemodynamically significant PDA is also challenging and important. This would promote targeted therapy and treatment strategies in a bid to reduce comorbidities, improve mortality rates, and promote positive neurodevelopmental outcomes.

Echocardiography remains the gold standard for the assessment of a preterm PDA, providing rapid, non-invasive bedside assessment of some of the most complex and fragile patients in our care.

In the absence of an international consensus, neonatal practice may vary between neonatal units—proactive use of medical therapy in some cases; proceeding to targeted medical therapy in the presence of a haemodynamically significant PDA; failure to wean from ventilatory support, or evidence of cardiac failure in others. If failure of medical management, it may be appropriate to involve the cardiac MDT to debate the merits of surgical or percutaneous closure, taking into account the comorbidities associated with prematurity; with a haemodynamically significant PDA and cardiac intervention in a very small and fragile infant. The decision between surgical ligation and percutaneous intervention may vary between institutions, depending on individual expertise of surgical versus percutaneous closure in low-birthweight infants.

References

1. Dix L et al. Cerebral oxygenation and echocardiographic parameters in preterm neonates with a patent ductus arteriosus: an observational study. *Arch Dis Child Fetal Neonatal Ed* 2016;101:F520–6.

2. El-Khuffash A et al. Biochemical markers may identify preterm infants with a patent ductus arteriosus at high risk of death or severe Intraventricular haemorrhage. *Arch Dis Child Fetal Neonatal Ed* 2008;93:F407–12.
3. Dice J, Bhatia J. Patent ductus arteriosus: an overview. *J Pediatr Pharmacol Ther* 2007;12:138–46.
4. Koch J et al. Prevalence of spontaneous closure of the ductus arteriosus in neonates at a birth weight of 1000 grams or less. *Pediatrics* 2006;117:1113.
5. Hamrick SE, Hansmann G. Patent ductus arteriosus of the preterm infant. *Pediatrics* 2010;125:1020–10.
6. Condo M et al Echocardiographic assessment of ductal significance retrospective comparison of two methods. *Arch Dis Child Fetal Neonatal Ed* 2012;97:F35 – 8.
7. Heuchan AM, Clyman RI. Managing the patent ductus arteriosus: current treatment options. *Arch Dis Child Fetal Neonatal Ed* 2014;99:F431–6.
8. Ohlsson A, Walia R, Shah SS. Ibuprofen for the treatment of patent ductus arteriosus in preterm or low birth weight (or both) infants. *Cochrane Database Syst Rev* 2015;2:CD003481.
9. Ohlsson A, Shah PS. Paracetamol (acetaminophen) for patent ductus arteriosus in preterm or low-birth-weight infants. *Cochrane Database Syst Rev* 2015;3:CD010061.
10. Wyllie JP, Gupta S. Prophylactic and early targeted treatment of patent ductus arteriosus. *Semin Fetal Neonatal Med* 2018;23:250–4.
11. Su B, Watanabe T, Shimizu M, Yanagisawa M. Echocardiographic assessment of patent ductus arteriosus shunt flow pattern in premature infants. *Arch Dis Childhood* 1997;77:F36–40.
12. Backes C et al. Percutaneous patent ductus arteriosus (PDA) closure in very preterm infants: feasibility and complications. *J Am Heart Assoc* 2016;5:e002923.
13. Kang SL et al. Outcome after transcatheter occlusion of patent ductus arteriosus in infants less than 6 kg: a national study from United Kingdom and Ireland. *Catheter Cardiovasc Interv* 2017;90:1135–44.
14. Mitra S et al. Effectiveness and safety of treatments used for the management of patent ductus arteriosus (PDA) in preterm infants: a protocol for a systematic review and network meta-analysis. *BMJ Open* 2016;6:e011271.
15. Hallik M et al. Population pharmacokinetics and dosing of milrinone after patent ductus arteriosus ligation in preterm infants. *Pediatr Crit Care Med* 2019;20:621–9.
16. Palder SB et al Management of patent ductus arteriosus: comparison of operative vs pharmacologic treatment. *J Pediatr Surg* 1987;22:1171–4.
17. Trus T et al. Optimum management of patent ductus arteriosus in neonate weighing less than 800 g. *J Pediatr Surg* 1993;28:1137–9.
18. Malviya MN, Ohlsson A, Shah SS Surgical versus medical treatment with cyclooxygenase inhibitors for symptomatic patent ductus arteriosus in preterm infants. *Cochrane Database Syst Rev* 2013;3:CD003951.
19. Benitz WE; Committee on Fetus and Newborn, American Academy of Paediatrics. Patent ductus arteriosus in preterm infants. *Pediatrics* 2016;137:e20153730.

CASE

18 Cardiac evaluation of a child with stridor

Louise Morrison

Expert commentary Brian A McCrossan

Case history

A 9-day-old baby, born via normal delivery at term and weighing 3.2 kg, was noted to have a murmur at his postnatal check. He attended for cardiology review and was feeding well at this stage, with no cardiovascular symptoms. Initial echocardiogram was challenging, as the patient was unsettled, but demonstrated a patent foramen ovale and a small muscular ventricular septal defect with an otherwise normal intracardiac anatomy. It was not possible to fully assess the aortic arch. At the time, there were no clinical concerns.

He presented to the paediatric intensive care unit (PICU) at 4 months of life, requiring ventilation for respiratory syncitial virus (RSV)-positive bronchiolitis. Chest X-ray demonstrated patchy changes, consistent with his condition and, in retrospect, a right-sided aortic arch (Figure 18.1). He was treated with steroids, and, on extubation, having been ventilated for 10 days, he was noted to have a stridulous cry. His parents reported that he had intermittently sounded like that at home in the weeks prior to his admission and had also been concerned that his feeding had begun to slow down. As such, he had also been reviewed by his general practitioner at 3 months of life due to 'noisy breathing' and was awaiting paediatric assessment. During his admission, following review, the ear, nose, and throat (ENT) team suggested an outpatient review would be appropriate once he was discharged.

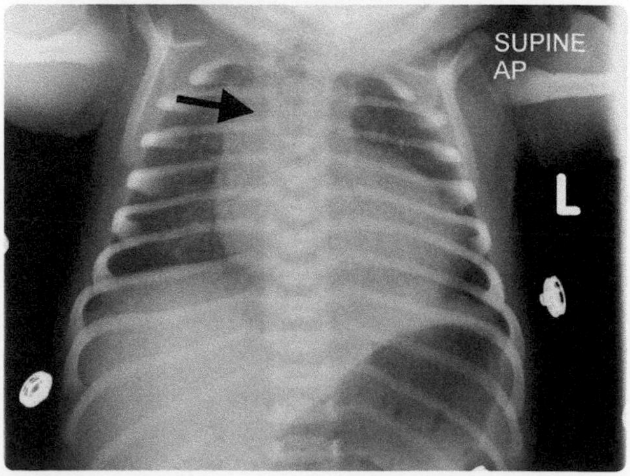

Figure 18.1 Chest X-ray showing changes consistent with bronchiolitis and a right-sided aortic arch, with the aortic knuckle apparent on the right side of the chest (arrow).

He re-presented to paediatric A & E a week later with worsening stridor and respiratory distress. He was readmitted to PICU and was reviewed by a member of the ENT team who performed a flexible bronchoscopy, demonstrating slightly bulky arytenoids, but no obvious strictures, and subglottic oedema thought to be due to prolonged intubation from his previous admission. He was commenced on a further course of steroids and supplemental nasogastric tube feeding. His symptoms persisted, and microlaryngoscopy and bronchoscopy (MLB) by the ENT consultant demonstrated compression of the trachea in the left postero-lateral segment. An inpatient cardiology review at this stage resulted in a repeat echocardiogram, which suggested a right-sided aortic arch.

A computed tomography (CT) angiogram under general anaesthesia demonstrated a right-sided aortic arch with a retro-oesophageal left subclavian artery. Airway views showed postero-lateral tracheal narrowing (Figure 18.2), confirming a vascular ring. He underwent division of his vascular ring and division of the left-sided ligamentum arteriosum with aortopexy, at the age of 8 months, through a left thoracotomy incision. There was an uneventful post-operative recovery and he is currently well and symptom-free.

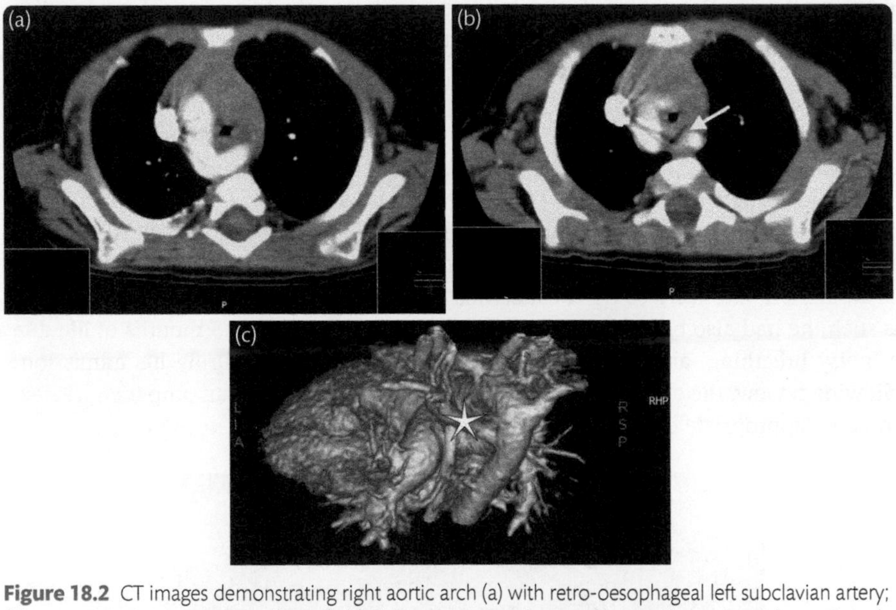

Figure 18.2 CT images demonstrating right aortic arch (a) with retro-oesophageal left subclavian artery; (b) causing airway compression (arrow). (c) Three-dimensional reconstruction illustrating right aortic arch with aberrant left subclavian artery (star).

Learning point Symptoms and clinical presentation

Clinical presentation of vascular rings is variable and is dependent on the site and degree of compression of adjacent structures such as the airway or oesophagus. The types of vascular ring that most frequently cause symptoms are a double aortic arch, a right aortic arch with left ductus, an aberrant subclavian artery, and an aberrant innominate artery. A pulmonary artery sling and rarer types of vascular sling can produce similar symptoms [1].

A high index of suspicion for vascular compression of the airway should be maintained in infants with recurrent respiratory distress, stridor, cough, apnoea, or recurrent respiratory infections, especially during the first year of life. Respiratory symptoms are reported in 70–97% of patients with vascular rings at presentation [2, 3]. Due to the fixed nature of the airway obstruction, symptoms are present throughout the respiratory cycle. As in this case, patients have often been treated for bronchiolitis, asthma, or recurrent lower respiratory tract infection, with a delay in their diagnosis [4]. As a general rule, neonates present with airway issues, whereas older children and adults may present with dysphagia or asthma-type symptoms that are refractory to treatment [5]. Occasionally, the diagnosis of a vascular ring is incidental during evaluation for other reasons.

Expert comment

Although there seemed a reasonable explanation for the stridor (prolonged intubation), a high index of suspicion should be maintained until investigations have definitively ruled out airway compression. The role of the cardiologist is to explain arch sidedness, head and neck vessel arrangement, and the presence of a left pulmonary artery sling and dilated cardiac structures, which could potentially compress the airway or oesophagus.

Clinical tip

With echocardiography, difficulty in demonstrating aortic arch sidedness should raise an index of suspicion for a right aortic arch. If all the head and neck vessels are not seen, rule out an aberrant subclavian artery. Difficulty showing the common carotid arteries in the same sweep could suggest a double aortic arch. If so, interrogate this further with a high parasternal short axis view. The first echocardiogram is an opportunity to delineate all cardiac structures, including the head and neck vessel arrangement. If not commented on, it may be assumed to be normal, and therefore, diagnosis and appropriate management may be delayed.

Learning point Investigations and assessment

Patients presenting with symptoms suggestive of airway compression require a comprehensive diagnostic workup and a multidisciplinary assessment. Appropriate investigations include the following.

Chest X-ray will demonstrate the location of the aortic arch in relation to the trachea and dilated pulmonary arteries. Unilateral hyperinflation of a lung may suggest a pulmonary artery sling or other lung pathology. Some authors suggest an entirely normal chest X-ray is strong evidence against a vascular ring, as most are associated with a right aortic arch, which may be identified on chest X-ray [6].

Echocardiography can demonstrate aortic arch and pulmonary artery anatomy, along with any associated congenital heart disease. An appreciation of aortic arch embryology is important in interpreting echocardiographic images. It permits bedside evaluation in the critically ill patient. However, echocardiography may be limited due to operator expertise and patient compliance, as demonstrated in this case.

Microlaryngoscopy and bronchoscopy (MLB) will document the location and extension of airway obstruction. MLB is useful for distinguishing between dynamic or static narrowing of the airways, which cannot be reliably identified by other means. Bronchoscopy can evaluate for other unexpected airway pathology such as tracheal rings or subglottic stenosis [7]. It can be repeated to follow up the resolution of airway malacia and also used to document vocal cord motion prior to, and after, surgical intervention [1, 5].

Although a vascular ring may be suspected by other investigations, its exact configuration may only be reliably defined by **cross-sectional imaging such as computed tomography (CT) or magnetic resonance imaging (MRI)**. Angiography permits accurate delineation of vascular anatomy and three-dimensional reconstruction, which can facilitate surgical planning. Associated static airway abnormalities may also be identified. Both techniques have a similar sensitivity. However, the advantages of CT include rapid acquisition, high resolution, and accessible imaging of both the vasculature and the airways without the need for general anaesthesia. Like echocardiography, an appreciation of aortic arch embryology is important in interpreting cross-sectional images.

Barium studies are often performed in children with feeding difficulties. They may suggest vascular compression by an extrinsic indentation of the oesophagus, the position of which may give a clue to the diagnosis [1].

A diagnostic algorithm for patients presenting with symptoms suggestive of airway compression is proposed in Figure 18.3 [1].

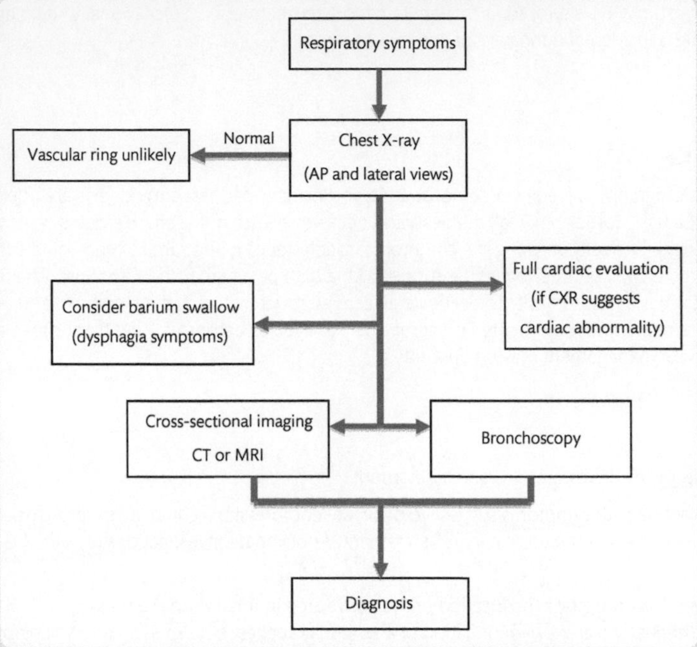

Figure 18.3 Diagnostic algorithm for patients presenting with symptoms suggestive of airway compression.

Expert comment

Plain X-ray may not be reliable for arch sidedness, and interpretation depends on the skill and experience of the viewer. Requesting a lateral chest X-ray suggests a degree of suspicion, and it would be better to opt for more reliable and detailed investigations such as echocardiography, bronchoscopy, and cross-sectional imaging. Either CT or MRI will demonstrate the anatomy. CT is probably preferable to MRI, despite exposure to ionizing radiation, as it provides better spatial resolution, usually does not require general anaesthesia, and is quicker. The severity of symptoms will determine the number and extent of investigations performed. If dysphagia is present, a barium swallow is indicated. Echocardiography and bronchoscopy are user-dependent, and if symptoms persist, it is reasonable to revisit these investigations.

Learning point Diagnosis in this case

The patient described had a right aortic arch with a retro-oesophageal left subclavian artery. This is the second most common type of vascular ring, accounting for 12–25% of cases [4]. The ring is completed by a left ligamentum arteriosum, which is a fibrous structure tethered inferiorly to the left pulmonary artery and not usually visible on CT or MRI scan, thus completely encircling the trachea and oesophagus (Figure 18.4). Treatment involves surgical division of the ligamentum. It is also necessary to excise the diverticulum of Kommerell, an outpouching of the descending aorta which is embryologically derived from ductus arteriosus tissue; if left intact, the diverticulum can cause late compression of the trachea or oesophagus [5]. It is, however, important to be aware that a right aortic arch with an aberrant left subclavian artery frequently is not associated with a vascular ring.

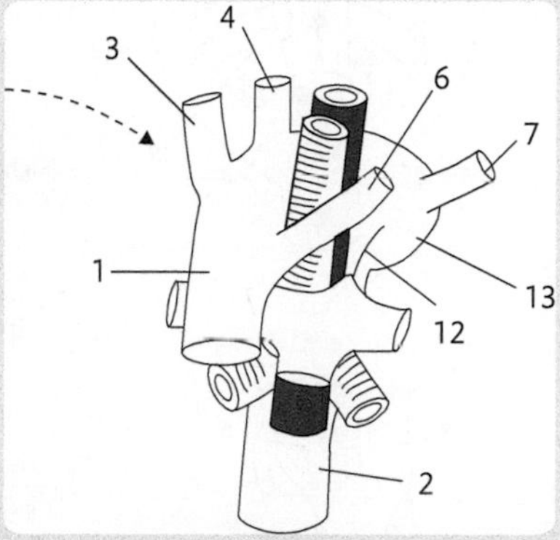

Figure 18.4 Drawing illustrating right aortic arch with aberrant left subclavian artery. Structures are: 1, ascending aorta; 2, descending aorta; 3, right common carotid artery; 4, right subclavian artery; 6, left common carotid artery; 7, left subclavian artery; 12, ductus arteriosus or ligamentum arteriosum; 13, aortic (Kommerell's) diverticulum.

Learning point Aortic arch development

Knowledge of the normal embryological development of the aortic arch and its related structures is vital in helping to understand the classification of vascular rings.

During fetal development, six pairs of primitive aortic arches sequentially form and regress, as each successive arch develops with the remnants contributing to the head and neck vessels [1].

The persistent arches are the fourth arch, which contributes to the left aortic arch and right subclavian artery, and the sixth arch, which becomes the mediastinal segment of the pulmonary arteries and their distal portions form the ductus arteriosus [8].

In 1948, Edwards in his definitive publication described a hypothetical double arch with bilateral 'ducti arteriosi', which explains most aortic arch malformations in terms of failure of regression or abnormal regression of the fourth aortic arch system at one or more of four common locations [4] (Figure 18.5). If no regression occurs at any location, a double aortic arch forms.

In normal arch development, regression occurs at (d), resulting in a left-sided arch, with the first branch passing to the right as the innominate artery, which gives rise to the right common carotid artery and right subclavian artery. Regression at (b) results in a left arch with an aberrant right subclavian artery.

Expert comment

An appreciation of the embryology, and particularly the double arch model, is essential to understand the various combinations of arch sidedness/head and neck vessel arrangement. Once the diagnosis of airway compression has been ascertained, it is important to explain how the vascular arrangement could potentially cause the compression (or not) and to guide the cardiac surgeon as to the best method for its relief, although surgical repair almost always is via left thoracotomy.

Regression at d′ results in a right-sided aortic arch with a mirror image-branching pattern to normal. A right aortic arch with an aberrant left subclavian artery is formed by regression at b′ (the diagnosis in this case).

If no regression occurs at any site, a double arch is formed.

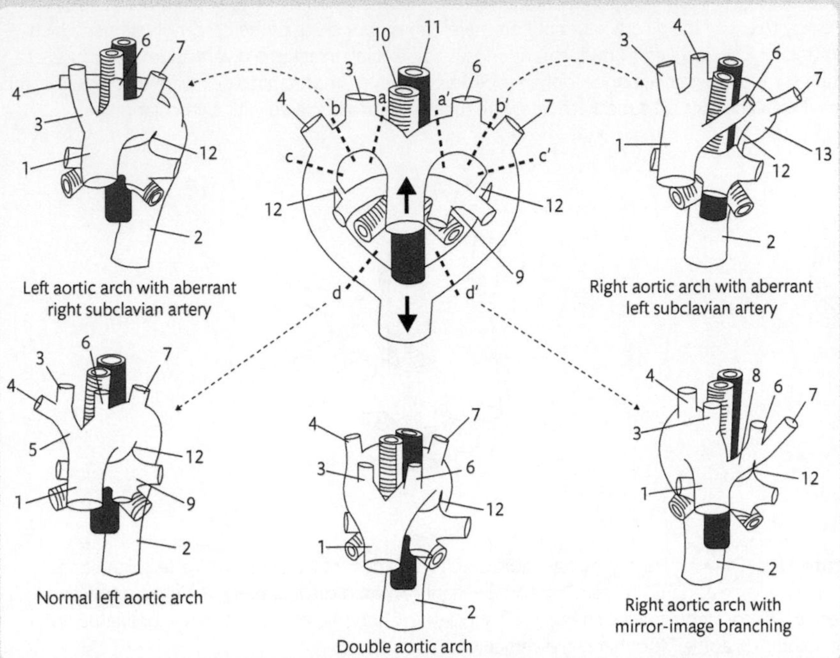

Figure 18.5 Drawing illustrating Edward's hypothetical double arch encircling the trachea and oesophagus. Regression at each of the dotted lines results in the development of a normal or a malformed aortic arch. Structures are: 1, ascending aorta; 2, descending aorta; 3, right common carotid artery; 4, right subclavian artery; 5, right innominate artery; 6, left common carotid artery; 7, left subclavian artery; 8, left innominate artery; 9, pulmonary artery; 10, trachea; 11, oesophagus; 12, ductus arteriosus; 13, aortic (Kommerell's) diverticulum).

M. Yorimitsu; Department of Radiology, Kyorin University School of Medicine, Tokyo, Japan.

Discussion

Post-mortem studies suggest that around 3% of the population have some form of aortic arch abnormality, although most remain asymptomatic throughout life [9]. Vascular rings and slings account for < 1% of all congenital heart disease but remain important and eminently treatable causes of airway or oesophageal compression [4].

The most prevalent vascular anomalies resulting in airway compression are a double aortic arch, a right aortic arch with an aberrant left subclavian artery, innominate artery compression, a left aortic arch with an aberrant right subclavian artery, and a pulmonary artery sling [3]. A left aortic arch with an aberrant right subclavian artery is common among the general population and considered a normal variant, rarely causing symptoms. A right aortic arch could cause a vascular ring in the presence of a left-sided ligamentum arteriosus to complete the ring [5].

True, complete vascular rings wholly encircle the trachea and oesophagus and may also affect the main bronchi. They include a double aortic arch, which is the most frequent cause of vascular airway compression in children, accounting for 50–60% of cases [3, 4], and a right aortic arch with an aberrant left subclavian artery, which is discussed in Learning point: Aortic arch development, p. 241.

A double aortic arch is formed by persistence of both fourth primitive arches (Figure 18.3). The right arch is usually larger or dominant, and the left arch is often hypoplastic or forms an atretic segment beyond the origin of the left common carotid or subclavian artery, tethering the left arch to the descending aorta [7]. A double aortic arch requires surgical correction by division of the smaller, non-dominant arch. It is imperative to accurately document the aortic arch anatomy preoperatively, as it will determine the surgical approach.

Other lesions causing vascular compression do not form true vascular rings. The innominate artery may cause pulsatile compression of the anterior trachea, just proximal to the carina, or compression of the right main bronchus—such findings will be visible on bronchoscopy and the diagnosis confirmed by cross-sectional imaging [5]. In mildly affected individuals, a conservative approach is sufficient as symptoms may improve with growth. However, more severely affected children may require aortopexy with suspension of the innominate artery and ascending aorta to the undersurface of the sternum.

In a pulmonary artery sling, the left pulmonary artery does not originate from the main pulmonary artery, but from the posterior aspect of the right pulmonary artery, passing leftward between the oesophagus and the trachea. It may cause compression of the right main bronchus, the distal trachea, and occasionally the left main bronchus, as well as the anterior aspect of the oesophagus. Pulmonary artery slings are rare and may be associated with other severe congenital abnormalities in 58–83% of cases; 50% of patients also have concomitant malformations of the trachea and 50% have congenital heart disease [4]. This highlights the need for a thorough multidisciplinary assessment of such children, including cross-sectional imaging and direct airway evaluation. Surgical repair of a pulmonary artery sling is difficult; translocation of the anomalous left pulmonary artery may result in stenosis at the anastomotic site, and complex tracheal reconstruction may also be needed.

A cervical aortic arch is rare and is found when the arch rises abnormally high into the neck, above the level of the clavicle, potentially as high as C2. Around half of affected patients have a symptomatic vascular ring, which presents as a pulsatile mass in the supraclavicular fossa or neck [4].

Airway compression may also occur as a direct result of complex congenital heart disease itself. Although rare, it is an often under-recognized cause of respiratory symptoms. The trachea, carina, and left main bronchus are closely related to the left atrium, pulmonary arteries, and pulmonary veins. Therefore, conditions leading to dilatation of these cardiac structures may precipitate airway compromise [5]. Cardiac problems leading to pulmonary artery enlargement include tetralogy of Fallot with an absent pulmonary valve, large ventricular septal defects, atrioventricular septal defects, and patent ductus arteriosus. Significant left-to-right shunts and mitral stenosis or regurgitation may cause left atrial enlargement. Massive cardiomegaly resulting from cardiomyopathy, anomalous left coronary artery arising from the pulmonary artery (ALCAPA), or end-stage congestive heart failure may itself impact on the airways [4]. Finally, intraluminal bronchial obstruction may result from enlarged bronchial vessels or lymphatics due to raised cardiac filling pressures. Management of airway compression in the setting of congenital heart disease requires that the underlying cardiac defect be addressed, if possible. If not, patients may require long-term palliation with a tracheostomy and ventilatory support.

Management of lesions causing vascular compression of the airway requires a multidisciplinary approach with collaboration between ENT specialists, paediatric cardiologists, respiratory physicians, intensivists, and cardiothoracic surgeons. Surgical repair aims to divide the vascular ring, as detailed, or to suspend the offending vessel to relieve airway or oesophageal compression, whilst maintaining normal perfusion of the aortic arch [4]. Surgery usually is performed through a left posterolateral thoracotomy or, more recently, by video-assisted thoracoscopy (VATS) [3, 4, 10]. Determination of arch sidedness is a critical step in preoperative assessment and will direct the surgical approach. The main post-operative complication is damage to the recurrent laryngeal nerve, which lies close to the ligamentum arteriosum and the descending aorta, and resultant vocal cord paralysis. Chylothorax has also been reported [10].

Early surgery will minimize damage to the airway and permit normal tracheobronchial growth. The majority of patients are successfully extubated following surgery. It is important to remember that successful surgery may not immediately relieve the obstruction and a proportion of patients may continue to exhibit symptoms of tracheobronchomalacia for several months, e.g. around 30% of those treated for double aortic arch [4]. Bronchoscopy at the end of the surgical procedure will not only document vocal cord motion, but also assess any residual dynamic airway obstruction. A minority of patients may require ongoing ventilatory support until their airway cartilage matures and regains stiffness and their symptoms resolve. Occasionally, reconstruction of the affected airway segment may be required, particularly if there is concomitant tracheal stenosis.

The role of stenting to overcome airway malacia is controversial in the paediatric population. It is generally only indicated in palliative situations or where there is no alternative treatment option. Stent placement may be complicated by vascular erosion, stent fracture, blockage, or migration, all of which may worsen the situation, compared to pre-intervention status. De Trey et al. described a complication rate of 33%, with the most prevalent complication being stent fracture [11].

In conclusion, cardiovascular causes of paediatric airway compression are an often under-recognized diagnosis. Although they are much less common than other causes of stridor, chronic airway compression in childhood from vascular malformations carries significant morbidity and mortality. They are readily treatable and should not be overlooked. Clinical presentation is variable and a high index of suspicion should be maintained to avoid delay in diagnosis. Although the diagnosis may be suggested on chest X-ray, barium studies, or echocardiography, cross-sectional imaging is usually required for accurate delineation, along with bronchoscopy, to identify dynamic versus static airway obstruction.

A final word from the expert

This case neatly illustrates some pitfalls in diagnosis. The initial echocardiogram was performed when there was a low index of suspicion for a vascular ring. The patient was unsettled. The aortic arch and head and neck vessels were not adequately defined. On 99% of occasions, this will be OK because of the low incidence of vascular rings. This case underlines the importance of a patient's initial echocardiogram, systematically looking for, and commenting on, all structures. If this is not done, something will be missed at some point! Despite this, the gold standard for investigation and planning management for this patient group are a combination of cross-sectional imaging and bronchoscopy.

References

1. Licari A, Manca E, Rispoli GA, et al. Congenital vascular rings: a clinical challenge for the pediatrician. *Pediatr Pulmonol* 2015;50:511–24.
2. Valletta EA, Pregarz M, Bergamo-Andreis IA, et al. Tracheosophageal compression due to congenital vascular anomalies (vascular rings). *Pediatr Pulmonol* 1997;24:93–105.
3. Shah RK, Mora BN, Bacha E, et al. The presentation and management of vascular rings:an otolaryngology perspective. *Int J Pediatr Otorhinolar* 2007;71:57–62.
4. Kussman B, Geva T, McGowan F. Cardiovascular causes of airway compression. *Pediatr Anesth* 2004;14:60–74.
5. Javia L, Harris MA, Fuller S. Rings, slings and other tracheal disorders in the neonate. *Semin Fetal Neonatal Med* 2016;21:277–84.
6. Pickhardt PJ, Siegel MJ, Gutierrez FR. Vascular rings in symptomatic children: frequency of chest radiographic findings. *Radiology* 1997;203:423–6.
7. McLaren CA, Elliott MJ, Roebuck DJ. Vascular compression of the airway in children. *Paed Resp Rev* 2008;9:85–94.
8. Kellenberger CJ. Aortic arch malformations. *Pediatr Radiol* 2010;40:876–84.
9. McLaughlin RB Jr, Wetmore RF, Tavill MA, et al. Vascular anomalies causing symptomatic tracheobronchial compression. *Laryngoscope* 1999;109:312–19.
10. Kogon BE, Forbess JM, Wulkan M, et al. Video-assisted thoracoscopic surgery: is it a superior technique for the division of vascular rings in children. *Congenit Heart Dis* 2007;2:130–3.
11. De Trey LA, Dudley J, Ismail-Koch H, et al Treatment of severe tracheobronchomalacia: ten-year experience. *Int J Pediatr Otorhinolaryngol* 2016;83:57–62.

CASE

19 Coronary artery fistula

Sophie Duignan and Colm Breatnach

Expert commentary Damien Kenny

Case history

A 14-year-old male presented to the emergency department systemically unwell with pyrexia, cough, and arthralgia. On examination, he was found to be pale, with a 2/6 continuous murmur loudest over the left sternal edge. His liver was distended 2 cm below the right subcostal margin. Blood tests revealed a C-reactive protein (CRP) level of 270, and three separate blood cultures were positive for meticillin-sensitive *Staphylococcus aureus*, following which he was commenced on intravenous antibiotics and treated for sepsis.

An electrocardiogram (ECG) demonstrated normal sinus rhythm and an incomplete right bundle branch block (Figure 19.1). There was cardiomegaly, with patchy consolidation of both lungs on chest X-ray, as well as confluent consolidation of the left base and associated left pleural effusion. A computed tomography pulmonary angiogram (CTPA) (Figure 19.2) was performed due to increased work of breathing, cough, and desaturations, which revealed multiple cavitating nodules throughout both lung fields, representing septic emboli.

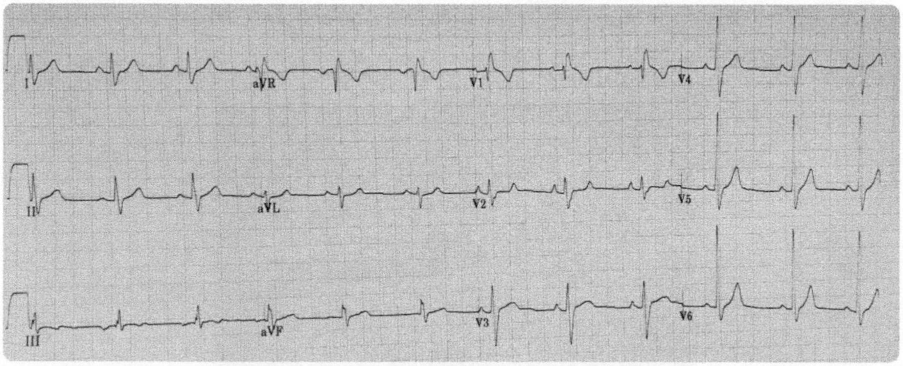

Figure 19.1 ECG demonstrating normal sinus rhythm with RSR in V1.

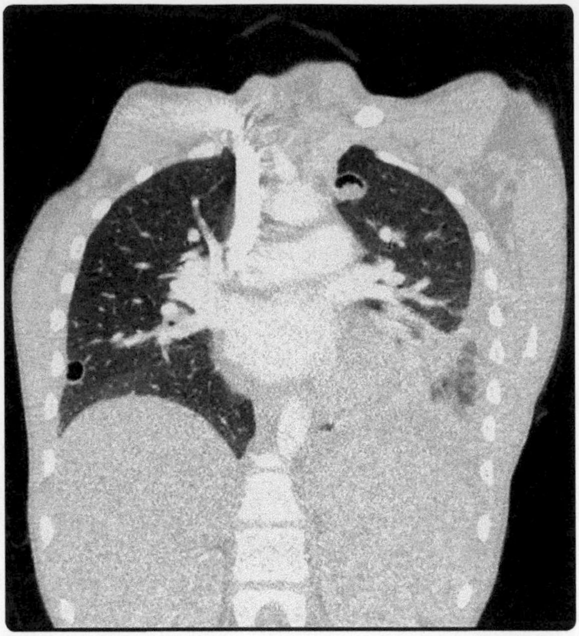

Figure 19.2 CTPA showing bilateral cavitating nodules representing septic emboli.

Echocardiography revealed a large (6cm × 2cm) pedunculated thrombus in the right atrium (Figure 19.3). There were no valvar vegetations. Additionally, there was proximal right coronary artery (RCA) dilatation (7 mm) and mild to moderate dilatation of the right heart, main pulmonary artery, and branch pulmonary arteries, suggestive of a coronary–cameral fistula from the RCA to the right atrium (RA) (see Learning point: Definition and types of coronary artery fistula, p. 249) (Figure 19.4). With the exception of a secundum atrial septal defect (ASD), the rest of the intracardiac anatomy was normal. The patient was at risk of cerebral emboli across the ASD. However, brain magnetic resonance imaging (MRI) scanning was performed and detected no abnormalities.

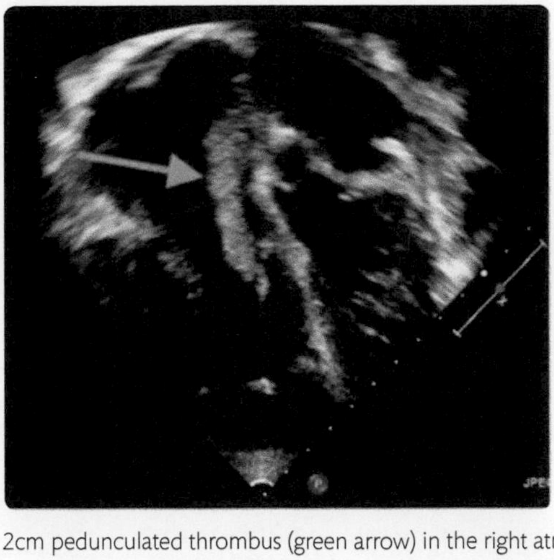

Figure 19.3 A 6cm × 2cm pedunculated thrombus (green arrow) in the right atrium on echocardiography.

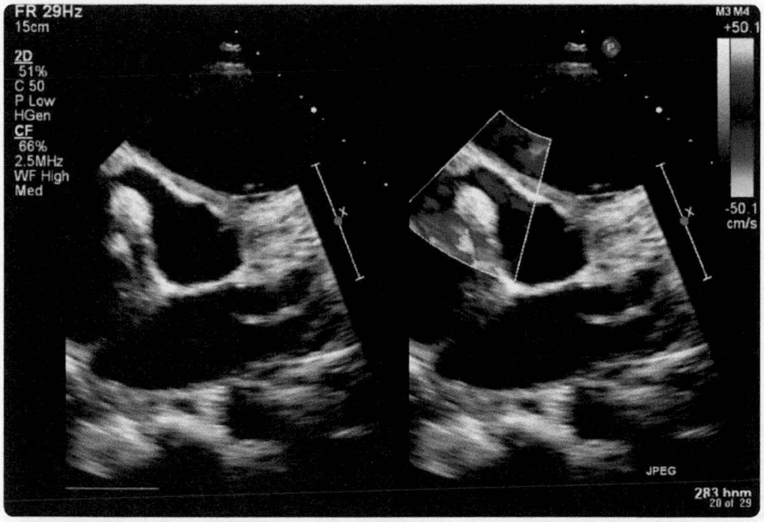

Figure 19.4 Echocardiography showing dilatation of the proximal right coronary artery on echocardiography.

Learning point Definition and types of coronary artery fistula

A coronary artery fistula is an abnormal connection that directly links one or more coronary arteries to a heart chamber or to major thoracic vessels without an interposed capillary bed [1]. Coronary artery anomalies can be divided into three categories, as per Greenberg et al.: anomalies of origin, anomalies of course, and anomalies of termination [2]. Coronary artery fistulae are considered anomalies of termination.

In addition, there are two main subtypes:

1. Coronary-cameral fistulae arise from a coronary artery and terminate into a chamber of the heart (usually the right side)
2. Coronary arteriovenous fistulae arise in a coronary artery and terminate into a vein.

The patient was slow to respond to intravenous antibiotics, and blood cultures taken 6 days after the start of treatment remained positive due to the septic nidus within the right atrium It was decided, following discussion with the haematology team, to initiate intravenous thrombolysis. He was transferred to the intensive care unit where tissue plasminogen activator was administered via a central line over 6 hours. Echocardiography post-thrombolysis demonstrated almost complete resolution of the thrombus.

The patient made a full recovery following a 6-week course of intravenous antibiotics. He also completed a 3-month course of low-molecular weight heparin injections. A repeat CTPA demonstrated resolution of the cavitating lesions.

The patient was discharged following a 6 week-long hospital stay on low-dose aspirin due to the history of right atrial thrombus. As infective endocarditis is an indication for coronary artery fistula closure, the patient underwent elective cardiac catheterization and transoesophageal echocardiography (TOE) a few months later. TOE showed a 16 mm × 18 mm inferior ASD, with an absent inferior vena cava (IVC) rim Selective right coronary angiography demonstrated a moderate-sized coronary artery fistula originating from the proximal right coronary artery and draining into the junction of the superior vena cava (SVC) and the RA (see Learning point: Morphology, p. 250) (Figure 19.5). The size of the fistula proximal to its exit to the RA measured 7 mm × 6 mm

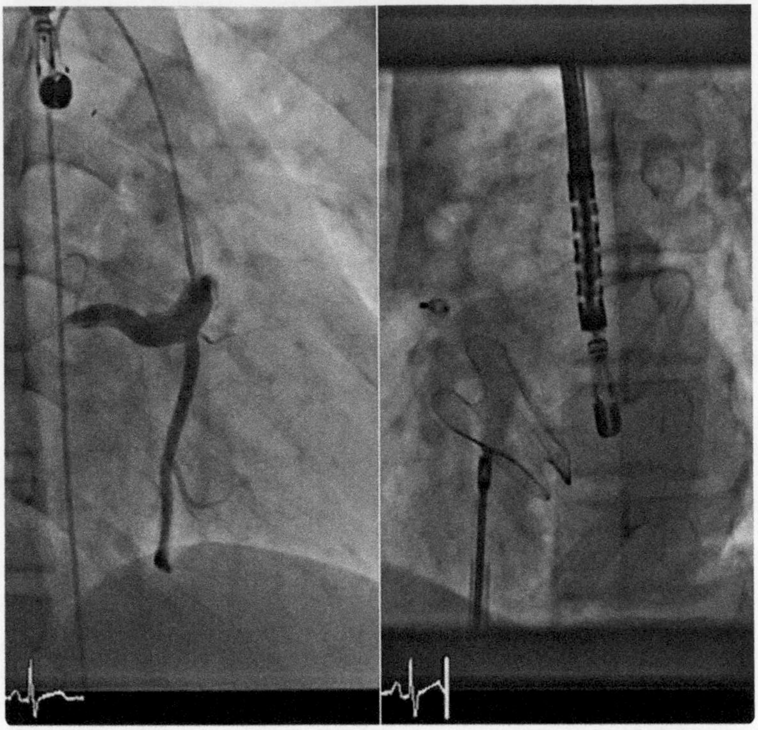

Figure 19.5 (a) Selective coronary angiography demonstrating a coronary artery fistula originating from the proximal right coronary artery. (b) AVP II device *in situ* in a coronary artery fistula.

Learning point Morphology

Coronary artery fistulae are defined as unilateral, bilateral, or multilateral, based on the number of donor coronary arteries. They are almost always unilateral (>90%). However, up to 7% are bilateral in the paediatric population [3]. The feeding artery of the fistula may drain from a main coronary artery or one of its branches. Just over half (50–60%) of coronary artery fistulae originate in the right coronary artery, 30% from the left anterior descending and the remaining 18% from the left circumflex [4–6]. Regardless of the point of origin, over 90% of fistulae drain into the right side of the heart; most frequently to the right ventricle (40%), followed by the right atrium, coronary sinus, and pulmonary trunk [4].

The fistula was crossed with a Terumo guidewire (Terumo Medical, Tokyo, Japan) from the coronary ostium and an arteriovenous guidewire loop was created. A 5-Fr-long delivery sheath was placed in the ascending aorta and a 10-mm Amplatzer™ Vascular Plug II (AVPII) (Abbott, IL, USA) was used to close the fistula; the proximal disc remained in the stump of the fistula and therefore did not protrude into the right coronary artery (Figure 19.5b). Following balloon sizing, the ASD was then closed with a 30-mm Occlutech Figulla Flex II device (Occlutech International AB, Helsingborg, Sweden). Although a deficiency of the IVC rim has traditionally been viewed as a contraindication to transcatheter device closure, recent data have shown the feasibility of this approach in the presence of a deficient posterior–inferior rim, the procedural success being related to the demonstration of an inferior indentation on the sizing balloon on lateral fluoroscopy [7]. Post-procedural echocardiography demonstrated both devices *in situ*, with no residual flow seen through the ASD. It was not possible to visualize the coronary artery fistula.

The patient was loaded with 300 mg each of aspirin and clopidogrel. He continued clopidogrel 75 mg once daily for 3 months and will continue on long-term aspirin at a dose of 75 mg once daily (see Learning point: Prevention of thrombosis following intervention, p. 251).

Learning point Prevention of thrombosis following intervention

Most centres use antithrombotic therapy to prevent thrombosis from extending from the coronary artery fistula into the coronary artery. Antiplatelet therapy is generally prescribed for approximately 6 months following the procedure; however, there is no consensus on this and some centres advocate the use of oral anticoagulation such as warfarin therapy.

Discussion

History of congenital artery fistula

The first description of a coronary artery fistula was made by the German anatomist Krause in 1865. A pathological account of this condition was not published until 1908 when Maude Abbott described this lesion. The first coronary artery fistula to undergo successful ligation was carried out by Bjork and Crafoord in 1947, but it was not until 1983 that a transcatheter approach was employed in the closure of one by Reidy et al. [8].

Incidence

There is an equal distribution of coronary artery fistulae in both sexes. The incidence is 0.002% among the general population [9] and 0.08–0.4% in the context of patients with congenital heart disease [10–14]. However, the true incidence is difficult to calculate due to the fact that approximately half are asymptomatic and, therefore, many are never diagnosed. An isolated congenital coronary artery fistula is considered as a major coronary artery malformation by Odgen's classification, and it represents 0.4% of all cardiac malformations [4].

Aetiology

The vast majority (80%) of coronary artery fistulae are congenital in origin and occur as an isolated defect in a structurally normal heart [15]. Congenital coronary artery fistulae may be due to the persistence of embryonic myocardial trabecular sinusoids [16]. Usually, myocardial sinusoids become narrowed and persist as Thebesian vessels in adults. However, if there is any interference in this process, a fistulous communication may persist between coronary arteries and a cardiac chamber. Fistulae that connect to the pulmonary artery are hypothesized to be the result of failure of involution of the aortopulmonary anlage [17]. Associated congenital cardiac anomalies have been reported in the literature in 5–30% of patients with coronary artery fistulae [18–21], including pulmonary atresia with an intact septum (see Clinical tip: Coronary artery fistula in pulmonary atresia with an intact septum, p. 251), tetralogy of Fallot, and both atrial and ventricular septal defects. Notably, our patient had an associated ASD.

Clinical tip Coronary artery fistula in pulmonary atresia with an intact septum

Coronary artery fistulae and right ventricular sinusoids are common in pulmonary atresia with an intact septum. They can be found in up to 50% of patients with a small hypertrophic subtype of pulmonary artery/intact septum and act as the only egress of blood. Right ventricular sinusoids are endothelial-lined channels within the myocardium that communicate with the right ventricular cavity. They are remnants of the sinusoidal spaces, which nourish the fetal myocardium. In this situation, the myocardium may have a right ventricle-dependent coronary circulation (10–20%), which must be established prior to attempted right ventricular decompression as a reduction in right ventricular pressures may be detrimental to myocardial perfusion [22].

Learning point Aetiology of iatrogenic coronary artery fistulae

Suspect if a new continuous murmur is audible post-operatively following:

- Heart transplant
- Mitral valve replacement
- Percutaneous coronary intervention
- Septal myectomy
- Permanent pacemaker insertion
- Transbronchial lung biopsy
- Closed chest ablations.

Iatrogenic fistulae should be suspected if there is a new continuous murmur audible post-operatively and have been reported following the procedures listed in Learning point: Aetiology of iatrogenic coronary artery fistulae, p. 252 [9, 23, 24]. Allen et al. reported that 95% of paediatric heart transplant recipients in a 100-patient cohort had non-cameral coronary artery fistulae detectable at first angiogram post-heart transplant. They drained predominantly into the ipsilateral pulmonary vasculature and correlated with graft ischaemic time. However, they were not associated with early graft loss or death. Traumatic fistulae can occur following penetrating or non-penetrating thoracic injuries and usually form a connection between the right coronary artery and the right chamber of the heart.

Pathophysiology

When a fistula drains into the right side of the heart (as in the majority of cases), the volume load is increased to the right heart and subsequently to the pulmonary vascular bed, the left atrium, and the left ventricle. Those that drain to the systemic veins or right atrium have a pathophysiology similar to an ASD, although volume loading occurs throughout the cardiac cycle, whilst those that drain to the pulmonary artery are haemodynamically similar to a patent ductus arteriosus. In contrast, fistulae draining to the left atrium cause volume loading similar to mitral regurgitation, and fistulae draining to the left ventricle are haemodynamically comparable to aortic regurgitation [25]. The degree of shunting is determined by the size of the fistula and the pressure gradient between the coronary artery and the chamber into which the fistula drains. Therefore, the largest shunts occur when the fistula drains into right-sided heart chambers (see Learning point: Complications, p. 252).

Learning point Complications

Complications of coronary artery fistulae include:

1. Impact of the shunt on the pulmonary circulation: moderate to large coronary artery fistulae with a distal anastomosis into the right cardiac structures may result in significant over-circulation of blood to the lungs and excessive venous return to the left atrium and ventricle. Ventricular dilatation and congestive cardiac failure may progress over time.
2. Effect of systemic steal: 'steal' of blood supply from the myocardium can result in myocardial ischaemia, arrhythmias, rupture, and infective endocarditis [5].
3. Specific complications to the coronary vasculature: include coronary artery dilatation, medial degeneration, aneurysm formation, calcification, side branch obstruction, and atherosclerosis. Thrombosis of the coronary artery fistula may occur with subsequent myocardial infarction and atrial or ventricular arrhythmias. Rupture of an aneurysmal fistula causing a haemo-pericardium has also been reported [26].

Clinical signs and symptoms

Our case study presented with infective endocarditis, an unusual complication in the setting of coronary artery fistula, occurring in approximately 1% of patients. It was relevant that the patient in our case study also had an ASD and a consequent risk for cerebral septic emboli.

Up to 79% of paediatric patients with coronary artery fistulae [3] are asymptomatic. In Said et al.'s cohort of 129 paediatric patients with coronary artery fistula, 8% presented with congestive heart failure, 8% with either chest pain or dyspnoea, 3% with palpitations, and 1.5% with infective endocarditis. Congestive heart failure tends to occur in neonates and infants in the setting of a large left-to-right shunt. The frequency of symptoms and complications associated with coronary artery fistulae increases with age, and in adults, it is common to present with exertional chest pain or dyspnoea. Angina may be due to coronary artery steal (see Clinical Tip: Symptoms in paediatric patients with coronary artery fistula, p. 253).

Investigation of a murmur is the most common presentation in the paediatric population. This is reported to be a continuous murmur in 54–69% of cases [3, 12, 27], and the main differential diagnosis is patent ductus arteriosus. However, the murmur is typically loudest at the left lower sternal edge, as opposed to beneath the left clavicle, and peaks in mid to late diastole, rather than systole. If the fistula terminates in the left ventricle, an early diastolic murmur, which mimics aortic insufficiency, may be heard (see Clinical tip: Murmur in coronary artery fistula (CAF), p. 253) (Table 19.1).

Clinical tip Symptoms in paediatric patients with coronary artery fistula

- Asymptomatic (80%)
- Congestive heart failure (8%)
- Chest pain or dyspnoea (8%)
- Palpitations (3%)
- Infective endocarditis (1.5%)

Clinical tip Murmur in coronary artery fistula

Table 19.1 Murmurs in coronary artery fistulae

Type of CAF	Murmur	Mimic
Haemodynamically insignificant CAF to right-sided heart chamber or vessel	Systolic murmur	Flow murmur, innocent murmur
Haemodynamically significant CAF to right-sided chamber or vessel	Continuous murmur	Patent ductus arteriosus
CAF terminating in left ventricle	Early diastolic murmur	Aortic insufficiency

CAF, coronary artery fistula.

Diagnosis

Basic investigations, such as ECG and chest X-ray, are usually unhelpful in making the diagnosis. An ECG may show volume overload or occasionally ischaemic changes. In our case, the ECG showed normal sinus rhythm with a complete right bundle branch block. A chest X-ray may show cardiomegaly or pulmonary congestion if the fistula drains to the right side of the heart. If the patient is old enough to undergo exercise stress testing, ischaemic ST changes may become apparent; however, this is more commonly seen in the adult population [28]. Our patient did not undergo exercise stress testing (see Clinical tip: Investigations in coronary artery fistula, p. 254).

Echocardiography

Echocardiography and colour Doppler flow techniques are extremely sensitive for the diagnosis of coronary artery fistulae. Echocardiography may show a dilated cardiac chamber and dilatation of the proximal segment of the involved coronary artery. Colour Doppler demonstrates abnormally high-velocity flow signal in the fistula and at its entry point.

A continuous-wave (CW) Doppler signal is seen when the entry site is into the right heart, pulmonary arteries, or left atrium [29]. However, if the entry point is the left ventricle, high-speed blood flow signals are only seen during diastole due to high left ventricular systolic pressures. Mild functional tricuspid regurgitation may be seen due to right heart volume overload. Smaller coronary artery fistulae are more difficult to detect, as there may be no dilatation of the affected coronary or the cardiac chambers with just high-velocity flow signals observed near the fistula. Advantages of echocardiography as a mode of diagnosis include the fact that it is non-invasive and inexpensive and has no side effects. It also accurately shows ventricular dilatation, abnormal ventricular wall motion, and decreased systolic function (see Learning point: First-line method for diagnosis, p. 254).

Cardiac catheterization

Catheterization with coronary angiography is considered the gold standard for diagnosis. It directly visualizes the morphology of the coronary arteries and their branches, the course of the coronary artery fistula and its connections with heart chambers or vessels. It is, however, invasive and expensive, and it carries the risks for exposure to both ionizing radiation and nephrotoxic contrast dye.

Radiological imaging

Multi-detector CT with reconstruction has been used as a non-invasive technique. Low-radiation CT scans and MRI scans can accurately delineate the anatomy of a fistula, as well as assess its haemodynamic relevance (see Expert Comment, p. 254).

Learning point First-line method for diagnosis

A recent paper reviewed the echocardiograms of 63 patients with coronary artery fistulae who had undergone catheterization and/or surgery [29]. Echocardiography correctly identified the diagnosis in over 95% of patients, and there was no statistically significant difference in diagnostic accuracy between echocardiogram and coronary arteriography. The authors recommended echocardiography as the first-line method for diagnosis of coronary artery fistulae.

Clinical tip Investigations in coronary artery fistula

(See Table 19.2.)

Table 19.2 Investigations in coronary artery fistulae

Basic investigations	ECG—volume overload, ischaemic changes Chest X-ray—cardiomegaly Exercise stress test—ischaemic changes
Imaging	Echocardiography—first line CT with reconstruction—superior to MRI Cardiac MRI
Interventional	Catheterization with coronary angiography

Learning point Antenatal diagnosis

Coronary artery fistulae may be diagnosed accurately antenatally. Sharland et al. reported five cases where the diagnosis was made between 19 and 22 weeks' gestation by cross-sectional and colour Doppler echocardiography. Signs of a coronary artery fistula on antenatal echocardiography include an abnormal jet of blood flow draining into one of the cardiac chambers, dilatation of the feeding coronary artery, cardiomegaly, and reversal of flow in the ascending aorta and transverse arch. In four of the cases, there was significant progression in size of the fistula during fetal life. Two cases developed congestive heart failure soon after birth and required early transcatheter closure. The authors suggested that prenatal presence of cardiomegaly and to-and-fro flow in the aorta were good predictors of congestive cardiac failure soon after birth.

Expert comment

The temporal and spatial resolution of CT is superior to MRI, and therefore, CT would be the imaging modality of choice. Its increasing use may eventually decrease the need for invasive diagnostic coronary angiography. However, coronary angiography may provide superior assessment of anatomical nuances to determine the suitability for transcatheter closure.

Management

The natural history of isolated congenital coronary artery fistulae is poorly defined. Both spontaneous regression and sudden death have been reported; therefore, the management of coronary artery fistulae in children is controversial and includes conservative, medical, catheterization, and surgical approaches.

Generally accepted indications for closure include volume overload, left ventricular dysfunction, evidence of myocardial ischaemia, and previous episode of infective endocarditis (see Clinical tip: American Heart Association guidelines, p. 255).

Expert comment Deciding to close a coronary artery fistula

An important point when considering interventional closure of a coronary artery fistula is the fact that some fistulae may recede with time. Therefore, in an asymptomatic child with a small, haemodynamically insignificant coronary artery fistula, an observant conservative approach may be appropriate.

Clinical tip American Heart Association guidelines

The 2011 American Heart Association (AHA) scientific statement for cardiac catheterization in paediatric cardiac disease recommends transcatheter occlusion for patients with symptomatic coronary artery fistulae, as a Class 1 recommendation.

There is a Class 2a recommendation based on Level C evidence, which states occlusion is also reasonable for patients with a moderate or large coronary artery, even without clinical symptoms.

Finally, there is a Class 3 recommendation that occlusion is not recommended for clinically insignificant coronary artery fistulae [30].

Some groups advocate for early closure of congenital artery fistulae in childhood, regardless of symptoms, due to the high incidence of complications and development of symptoms in adolescence and adulthood [31]. A review of 174 patients by Liberthson et al. found, in those aged ≥20 years with congenital artery fistula, 55% were symptomatic and 63% had complications [11]. Others, however, adopt a more conservative approach. This is considered a reasonable option in paediatric patients more often than in adults, as the likelihood of spontaneous closure is higher, reportedly as high as 20–39% [32]; coronary artery fistulae are also more likely to be asymptomatic in children and less likely to cause complications. Symptoms and complications in patients ≤20 years were found in 9% and 19%, respectively, in the same review by Liberthson et al. (see Expert comment: Deciding to close a coronary artery fistula, p. 255).

Surgical management

Surgical obliteration of coronary artery fistulae is performed via median sternotomy and achieved by direct suture or path closure. Ligation may be safely performed without cardiopulmonary bypass in the majority of cases, particularly when the fistula represents the termination of a coronary artery branch. The approach may be epicardial or intracardiac and transcoronary, transcameral, or transpulmonary. Intraoperatively, temporary occlusion with ECG monitoring is performed to prevent myocardial ischaemia after ligation.

Recanalization is unfortunately a problem, particularly with epicardial ligation, and therefore, patients require careful follow-up. Other complications include arrhythmias, ischaemic electrocardiographic changes, stroke, and thrombosis of the parent coronary artery. Overall morbidity and mortality from surgical ligation in children approaches zero [3, 33]. However, the rate of surgical complications increases with age in adult patients, and for this reason, some centres advocate early intervention, regardless of symptoms (see Expert comment: When to consider a surgical approach, p. 255).

Learning point Beating heart endoscopic coronary artery surgery

Advances in minimally invasive thoracic surgery over the past two decades have led to cases of closed-chest beating heart endoscopic coronary artery surgery in adults [34, 35]. These patients did not require intensive care stay post-operatively and none of the three reported suffered from early post-operative complications. This technology has the potential to revolutionize the management of coronary artery fistulae, particularly in the asymptomatic patient.

Expert comment When to consider a surgical approach

A surgical approach may be favoured over a transcatheter approach for large-sized fistulae with multiple communications, for diffuse or multiple fistulae, if the feeding coronary artery is very tortuous, or if the heart has an anomaly that will require concomitant repair. Patient size is also a factor in the paediatric population. It is preferable to perform transcatheter closure once the patient has reached 10 kg, as it is a technically easier procedure, although successful closure in smaller symptomatic infants has been reported. In addition, if the feeding coronary artery gives rise to branches near the drainage site, there is a risk for the occlusion device compromising distal flow.

Learning point Complications of transcatheter occlusion

- Retrograde coronary artery thrombosis
- Coronary artery spasm or dissection
- Myocardial ischaemia and infarction
- Device migration
- Tricuspid valve injury
- Residual flow
- Failure of procedure
- Late recanalization

Transcatheter management

Increasingly, transcatheter closure of coronary artery fistulae is carried out as an alternative to surgical closure. Advantages of closure via cardiac catheterization include avoidance of cardiopulmonary bypass and quicker post-procedural recovery.

The approach can be retrograde arterial, antegrade venous, or retrograde arterial after creation of an arteriovenous loop. Early procedures favoured detachable balloons; however, plugs, duct occluders, and coils are now the devices of choice for fistula occlusion. In patients with tortuous fistulae, a microcatheter may be used to cross the distal part of the fistula and facilitate the placement of microcoils. Selective coronary angiography is performed to delineate the anatomy of the fistula and its drainage site and to identify distal coronary branches and post-procedurally to assess the presence of residual flow and coronary perfusion. Sometimes temporary balloon occlusion with distal angiography is necessary to ensure all distal coronary branches have been identified.

Complications include retrograde coronary artery thrombosis, dissection, or coronary spasm and may result in persistent ischaemic changes on ECG and myocardial infarction. Device migration and tricuspid valve injury may also occur. The main complication in the peri-procedural period is myocardial ischaemia. This occurs more frequently with distal coronary artery fistulae. Residual flow may, in some cases, necessitate re-intervention. This is usually detectable in the early post-procedural period; however, late recanalization may also occur. Failure of the procedure may occur if the fistula is very large, if the vessel is tortuous, or if the distal coronary artery branches are near the fistula drainage site due to occlusion of branch flow by the device (see Learning Point: Complications of transcatheter occlusion, p. 256).

The largest paediatric cohort published to date of patients who have undergone transcatheter coronary artery fistula occlusion included 61 patients and had an incomplete occlusion rate of 21% [36].

Follow-up post-closure

Patients require long-term follow-up after an intervention to close a coronary artery fistula. In general, large, complete long-term follow-up studies are lacking and efforts are ongoing to create an international registry. Echocardiography is used to assess for residual shunt, late recanalization, and evidence of ischaemia (regional wall motion abnormalities, decreased left ventricular systolic function). Generally, the affected coronary artery diameter significantly reduces in the long term, following catheter occlusion of the fistula.

Learning point Beta-blocker therapy in coronary artery fistula

A recent case report described successful resolution of multiple congenital coronary artery–left ventricle microfistulae with treatment with propranolol over the course of 6 months at a dose of 2 mg/kg/day [37]. The authors highlighted the potential use of propranolol in diffuse congenital coronary artery fistulae where surgical or catheter intervention is not an option.

Conclusions

High-resolution modern echocardiography is leading to increasing diagnosis of coronary artery fistulae that, in the past, may have been undiagnosed due to a lack of clinical symptoms.

The majority of paediatric patients with small coronary artery fistulae are asymptomatic and are unlikely to develop complications in the first two decades of life. Also many small fistulae undergo spontaneous closure. However, the likelihood of symptoms and complications increases with increasing age, as does the rate of interventional morbidity and mortality. Therefore, elective closure of clinically apparent lesions is generally advocated in children.

A final word from the expert

This is a rare and heterogenous lesion with the potential to regress through childhood. Indications to intervene should be clear, as consequences of coronary artery thrombosis are potentially catastrophic. Detailed pre-procedural imaging to facilitate a complete understanding of the anatomy and a strategic approach, along with collaboration with adult coronary interventionalists, will increase the potential for a successful outcome. Results from an international registry evaluating long-term outcomes are eagerly awaited to guide future management.

References

1. Ashraf SS, Shaukat N, Fisher M, Clarke B, Keenan DJ. Bicoronary-pulmonary fistulae with coexistent mitral valve prolapse: a case report and literature review of coronary-pulmonary fistula. *Eur Heart J* 1994;15:571–4.
2. Greenberg MA, Fish BG, Spindola-Franco H. Congenital anomalies of the coronary arteries. Classification and significance. *Radiol Clin North Am* 1989;27:1127–46.
3. Said SA, Lam J, van der Werf T. Solitary coronary artery fistulas: a congenital anomaly in children and adults. A contemporary review. *Congenit Heart Dis* 2006;1:63–76.
4. Dodge-Khatami A, Mavroudis C, Backer CL. Congenital Heart Surgery Nomenclature and Database Project: anomalies of the coronary arteries. *Ann Thorac Surg* 2000;69(4 Suppl):S270–97.
5. Qureshi SA. Coronary arterial fistulas. *Orphanet J Rare Dis* 2006;1:51.
6. Tiryakioglu SK, Gocer H, Tiryakioglu O, Kumbay E. Multiple coronary-cameral fistulae. *Tex Heart Inst J* 2010;37:378–9.
7. Papa M, Gaspardone A, Fragasso G, et al. Feasibility and safety of transcatheter closure of atrial septal defects with deficient posterior rim. *Catheter Cardiovasc Interv* 2013;81:1180–7.
8. Reidy JF, Sowton E, Ross DN. Transcatheter occlusion of coronary to bronchial anastomosis by detachable balloon combined with coronary angioplasty at same procedure. *Br Heart J* 1983;49:284–7.
9. Luo L, Kebede S, Wu S, Stouffer GA. Coronary artery fistulae. *Am J Med Sci* 2006;332:79–84.
10. Farooki ZQ, Nowlen T, Hakimi M, Pinsky WW. Congenital coronary artery fistulae: a review of 18 cases with special emphasis on spontaneous closure. *Pediatr Cardiol* 1993;14:208–13.
11. Liberthson RR, Sagar K, Berkoben JP, Weintraub RM, Levine FH. Congenital coronary arteriovenous fistula. Report of 13 patients, review of the literature and delineation of management. *Circulation* 1979;59:849–54.
12. Wong KT, Menahem S. Coronary arterial fistulas in childhood. *Cardiol Young* 2000;10:15–20.
13. Burch GH, Sahn DJ. Congenital coronary artery anomalies: the pediatric perspective. *Coron Artery Dis* 2001;12:605–16.
14. Mavroudis C, Backer CL, Rocchini AP, Muster AJ, Gevitz M. Coronary artery fistulas in infants and children: a surgical review and discussion of coil embolization. *Ann Thorac Surg* 1997;63:1235–42.
15. Wilde P, Watt I. Congenital coronary artery fistulae: six new cases with a collective review. *Clin Radiol* 1980;31:301–11.
16. Mangukia CV. Coronary artery fistula. *Ann Thorac Surg* 2012;93:2084–92.
17. Heifetz SA, Robinowitz M, Mueller KH, Virmani R. Total anomalous origin of the coronary arteries from the pulmonary artery. *Pediatr Cardiol* 1986;7:11–18.
18. Hobbs RE, Millit HD, Raghavan PV, Moodie DS, Sheldon WC. Coronary artery fistulae: a 10-year review. *Cleveland Clinic Quarterly* 1982;49:191–7.
19. Gillebert C, Van Hoof R, Van de Werf F, Piessens J, De Geest H. Coronary artery fistulas in an adult population. *Eur Heart J* 1986;7:437–43.
20. Upshaw CB, Jr. Congenital coronary arteriovenous fistula. Report of a case with an analysis of seventy-three reported cases. *Am Heart J* 1962;63:399–404.

21. Wang S, Wu Q, Hu S, et al. Surgical treatment of 52 patients with congenital coronary artery fistulas. *Chin Med J* 2001;114:752–5.
22. Hanley FL, Sade RM, Blackstone EH, Kirklin JW, Freedom RM, Nanda NC. Outcomes in neonatal pulmonary atresia with intact ventricular septum. A multiinstitutional study. *J Thorac Cardiovasc Surg* 1993;105:406–23, 24–7; discussion 23–4.
23. Chiu SN, Wu MH, Lin MT, Wu ET, Wang JK, Lue HC. Acquired coronary artery fistula after open heart surgery for congenital heart disease. *Int J Cardiol* 2005;103:187–92.
24. Allen KY, Goldstein BH, Pahl E, et al. Non-cameral coronary artery fistulae after pediatric cardiac transplantation: a multicenter study. *J Heart Lung Transplant* 2012;31:744–9.
25. Latson LA. Coronary artery fistulas: how to manage them. *Catheter Cardiovasc Interv* 2007;70:110–16.
26. Bauer HH, Allmendinger PD, Flaherty J, Owlia D, Rossi MA, Chen C. Congenital coronary arteriovenous fistula: spontaneous rupture and cardiac tamponade. *Ann Thorac Surg* 1996;62:1521–3.
27. Schumacher G, Roithmaier A, Lorenz HP, et al. Congenital coronary artery fistula in infancy and childhood: diagnostic and therapeutic aspects. *Thorac Cardiovasc Surgeon* 1997;45:287–94.
28. Oshiro K, Shimabukuro M, Nakada Y, et al. Multiple coronary LV fistulas: demonstration of coronary steal phenomenon by stress thallium scintigraphy and exercise hemodynamics. *Am Heart J* 1990;120:217–19.
29. Xie M, Li L, Cheng TO, et al. Coronary artery fistula: comparison of diagnostic accuracy by echocardiography versus coronary arteriography and surgery in 63 patients studied between 2002 and 2012 in a single medical center in China. *Int J Cardiol* 2014;176:470–7.
30. Feltes TF, Bacha E, Beekman RH, 3rd, et al. Indications for cardiac catheterization and intervention in pediatric cardiac disease: a scientific statement from the American Heart Association. *Circulation* 2011;123:2607–52.
31. Sunder KR, Balakrishnan KG, Tharakan JA, et al. Coronary artery fistula in children and adults: a review of 25 cases with long-term observations. *Int J Cardiol* 1997;58:47–53.
32. Welisch E, Norozi K, Burrill L, Rauch R. Small coronary artery fistulae in childhood: a 6-year experience of 31 cases in a tertiary paediatric cardiac centre. *Cardiol Young* 2016;26:738–42.
33. Yim D, Yong MS, d'Udekem Y, Brizard CP, Konstantinov IE. Early surgical repair of the coronary artery fistulae in children: 30 years of experience. *Ann Thorac Surg* 2015;100:188–94.
34. Watanabe G, Takahashi M, Misaki T, Kotoh K, Doi Y. Beating-heart endoscopic coronary artery surgery. *Lancet* 1999;354:2131–2.
35. Nishida S, Watanabe G, Ishikawa N, Kikuchi Y, Takata M, Ushijima T. Beating-heart totally endoscopic coronary artery bypass grafting: report of a case. *Surg Today* 2010;40:57–9.
36. Mottin B, Baruteau A, Boudjemline Y, et al. Transcatheter closure of coronary artery fistulas in infants and children: a French multicenter study. *Catheter Cardiovasc Interv* 2016;87:411–18.
37. Hernandez M, Carretero JM, Prada F. Propranolol as a treatment for multiple coronary artery micro-fistulas. *Cardiol Young* 2015;25:380–3.

CASE

20 Arrhythmias in congenital heart disease

Alexander Van De Bruaene and Shouvik Haldar

Expert commentary Krishnakumar Nair

Case history 1

A 45-year-old female presented to the emergency department with a 24-hour history of palpitations. She described the palpitations as a faster heart rate, regular and associated with shortness of breath on exertion and dizziness, but no syncope. Apart from palpitations, mild exercise intolerance with shortness of breath on exertion, and dizziness, she did not report chest discomfort, lower limb oedema, or orthopnoea.

The patient had a past medical history of transposition of the great arteries, for which she underwent a Mustard operation in 1972. In terms of heart function, she had moderate dilatation of the subaortic right ventricle, with moderate systolic dysfunction and moderate to severe tricuspid valve regurgitation. She underwent dual-chamber pacemaker implantation for sick sinus syndrome 4 years ago. She had previous intra-atrial re-entry tachycardia in 2011 and 2014, requiring DC cardioversion and overdrive pacing, respectively. She was a lifelong non-smoker, drank alcohol and coffee occasionally and had no other relevant history of note. Her chronic medications included aspirin 75 mg once daily (od), candesartan 8 mg od, and bisoprolol 10 mg od.

Learning point Transposition of the great arteries and Mustard operation

Transposition of the great arteries represents 3–7% of congenital heart diseases [1]. In patients with transposition of the great arteries, there is atrioventricular (AV) concordance and ventriculo-arterial discordance, with the pulmonary and systemic circulations connected in parallel, rather than in series. Following birth and after closure of the ductus arteriosus, survival depends on mixing of both circulations—either naturally [presence of an atrial or a ventricular septal defect or patent ductus arteriosus (PDA)] or interventionally (Blalock–Hanlon atrial septectomy or Rashkind balloon atrial septostomy). Almost all patients underwent repair with an atrial switch procedure (Senning or Mustard operation) or an arterial switch procedure (Jatene procedure) or Rastelli repair.

Our patient underwent an atrial switch operation in which blood is redirected at the atrial level using baffles made of Dacron or the pericardium (Mustard operation) (Figure 20.1) or atrial flaps (Senning operation). Hence systemic venous return is redirected through the mitral valve into the subpulmonary morphological left ventricle, and pulmonary venous blood is redirected through the tricuspid valve into the morphological right ventricle [2].

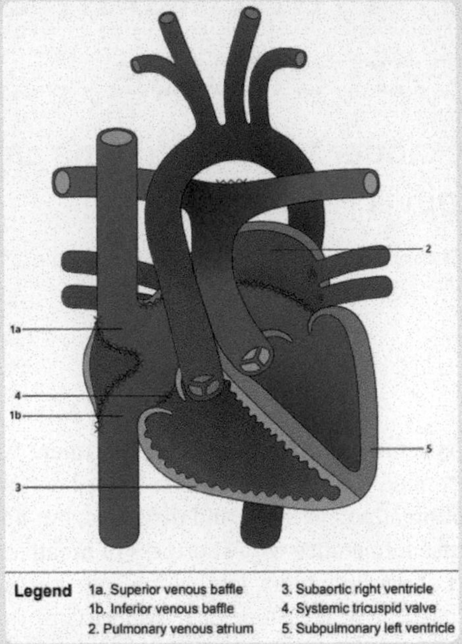

Figure 20.1 Transposition of the great arteries and Mustard operation. 1a, superior venous baffle; 1b, inferior venous baffle; 2, pulmonary venous atrium; 3, subaortic right ventricle; 4, systemic tricuspid valve; 5, subpulmonary left ventricle.

On arrival, the patient was haemodynamically stable. She was evaluated by an emergency doctor who conducted a thorough history-taking and examination, ordered a chest X-ray (CXR), an electrocardiogram (ECG), and routine blood work. Her blood pressure on admission was 90/50 mmHg, with a heart rate of 100 bpm. Her oxygen saturation was 99% on room air. She had a normal first heart sound, with a narrowly split second heart sound and a grade 2/6 pan-systolic murmur best heard at the left lower sternal border and at the apex. Chest auscultation was clear to the bases bilaterally. The jugular venous pressure (JVP) was not elevated, and there was no evidence of lower limb oedema (Table 20.1).

Table 20.1 Routine blood results and observations in the emergency department

Haematology		Biochemistry		Observations	
Hb	136 g/l	Na	141 mmol/l	BP	90/50 mmHg
WCC	8.6 × 10^9/l	K	4.5 mmol/l	Saturations	99% RA
Platelets	206 × 10^9/l	Creat	90 μmol/l	Temperature	36.5°C
INR	1.01	GFR	66 ml/min/kg		
		TSH	1.92 mIU/l		
		BNP	179 pg/ml		

BNP, brain natriuretic peptide; BP, blood pressure; Creat, creatinine; GFR, glomerular filtration rate; Hb, haemoglobin; INR, international normalized ratio; K, potassium; Na, sodium; RA, room air; TSH, thyroid-stimulating hormone; WCC, white cell count.

The postero-anterior and lateral CXRs on presentation are depicted in Figure 20.2. In the emergency department, her ECG was initially interpreted as sinus tachycardia (Figure 20.3).

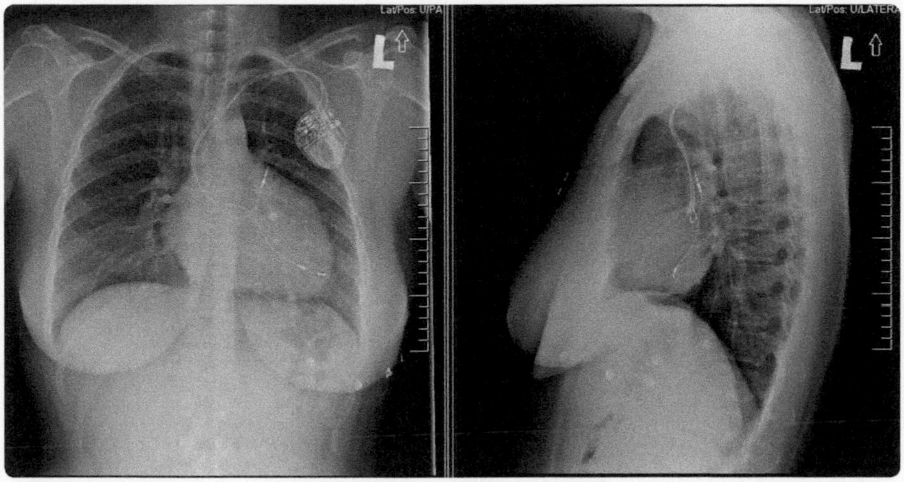

Figure 20.2 Postero-anterior and lateral CXRs on presentation. There is situs solitus based on the branching pattern of the bronchi, with a long, late-bifurcating left bronchus and a shorter, early-bifurcating right bronchus. The apex of the heart points to the left (levocardia). A narrow vascular pedicle with an oblong cardiac silhouette was noted (egg-on-its-side), which is common in patients who underwent atrial switch procedure [2]. The atrial pacemaker lead is located in the pulmonary venous baffle, whereas the ventricular lead is located in the subpulmonic morphological left ventricle.

(a)

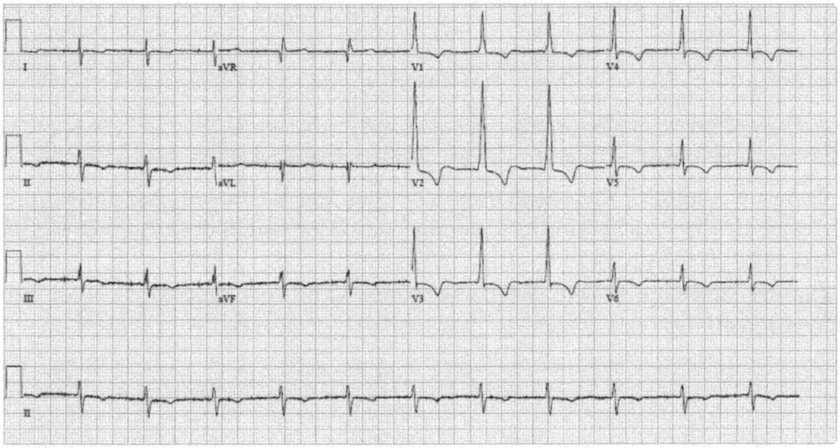

Figure 20.3 Continued

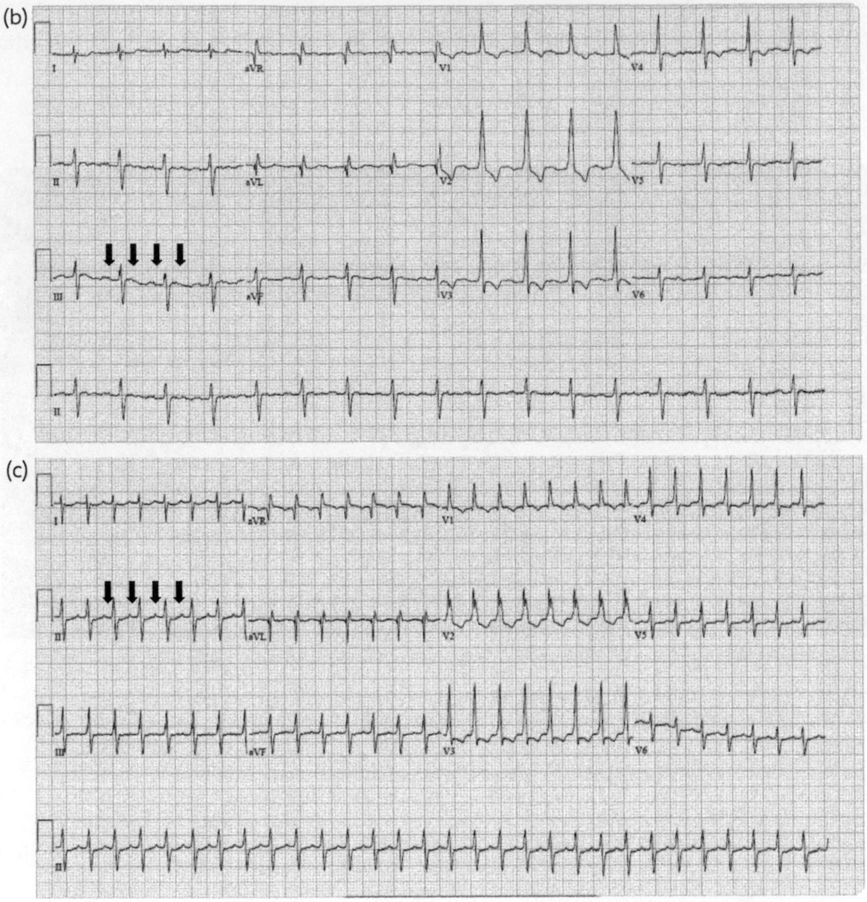

Figure 20.3 (a) A 12-lead ECG on the patient's last clinic visit. The patient is atrially paced. There is right ventricular hypertrophy, with a QRS duration of 112 ms, and T wave inversion in V1–V4. (b) A 12-lead ECG on presentation in the emergency department. There is intra-atrial re-entry tachycardia with 2:1 conduction and ventricular rate of 103 bpm. (c) A 12-lead ECG when the patient was not feeling well in the emergency department. There is regular narrow complex tachycardia at 181 bpm.

Review of the ECG on presentation indicated that the patient had intra-atrial re-entry tachycardia (IART) with a 2:1 conduction (cycle length of the circuit 300 ms or an atrial rate of 200 bpm).

She was started on low-molecular weight heparin, according to her body weight (enoxaparin 60 mg every 12 hours).

A few hours after being admitted to the emergency department, the patient suddenly felt unwell and was diaphoretic, hypotensive, and tachycardic. Her heart rate was 181 bpm, with a blood pressure of 70/40 mmHg. Her ECG showed a narrow complex tachycardia with a ventricular rate of 181 bpm (Figure 20.3c). She responded well to an intravenous (IV) bolus of metoprolol 5 mg and her heart rate slowed down to 100 bpm.

Clinical tip Comparison with previous ECGs

In patients with transposition of the great arteries who have undergone an atrial switch procedure, IART is the most common atrial arrhythmia. Its presentation on ECG is variable and can often be misinterpreted as sinus rhythm. Careful evaluation and comparison of atrial activity with previous ECGs (when the patient was in sinus rhythm) often show the diagnosis.

Learning point Transposition of the great arteries post-atrial switch procedure—a preload-dependent circulation

Derrick et al. performed an elegant study, published in 2000, evaluating the haemodynamic responses to exercise and dobutamine stress in patients after the Mustard operation to assess determinants of exercise limitation in this patient population. One of the most intriguing findings was that stroke volume fell with increasing heart rate (decreased diastolic filling time). As there was no evidence of systolic or diastolic dysfunction, impaired capacitance and conduit function of the baffles are the most likely explanation for exercise limitation. Therefore, the absence of atria (which have been replaced with baffles) will limit ventricular filling and decrease cardiac output, and may eventually cause cardiac arrest in patients post-atrial switch procedure [3]. Therefore, patients with a preload-dependent circulation (such as Fontan patients lacking a subpulmonary ventricle, as well as patients with transposition of the great arteries following an atrial switch procedure) should be monitored closely when they present with an atrial arrhythmia and a fast ventricular response.

Expert comment

One of the challenges in the management of these patients is the actual recognition of atrial arrhythmia. As discussed, comparison with the sinus rhythm ECG is critical. Subtle changes in QRS morphology could indicate flutter waves overlapped on the QRS. One should look for flutter waves in transition zones like at the onset of tachycardia and in zones with a change in ventricular rate, as in areas with AV block.

A transoesophageal echocardiogram was conducted which excluded intracardiac thrombi, allowing to proceed to DC cardioversion. Cardioversion was successful using one shock at 200 J biphasic. As her last atrial arrhythmia was 2 years ago, she was continued on bisoprolol 10 mg od. Since she had a complex congenital heart defect, she was started on warfarin, with a target international normalized ratio (INR) of 2.0–4.0. Her CHA2DS2Vasc score and HASBLED score were 0.

Learning point Assessment of stroke (CHA2DS2-Vasc) and bleeding (HASBLED) risk in patients with atrial fibrillation

The CHA2DS2-Vasc score assigns 1 point to congestive heart failure, hypertension, age 65–74 years, diabetes mellitus, vascular disease (aortic plaque, prior myocardial infarction, peripheral artery disease), and female gender. Two points are assigned if age is ≥75 years or if there is a history of stroke, transient ischaemic attack, or thromboembolism [4]. The HASBLED score, on the other hand, estimates bleeding risk and assigns 1 point for the presence of each of the following: hypertension (uncontrolled systolic blood pressure >160 mmHg), abnormal renal and/or liver function, previous stroke, bleeding history or predisposition, labile INR, elderly, and concomitant drugs and/or alcohol excess [5].

The use of both scores can help the clinician in estimating stroke and bleeding risk in, as well as the indication for anticoagulant therapy and management of, patients with atrial fibrillation.

However, the CHA2DS2-Vasc and HASBLED scores have not been validated in patients with congenital heart disease.

Expert comment

Patients may also remain asymptomatic in atrial flutter with AV block at baseline, and may become symptomatic only with a 1:1 AV conduction. Therefore, one cannot rely on the time of onset of atrial flutter from the patient history alone. This has implications in deciding on the need for a transoesophageal echocardiogram prior to cardioversion.

Over the course of the next 2 months, she was admitted four times with a recurrence of IART. Unfortunately, despite adding amiodarone to her therapy, she continued to have recurrences of her atrial arrhythmia.

Finally, she underwent successful radiofrequency ablation of the atrial arrhythmia. She underwent baffle puncture with mapping of the pulmonary venous baffle. Two separate circuits, one at a cycle length of 440 ms (atrial rate of 136 bpm) and one at 620 ms (atrial rate of 97 bpm), were identified and successfully ablated.

Expert comment

The arrhythmia substrate for atrial arrhythmias following atrial switch surgery (Mustard or Senning) for classic transposition of the great arteries may be partially or completely based in the pulmonary venous atrium (PVA). Access to the PVA may be obtained via different techniques:

1. Retrograde transaortic approach: this involves the catheter traversing multiple turns and bends, and catheter stability is sometimes an issue.
2. Stereotaxis: catheter navigation is much easier; however, multielectrode mapping with a PentaRay® catheter is not feasible.
3. Baffle puncture: both catheter stability and multielectrode mapping are possible; the puncture itself may be technically challenging and often requires serial balloon dilatations and sometimes even a radiofrequency wire or a cutting balloon.

Discussion

Atrial arrhythmias are common in patients with congenital heart disease. An epidemiological study indicated a 15% prevalence of atrial arrhythmias in patients with congenital heart disease, with 50% of patients having complex congenital heart disease developing atrial arrhythmias by the age of 65 [6]. Cavo-tricuspid isthmus-dependent flutter is common, but IART involving areas of slow conduction from fibrosis around atriotomy scars or patches is even more common [7].

In patients with transposition of the great arteries who underwent an atrial switch procedure, both brady- and tachyarrhythmias are common [6]. Hardly any patients with Mustard or Senning repair remain in reliable sinus rhythm 10 years after surgery [8, 9], and the presence of a pacemaker has been related with increased mortality in long-term follow-up [10]. On the other hand, patients are also predisposed to develop atrial tachyarrhythmias, which occur in 10–30% of patients over 10–20 years of follow-up [8, 11].

Current management is based on the management of atrial arrhythmias in the general population [7]. On admission, anticoagulation is started to prevent thromboembolic complications and a beta-blocker can be added for rate control. Usually, patients who underwent an atrial switch procedure do not tolerate atrial arrhythmias and a more aggressive approach towards rhythm control is adopted. When considering cardioversion, there is a low threshold for transoesophageal echocardiography or gated cardiac tomography to exclude intracardiac thrombi. Unless the patient is haemodynamically unstable, cardioversion should be performed in an environment with the ability to externally pace (risk of bradycardia in the setting of sinus node dysfunction) or resuscitate (haemodynamic compromise due to ventricular or fast atrial tachycardia).

After the initial management, a medium- and long-term management plan should be discussed in terms of anti-arrhythmic medication and anticoagulation. In the case of a first episode, the patient is usually started on a beta-blocker. In the case of recurrence, other options have to be discussed. In terms of medical management, there is limited evidence in patients with congenital heart disease. Sotalol has been shown to be moderately effective in patients with congenital heart disease [12], although it should be used cautiously as these patients have a structurally abnormal heart and often have systolic dysfunction of the subaortic ventricle. Amiodarone is usually more effective [13], but its use is hampered by the risk for non-cardiac toxicities in young patients.

Interestingly, a recent study evaluated the risk of thromboembolic events and the value of established risk scores (CHADS2 and CHA2DS2-Vasc) in patients with congenital heart disease. Whereas both the CHADS2 and CHA2DS2-Vasc scores were low, giving a misleading assessment of the thromboembolism risk, the occurrence of a thromboembolic event was mainly related to the complexity of the underlying defect. This is not surprising, given that the CHADS2 and CHA2DS2-Vasc scores were derived from non-congenital populations which are inherently different (in terms of the underlying complexity of anatomy and younger age of the patients). Therefore, the study supports current guidelines that long-term anticoagulation is indicated in adults with severe complexity of the underlying congenital heart defect [13].

Expert comment

Though sotalol is used extensively in patients with no significant structural heart disease, the safety of this medication in adult congenital heart disease has been questioned in a meta-analysis of 12 clinical trials. The authors showed that all-cause mortality doubles with sotalol [12, 14–16]. As such, use of sotalol has a Class IIB indication (level of evidence B) in the maintenance of sinus rhythm in atrial arrhythmias with congenital heart disease [13].

Although important progress has been made, ablation of IART in patients who underwent the atrial switch procedure remains challenging because of the complexity of post-surgical atrial anatomy [17]. Essentially, the Mustard operation divides the two atria into a systemic venous baffle and a pulmonary venous baffle. Often, right atrial tissue, surgical scarring, and part of the cavo-tricuspid isthmus are located within the pulmonary venous baffle and therefore require a trans-septal puncture of the atrial baffle in order to successfully ablate the arrhythmia.

Ablation in these complex congenital hearts is time-consuming and requires significant expertise to conduct the transbaffle puncture, to manipulate catheters around complex anatomy, and to collect and assimilate large numbers of activation points to understand complex scar-related arrhythmia circuits. Compared to the retrograde, transaortic approach, the antegrade technique via a transbaffle puncture is preferred as it allows more precise catheter manipulation. Furthermore, these patients often have significant biventricular dysfunction, so it is important to minimize time under sedation and/or general anaesthesia, and multielectrode mapping may provide one way to shorten the procedural time.

Finally, it is important to consider that the presence of atrial arrhythmias in patients who underwent an atrial switch procedure is related with ventricular dysfunction in patients with transposition of the great arteries and atrial switch procedure [11] and may be a marker of sudden cardiac death [18]. Clinical, radiographic, and echocardiographic evaluation to exclude heart failure is crucial. Brain natriuretic peptide may be elevated due to the presence of arrhythmia but could also indicate a decline in overall haemodynamic status of the patient. In patients older than 40 years, diagnostic catheterization to evaluate intracardiac pressures and the presence/absence of pulmonary hypertension in patients with transposition of the great arteries who underwent an atrial switch procedure is indicated.

A final word from the expert

Atrial arrhythmias occur commonly during the natural history of post-atrial switch patients. Recognition of atrial arrhythmias may be difficult. Comparison with sinus rhythm ECGs is important. Patient history may not be reliable in identifying the precise time of onset of atrial flutter since patients may be asymptomatic in chronic 2:1 atrial flutter and become symptomatic only with 1:1 conduction. The unique challenge to catheter ablation in post-Mustard and Senning patients is access to the pulmonary venous atrium. Different techniques are available. Our preference is the baffle puncture technique, which allows use of automated algorithms permitting rapid multielectrode mapping and also affords catheter stability.

Case history 2

A 50-year old gentleman with a past medical history of tetralogy of Fallot, who underwent surgical repair [pulmonary valvectomy, infundibulectomy, and ventricular septal defect (VSD) closure] in 1972, was seen in the outpatient clinic. In 2014, he presented with a type 2 AV block (Möbitz II) on ECG (Figure 20.4). Holter monitoring indicated intermittent AV block with a broad QRS escape rhythm, episodes of sinus arrest, and non-sustained ventricular tachycardia (VT). He eventually underwent cardiac resynchronization therapy defibrillator (CRT-D) implantation in 2014, as he had reduced left ventricular (LV) systolic function and a broad right bundle branch block (RBBB), with a QRS duration of 194–200 ms, in addition to intermittent AV block and non-sustained VT.

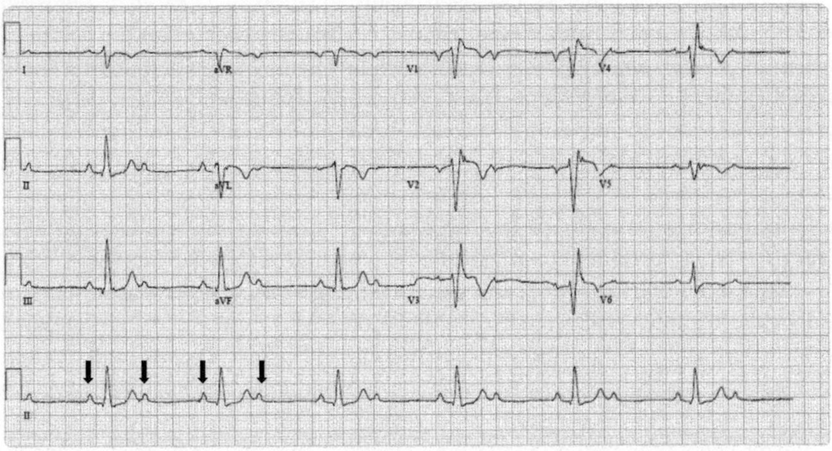

Figure 20.4 On 12-lead ECG, there is 2:1 AV block with two P waves for every conducted QRS complex. Conducted QRS complexes have a broad right bundle branch block morphology with a QRS duration of 196 ms. Right bundle branch block is probably the result of a combined effect of surgical injury on the myocardium and right bundle branch and of right ventricular enlargement.

Learning point Tetralogy of Fallot

Tetralogy of Fallot is the most common form of cyanotic congenital heart disease, occurring in three in every 1000 live births. It is the result of an antero-cephalad deviation of the developing outlet ventricular septum, in combination with hypertrophied septoparietal trabeculations, resulting in right ventricular outflow tract (RVOT) obstruction. The deviation of the outlet septum is responsible for the malalignment VSD and overriding of the aorta, and the RVOT obstruction will result in hypertrophy of the right ventricle [2].

Clinical management is guided by the degree of RVOT obstruction and the preference of the centre for the timing of surgical intervention. In patients with insufficient pulmonary blood flow, a palliative procedure to secure pulmonary blood flow whilst awaiting complete repair may be performed. Palliative shunts include the modified Blalock–Taussig shunt, which almost always involves an interposition prosthetic tube from the subclavian artery to the ipsilateral pulmonary artery. Shunts close to the pulmonary bifurcation are sometimes known as a central shunt. The Waterston and Potts shunts (ascending aorta to right pulmonary artery and descending aorta to left pulmonary artery, respectively) are rarely performed in the current or recent era. During early infancy, an alternative to the palliative shunt is percutaneous stenting of the RVOT and the main pulmonary artery and/or stenting of the arterial duct.

Complete repair involves closure of the VSD and relief of the RVOT obstruction (resection of infundibular muscle, RVOT ± pulmonary artery patch or transannular patch) [2].

Expert comment

Cardiac resynchronization therapy (CRT) is a Class I indication in adults with CHD with a systemic LV ejection fraction of ≤35%, sinus rhythm, New York Heart Association (NYHA) class II–IV (ambulatory) symptoms, and complete RBBB, with a QRS complex of ≥150 ms (spontaneous or paced) [13].

Indications for CRT have also been extended to patients with a systemic right ventricle and a single ventricle. In addition, even patients with a narrow QRS and an anticipated requirement for significant (>40%) pacing may benefit from CRT.

Learning point Risk and risk factors for sudden cardiac death in patients with tetralogy of Fallot

The incidence of sudden cardiac death in patients with tetralogy of Fallot has been estimated to be between 0.5% and 6.0%, with most events related to sustained VT [19]. Although risk stratification remains problematic, several clinical risk factors for sudden cardiac death have been identified (Table 20.2). Surgical scars related to the ventriculotomy allow for macro-re-entrant pathways in the right ventricle, although right ventricular (RV) remodelling with ventricular dilation and increased wall stress is also a contributor.

Table 20.2 Risk factors associated with sudden cardiac death in patients with tetralogy of Fallot (factors present at the time of ICD implantation in our patient are highlighted in red)

Older age at time of repair [20]	Severe RV enlargement [21]
Prior large palliative shunts [22]	Depressed LV function [21, 23]
Older age [22]	High-grade ventricular ectopy on Holter or exercise testing
Recurrent syncope	Prolonged QRS duration (>180 ms) [9]
Pulmonary regurgitation [8]	Positive electrophysiological study [24]
Depressed RV function [21, 23]	Atrial arrhythmia [23]

The patient was doing well from a cardiovascular perspective without exercise limitation, shortness of breath, palpitations, or syncope when he had two implantable cardioverter–defibrillator (ICD) shocks while skating in December 2015. On clinical examination, he had a mild RV heave, a grade 2/6 systolic ejection murmur, and an early decrescendo diastolic murmur on the left upper parasternal border. His blood pressure was slightly elevated at 144/92 mmHg. Chest auscultation was clear and the JVP not elevated, and there was no lower limb oedema On pacemaker interrogation, device and lead function was normal. He was atrial-paced 16% of the time and biventricular-paced 99% of the time. There was monomorphic VT detected with antitachycardia pacing before charging. A first 36 J shock accelerated the VT, whilst the second 40 J shock terminated the VT. A strip of his pacemaker interrogation and his ECG are shown in Figure 20.5, and his chest X-ray in Figure 20.6. His blood work was unremarkable (Table 20.3).

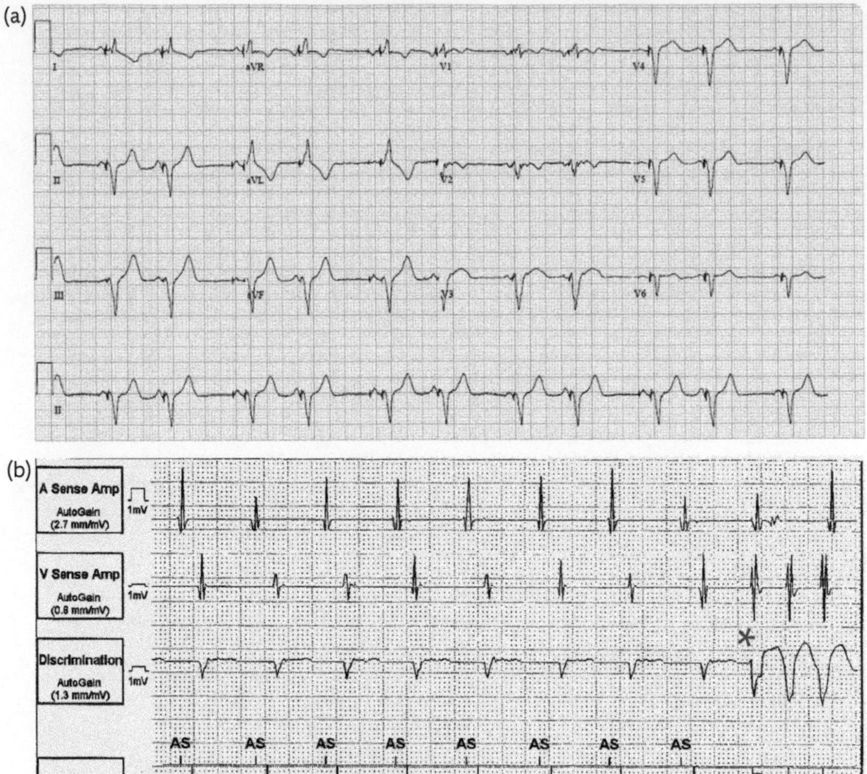

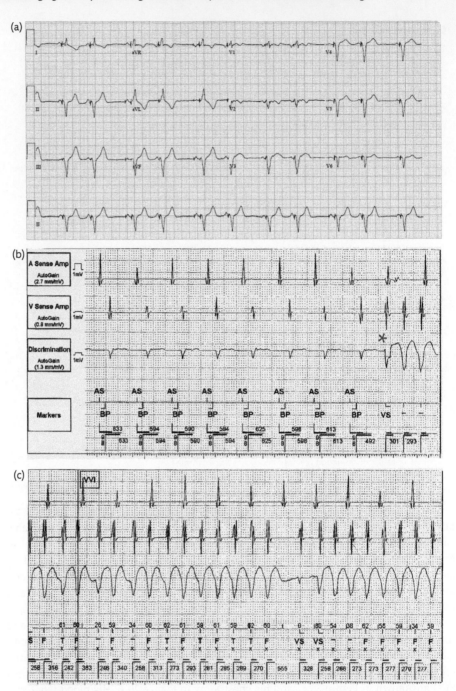

Figure 20.5 Continued

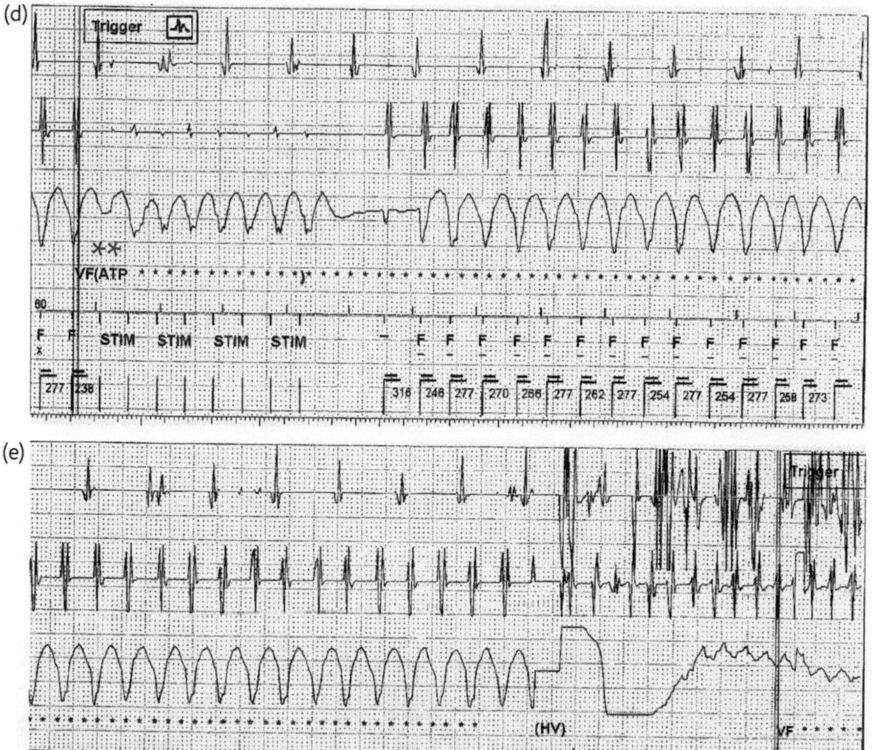

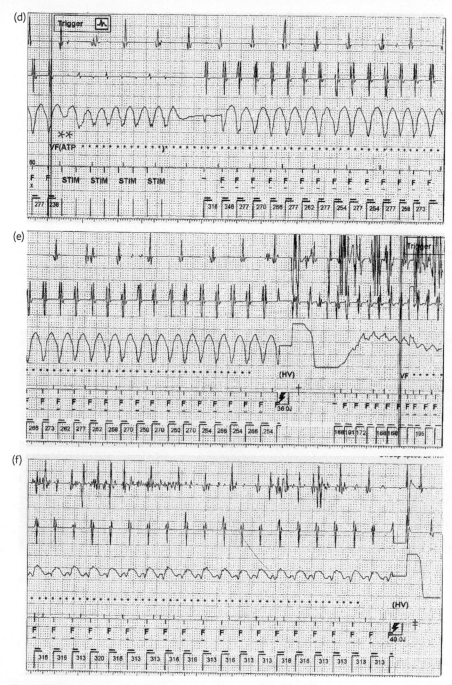

Figure 20.5 Continued

(g)

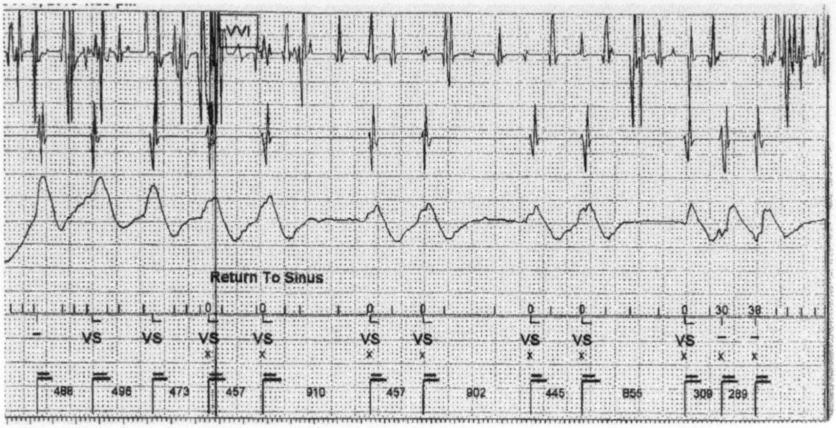

Figure 20.5 In (a), a 12-lead ECG indicates atrial sensing with biventricular pacing. Note that the QRS duration has shortened, when compared to the ECG prior to CRT implantation. In (b), the pacemaker strip indicates initiation of sustained ventricular tachycardia (more V signals than A signals) at 218 bpm, cycle length 275 ms (*), failed anti-tachycardic pacing (**), failed first DC shock at 36 J (†) with the patient going into ventricular fibrillation, and successful second DC shock at 40 J (‡) with return to sinus rhythm.

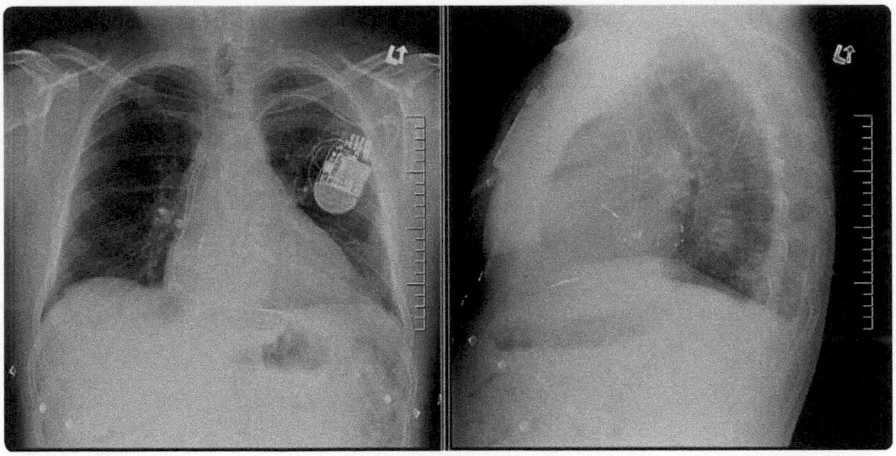

Figure 20.6 Postero-anterior and lateral CXRs. There is situs solitus based on the branching pattern of the bronchi, with a long, late-bifurcating left bronchus and a shorter, early-bifurcating right bronchus. The apex of the heart points to the left (levocardia). There is enlargement of the right ventricular silhouette and cardiomegaly. There is a pacemaker battery in the left subclavian position, with leads in the right atrium and right ventricle and to the left ventricle.

Table 20.3 Routine blood results and observations in the emergency department

Haematology		Biochemistry		Observations	
Hb	153 g/l	Na	141 mmol/l	BP	144/92 mmHg
WCC	8.0 × 10^9/l	K	4.6 mmol/l	Saturations	98% RA
Platelets	203 × 10^9/l	Creat	80 µmol/l	Temperature	36.0°C
INR	0.97	GFR	89 ml/min/kg		
		TSH	6.75 mIU/l		

BP, blood pressure; Creat, creatinine; GFR, glomerular filtration rate; Hb, haemoglobin; INR, international normalized ratio; K, potassium; Na, sodium; RA, room air; TSH, thyroid-stimulating hormone; WCC, white cell count.

Clinical tip Auscultation

Careful clinical examination, including auscultation, may already provide all, or part of, the information that further imaging will demonstrate.

His echocardiogram indicated a normal-sized left ventricle, with mild to moderately decreased LV systolic function. His right ventricle was severely enlarged, with moderately reduced RV systolic function. Aortic, mitral, and tricuspid valves indicated only minor regurgitation. There was mild to moderate pulmonary valve regurgitation, without evidence of pulmonary valve stenosis. Although pulmonary regurgitation appeared to be mild to moderate on echocardiography, cardiac magnetic resonance (CMR) imaging completed in November 2014 revealed progressive RV dilatation [RV end-diastolic volume index (RVEDVi) 171 ml/m^2 from 159 ml/m^2) with a moderate degree of pulmonary valve regurgitation (Figure 20.7). His case was presented at the multidisciplinary conference, and it was decided to proceed with surgical intervention with peri-procedural ablation (progressive RV dilatation, moderate pulmonary regurgitation, and VT).

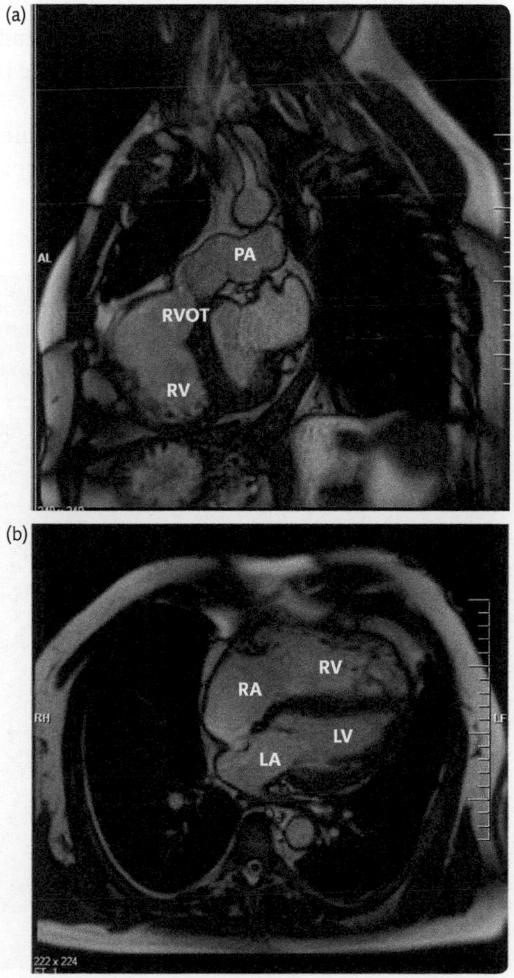

Figure 20.7 In (a), a sagittal oblique view parallel to the RVOT and proximal pulmonary artery. An ECG-gated cine SSFP image indicates patency of the RVOT and main pulmonary artery, the presence or absence of pulmonary valve tissue, wall motion abnormalities, and a qualitative assessment of the degree of pulmonary regurgitation. PA, pulmonary artery; RV, right ventricle; RVOT, right ventricular outflow tract. In (b), a four-chamber view indicating a severely enlarged right ventricular end-diastolic volume. End-diastolic volume, indexed for body surface area, was estimated at 171 ml/m^2. LA, left atrium; LV, left ventricle; RA, right atrium; RV, right ventricle.

Learning point CMR and tetralogy of Fallot

CMR imaging has become a cornerstone in the evaluation of patients with tetralogy of Fallot. CMR is the gold standard for accurate quantitative assessment of RV and LV volumes, mass, and ejection fraction. It also provides information on the degree of pulmonary regurgitation, the pulmonary-to-systemic flow ratio, and the anatomy of the RV outflow tract and pulmonary arteries.

Usually CMR is repeated every 3 years, unless indicated otherwise clinically.

Learning point Electrophysiological study in tetralogy of Fallot

The electrophysiological study is a popular method thought to be helpful for risk stratification in patients with tetralogy of Fallot. Inducible sustained VT has been shown to be an independent risk factor for VT/sudden cardiac death, with reasonable sensitivity but low specificity [24]. It is insufficiently predictive to be recommended as a screening tool for all patients with repaired tetralogy of Fallot but should be reserved for patients with additional risk factors [13].

Expert comment

The diagnostic and predictive value of electrophysiological testing has been proven to be of value in risk-stratifying patients following tetralogy of Fallot repair in a multi-centre trial [24]. The value of the VT induction study is greatest in those at moderate risk of sudden death [25]. The invasive ventricular stimulation protocol at our centre is performed at two drive cycle lengths of 400 ms and 600 ms from the RV apex, with five ventricular extra stimuli down to the ventricular effective refractory period or 200 ms, depending on whichever occurs later. Those with inducible VT receive an ICD. Those who do not develop inducible VT do not receive an ICD, unless they had presented with haemodynamically unstable VT.

He underwent an electrophysiological study prior to surgery. Programmed ventricular pacing induced two different monomorphic VTs. Subsequently, the anatomy of the right ventricle was delineated; specifically the VSD patch and the pulmonary valve were tagged. Scars were demonstrated in the infundibular patch and in the VSD patch area. Areas of late potentials were predominantly located near the borders of the scar and between the VSD patch and inferior to the pulmonary valve. An ablation line was performed between the pulmonary valve and the VSD patch (Figure 20.8), which was the most common critical isthmus seen in our intraoperative mapping experience and in previously published studies.

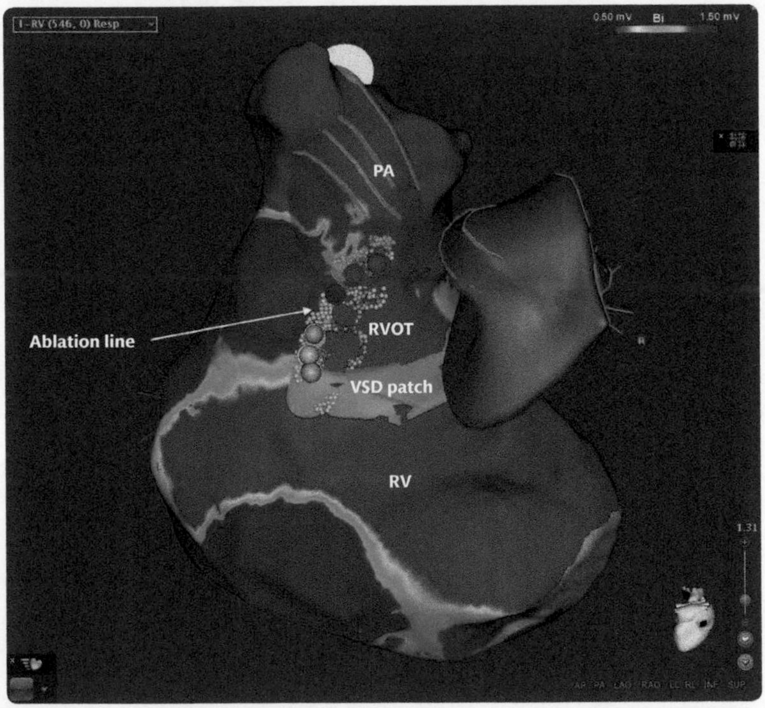

Figure 20.8 Three-dimensional electroanatomical CARTO map showing postero-anterior view of the ablation line conducted between the pulmonary valve and the VSD patch. The infundibular patch is not seen clearly here, as it is on the anterior aspect of the right ventricular outflow tract. PA, pulmonary artery; RV, right ventricle; RVOT, right ventricular outflow patch; VSD patch, ventricular septal defect patch.

Learning point Critical isthmuses in repaired tetralogy of Fallot patients

The four most common isthmuses in repaired tetralogy of Fallot include the following (Figure 20.9):

- Isthmus 1—bordered by the tricuspid annulus and a previous RV incision/RVOT patch
- Isthmus 2—between previous RV incision and the pulmonary valve
- Isthmus 3—bordered by the pulmonary valve and VSD patch
- Isthmus 4—bordered by the VSD patch and tricuspid annulus.

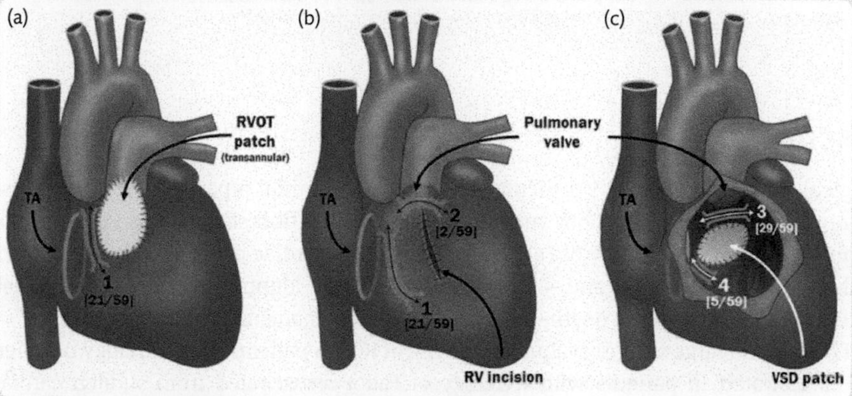

Figure 20.9 Critical isthmuses in repaired tetralogy of Fallot patients.
Reproduced from Kapel, G., Reichlin, T., Wijnmaalen, A., Re-Entry Using Anatomically Determined Isthmuses (A Curable Ventricular Tachycardia in Repaired Congenital Heart Disease), *Circulation: Arrhythmia and Electrophysiology*. 2015;8:102–109, with permission from Wolters Kluwer.

Expert comment

Though polymorphic ventricular arrhythmias may occur in tetralogy of Fallot, monomorphic VT is the most common VT in tetralogy of Fallot and has been shown to involve a distinct number of critical pathways. Catheter ablation is therefore feasible. Activation mapping is performed for haemodynamically tolerated VT. In haemodynamically unstable VT, the arrhythmia is terminated with overdrive pacing or cardioversion, and substrate mapping and catheter ablation of anatomic isthmuses in sinus rhythm are performed. Cryoablation with or without intraoperative mapping at the time of pulmonary valve replacement is a strategy that has been used effectively at the University Health Network in Toronto.

Based on the maps provided by the electrophysiology team, cryoablation lesion sets targeting all four critical isthmuses using the −160°C argon cryoablation probe were made. The patient underwent pulmonary valve replacement with a 29-mm bioprosthetic valve, and the anterior outflow tract was reconstructed with bovine pericardium.

Since his operation, the patient is doing clinically well, with no recurrences of the arrhythmia.

Learning point Ventricular arrhythmias in congenital heart disease

Ventricular arrhythmias are an important cause of late morbidity and mortality in the growing population of adults with repaired congenital heart disease. The majority of these ventricular arrhythmias are fast, monomorphic, and thereby life-threatening VT. Small studies have demonstrated that the VT substrate in repaired congenital heart disease often includes anatomic isthmuses that can be transected by radiofrequency catheter ablation, with favourable outcome. Recent data showed that in a large group of repaired congenital heart disease patients, transection of VT-associated anatomic isthmuses by radiofrequency catheter ablation was feasible in 74% of the patients and was highly effective in preventing VT recurrence during long-term follow-up.

In selected patients with repaired congenital heart disease, with preserved LV and RV function and anatomic isthmus-dependent re-entry VT in whom other ventricular arrhythmia mechanisms are unlikely, isthmus ablation may be reasonable as an alternative therapy to ICDs which do not prevent ventricular arrhythmias and are frequently associated with device-related complications and inappropriate therapy in repaired congenital heart disease [26].

Discussion

Surgical scarring related to ventriculotomy during the initial repair, as well as adverse RV remodelling with dilatation, ventricular stretch, and fibrosis, forms a substrate for VT in patients with tetralogy of Fallot. Hence, sudden cardiac death is a major concern in this patient population and—although studies have identified several clinical risk factors for sudden cardiac death—risk stratification remains difficult.

There are no large studies evaluating the use of ICD in patients with tetralogy of Fallot. ICD is indicated in patients with tetralogy of Fallot resuscitated from sudden cardiac death and in those with spontaneous sustained VT, after a careful workup to exclude reversible causes [27]. In primary prevention, ICD therapy is indicated if LV ejection fraction of ≤35% and NYHA classes II–III [13]. ICD therapy is reasonable in selected patients with multiple risk factors, as listed in Table 20.2, or in patients with unexplained syncope and inducible haemodynamically significant VT at electrophysiological study [18].

Pulmonary valve regurgitation is a classic late complication after tetralogy of Fallot repair, with a significant proportion of patients requiring pulmonary valve replacement at some point during follow-up [28]. The indication and timing of pulmonary valve replacement in asymptomatic patients remain a matter of controversy [29]. Progressive RV dilatation secondary to pulmonary valve regurgitation will increase wall stress and cause electrical instability. Pulmonary valve replacement will result in less pulmonary regurgitation, RV volume unloading, and RV reverse remodelling. Although there is a general consensus with regard to this approach, it remains difficult to assess how efficient pulmonary valve replacement is in reducing arrhythmia burden [30]. It has been suggested that pulmonary valve replacement with cryoablation is more effective in reducing arrhythmia burden post-operatively [31].

Although acute success rate for catheter ablation is now approximately 90%, there is a significant recurrence rate after ablation, estimated at around 18% [32]. Therefore, VT ablation is mainly reserved to reduce the number of appropriate shocks in patients who have already received an ICD for the prevention of sudden cardiac death.

A final word from the expert

CRT has emerged as an important therapeutic option in congenital heart disease. In patients without transvenous access to the systemic ventricle, an epicardial lead may have to be implanted.

Patients who have had ventriculotomies remain at risk for late ventricular arrhythmias. Re-entrant monomorphic VT seems to be the dominant ventricular arrhythmia in tetralogy of Fallot with four identifiable critical isthmuses. These could be targeted by activation mapping during VT and by substrate mapping in sinus rhythm. Catheter ablation may be limited by complexities of the anatomy, and surgical cryoablation remains an option, especially in patients who undergo pulmonary valve replacement.

References

1. Moons P, Sluysmans T, De Wolf D, et al. Congenital heart disease in 111 225 births in Belgium: birth prevalence, treatment and survival in the 21st century. *Acta Paediatr* 2009;98:472–7.
2. Gatzoulis M, Swan L, Therrien J, Panteley G. *Adult Congenital Heart Disease: A Practical Guide.* Oxford: Blackwell Publishing, 2005.
3. Derrick GP, Narang I, White PA, et al. Failure of stroke volume augmentation during exercise and dobutamine stress is unrelated to load-independent indexes of right ventricular performance after the Mustard operation. *Circulation* 2000;102:III154–9.
4. Lip GY, Nieuwlaat R, Pisters R, Lane DA, Crijns HJ. Refining clinical risk stratification for predicting stroke and thromboembolism in atrial fibrillation using a novel risk factor-based approach: the Euro Heart Survey on atrial fibrillation. *Chest* 2010;137:263–72.
5. Pisters R, Lane DA, Nieuwlaat R, de Vos CB, Crijns HJ, Lip GY. A novel user-friendly score (HAS-BLED) to assess 1-year risk of major bleeding in patients with atrial fibrillation: the Euro Heart Survey. *Chest* 2010;138:1093–100.
6. Bouchardy J, Therrien J, Pilote L, et al. Atrial arrhythmias in adults with congenital heart disease. *Circulation* 2009;120:1679–86.
7. Darby AE, Dimarco JP. Management of atrial fibrillation in patients with structural heart disease. *Circulation* 2012;125:945–57.
8. Hayes CJ, Gersony WM. Arrhythmias after the Mustard operation for transposition of the great arteries: a long-term study. *J Am Coll Cardiol* 1986;7:133–7.
9. Flinn CJ, Wolff GS, Dick M, 2nd, et al. Cardiac rhythm after the Mustard operation for complete transposition of the great arteries. *N Engl J Med* 1984;310:1635–8.
10. Vejlstrup N, Sorensen K, Mattsson E, et al. Long-term outcome of Mustard/Senning correction for transposition of the great arteries in Sweden and Denmark. *Circulation* 2015;132:633–8.
11. Gatzoulis MA, Walters J, McLaughlin PR, Merchant N, Webb GD, Liu P. Late arrhythmia in adults with the mustard procedure for transposition of great arteries: a surrogate marker for right ventricular dysfunction? *Heart* 2000;84:409–15.
12. Miyazaki A, Ohuchi H, Kurosaki K, Kamakura S, Yagihara T, Yamada O. Efficacy and safety of sotalol for refractory tachyarrhythmias in congenital heart disease. *Circ J* 2008;72:1998–2003.
13. Khairy P, Van Hare GF, Balaji S, et al. PACES/HRS expert consensus statement on the recognition and management of arrhythmias in adult congenital heart disease: developed in partnership between the Pediatric and Congenital Electrophysiology Society (PACES) and the Heart Rhythm Society (HRS). Endorsed by the governing bodies of PACES, HRS, the American College of Cardiology (ACC), the American Heart Association (AHA), the European Heart Rhythm Association (EHRA), the Canadian Heart Rhythm Society (CHRS), and the International Society for Adult Congenital Heart Disease (ISACHD). *Can J Cardiol* 2014;30:e1–63.
14. Koyak Z, Kroon B, de Groot JR, et al. Efficacy of antiarrhythmic drugs in adults with congenital heart disease and supraventricular tachycardias. *Am J Cardiol* 2013;112:1461–7.
15. Beaufort-Krol GC and Bink-Boelkens MT. Sotalol for atrial tachycardias after surgery for congenital heart disease. *Pacing Clin Electrophysiol* 1997;20:2125–9.
16. Lafuente-Lafuente C, Longas-Tejero MA, Bergmann JF, Belmin J. Antiarrhythmics for maintaining sinus rhythm after cardioversion of atrial fibrillation. *Cochrane Database Syst Rev* 2012;5:CD005049.
17. Jones DG, Jarman JW, Lyne JC, Markides V, Gatzoulis MA, Wong T. The safety and efficacy of trans-baffle puncture to enable catheter ablation of atrial tachycardias following the Mustard procedure: a single centre experience and literature review. *Int J Cardiol* 2013;168:1115–20.

18. Kammeraad JA, van Deurzen CH, Sreeram N, et al. Predictors of sudden cardiac death after Mustard or Senning repair for transposition of the great arteries. *J Am Coll Cardiol* 2004;44:1095–102.
19. Roos-Hesselink J, Perlroth MG, McGhie J, Spitaels S. Atrial arrhythmias in adults after repair of tetralogy of Fallot. Correlations with clinical, exercise, and echocardiographic findings. *Circulation* 1995;91:2214–19.
20. Gatzoulis MA, Balaji S, Webber SA, et al. Risk factors for arrhythmia and sudden cardiac death late after repair of tetralogy of Fallot: a multicentre study. *Lancet* 2000;356:975–81.
21. Knauth AL, Gauvreau K, Powell AJ, et al. Ventricular size and function assessed by cardiac MRI predict major adverse clinical outcomes late after tetralogy of Fallot repair. *Heart* 2008;94:211–16.
22. Deanfield JE, McKenna WJ, Presbitero P, England D, Graham GR, Hallidie-Smith K. Ventricular arrhythmia in unrepaired and repaired tetralogy of Fallot. Relation to age, timing of repair, and haemodynamic status. *Br Heart J* 1984;52:77–81.
23. Valente AM, Gauvreau K, Assenza GE, et al. Rationale and design of an International Multicenter Registry of patients with repaired tetralogy of Fallot to define risk factors for late adverse outcomes: the INDICATOR cohort. *Pediatr Cardiol* 2013;34:95–104.
24. Khairy P, Landzberg MJ, Gatzoulis MA, et al. Value of programmed ventricular stimulation after tetralogy of fallot repair: a multicenter study. *Circulation* 2004;109:1994–2000.
25. Khairy P, Dore A, Poirier N, et al. Risk stratification in surgically repaired tetralogy of Fallot. *Expert Rev Cardiovasc Ther* 2009;7:755–62.
26. Kapel GF, Reichlin T, Wijnmaalen AP, et al. Re-entry using anatomically determined isthmuses: A curable ventricular tachycardia in repaired congenital heart disease. *Circ Arrhythm Electrophysiol* 2015;8:102–9.
27. Epstein AE, DiMarco JP, Ellenbogen KA, et al.; American College of Cardiology Foundation; American Heart Association Task Force on Practice Guidelines; Heart Rhythm Society. 2012 ACCF/AHA/HRS focused update incorporated into the ACCF/AHA/HRS 2008 guidelines for device-based therapy of cardiac rhythm abnormalities: a report of the American College of Cardiology Foundation/American Heart Association Task Force on Practice Guidelines and the Heart Rhythm Society. *J Am Coll Cardiol* 2013;61:e6–75.
28. Ammash NM, Dearani JA, Burkhart HM, Connolly HM. Pulmonary regurgitation after tetralogy of Fallot repair: clinical features, sequelae, and timing of pulmonary valve replacement. *Congenit Heart Dis* 2007;2:386–403.
29. Wald RM, Altaha MA, Alvarez N, et al. Rationale and design of the Canadian Outcomes Registry Late After Tetralogy of Fallot Repair: the CORRELATE study. *Can J Cardiol* 2014;30:1436–43.
30. Harrild DM, Berul CI, Cecchin F, et al. Pulmonary valve replacement in tetralogy of Fallot: impact on survival and ventricular tachycardia. *Circulation* 2009;119:445–51.
31. Therrien J, Siu SC, Harris L, et al. Impact of pulmonary valve replacement on arrhythmia propensity late after repair of tetralogy of Fallot. *Circulation* 2001;103:2489–94.
32. Sherwin ED, Triedman JK, Walsh EP. Update on interventional electrophysiology in congenital heart disease: evolving solutions for complex hearts. *Circ Arrhythm Electrophysiol* 2013;6:1032–40.

CASE

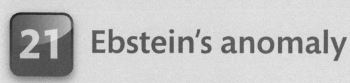

21 Ebstein's anomaly

Laura Vazquez-Garcia

Expert commentary Michael Rigby

Case history

A newborn infant with a prenatal diagnosis of Ebstein's anomaly (EA) was born in poor condition, deeply cyanosed and with signs of low cardiac output. He was immediately intubated and started on prostaglandin E1 (PGE1) and dopamine infusions. A transthoracic echocardiogram confirmed EA with severe tricuspid regurgitation (TR). The right atrium (RA) was severely dilated and there was a large oval fossa atrial septal defect (ASD) with shunting from right to left. There was no forward flow across a normal pulmonary valve, and the arterial duct was open with a left-to-right shunt. A 12-lead electrocardiogram showed pre-excitation, and the chest radiograph severe cardiomegaly, with a cardiothoracic ratio of 0.87.

On day 1 of life, he developed ventricular tachycardia (VT), with loss of cardiac output and required cardiopulmonary resuscitation with DC cardioversion and amiodarone infusion He remained on intravenous inotropic support and mechanical ventilation for 10 days, with gradual recovery. He was finally discharged from the hospital at 4 weeks of age, having an oxygen saturation of 87% on air, good systolic biventricular function, a right-to-left atrial shunt, normal forward flow across the pulmonary valve and a closed arterial duct.

Learning point Anatomy

The normal tricuspid valve (TV) has three leaflets—anterior, postero-inferior (mural) and septal—each having the hinge points at the atrioventricular junction. Normally, there are chordal insertions to three right ventricular (RV) papillary muscles. The leaflets develop from a process of delamination of the primitive RV myocardium during embryologic development, starting at the tip of the leaflets and progressing towards the atrioventricular junction. In Ebstein's anomaly delamination fails so that the leaflets remain tethered to the myocardium and the hinge points are displaced from the atrioventricular junction into the RV cavity in a rotational or spiral fashion, affecting mainly the septal and postero-inferior leaflets. There is characteristically severe tethering of the septal and posterior leaflets, with restriction to motion. The anterior leaflet is, however, usually enlarged and has adequate mobility, although it can also have tethering with apical displacement. The TV orifice is displaced downwards and anteriorly into the mid cavity or even into the right ventricular outflow tract (RVOT) in the most severe cases. Due to downward displacement of the effective TV annulus, the RV appears divided; the inlet component becomes functionally part of the RA, so-called 'RV atrialization', and the RA then appears dilated; the trabecular and outlet portions constitute the functional RV with relative hypoplasia. There is a wide anatomical spectrum in EA, and the degree of RV hypoplasia and RV atrialization will depend upon the severity of the downward displacement of the leaflets that can vary from minimal to severe [1–4].

Most cases have some degree of TR, from mild to severe. The severity of regurgitation is probably the most important factor contributing to clinical severity and results from various mechanisms, including inadequate leaflet size and restricted motion, favouring a lack of coaptation. Less frequently,

Expert comment

It is important to be aware that displacement of the attachment of the septal and inferior leaflets of the TV results in the orifice being displaced downwards and anteriorly into the cavity or outflow tract of the RV. As such, the RV becomes divided into the so-called 'atrialized' portion and the true functional RV, which will determine the prognosis and surgical management, together with the degree of TV regurgitation and/or stenosis.

leaflet fenestrations may be present and contribute to regurgitation. Rarely, the TV may be stenotic or even imperforate. The TV leaflets, especially the anterior one, might also be redundant and this can contribute to the development of RVOT obstruction [1–4].

Thus, EA is not limited only to the TV itself, but it also affects the RV and even the left ventricular (LV) myocardium. The RV myocardium is thinner than that of a normal heart, especially at the atrialized portion, and more trabeculated with frequent fibrosis. Fibrosis and hypertrabeculation may also affect the left ventricle, sometimes meeting the criteria for non-compaction [5]. It is not surprising therefore that some patients develop biventricular dysfunction.

Invariably, there is an associated secundum ASD or a patent foramen ovale. Approximately 50% have other cardiac defects [6], including tetralogy of Fallot, ventricular septal defect (VSD), coarctation of the aorta, mitral valve anomalies and atrioventricular discordance. However, the most common association is pulmonary stenosis or atresia, which likely develop secondary to low antenatal anterograde flow and progressive hypoplasia of the RVOT.

Apical displacement of the septal and postero-inferior leaflets is associated with a lack of continuity of the fibrous skeleton at the atrioventricular junction, so that muscular connections between the atria and the ventricles can be present, creating an important substrate for accessory pathways [7].

Expert comment Pathophysiology

EA is characterized by reduced pulmonary blood flow. The effective RV volume and filling are reduced, whereas the RA pressure is increased because of significant TR, sometimes associated with stenosis. Furthermore, during atrial relaxation, there is simultaneous contraction of the atrialized RV, which contributes to increasing the RA pressure and favours a right-to-left shunt through the ASD. On the other hand, when the RA contracts, the atrialized RV relaxes, behaving like an aneurysm or sump, so that part of the blood remains in the RA. However, as the RA becomes dilated, the pressure may remain normal. When all these anomalies are severe, the right heart output is significantly reduced and, if there is associated pulmonary valve stenosis, the output is even lower and pulmonary blood flow may be severely compromised. Additionally, RV dilatation compresses the left ventricle and alters the geometry and function of the left heart chambers. Underlying arrhythmias might also be present, contributing to low cardiac output.

In a significant minority of cases, EA is poorly tolerated in the neonatal period, probably because of the high pulmonary vascular resistance (PVR) present at birth, which contributes to the reduced anterograde flow across the pulmonary valve. In these cases, PGE1 infusion is often required to maintain an adequate pulmonary blood flow via the arterial duct until the PVR drops.

Learning point Incidence, aetiology, and clinical presentation

EA represents approximately 1% of all congenital cardiac conditions. It is the most common primary anomaly of the TV, with an incidence of around 100 cases per million live births, affecting males and females equally [8]. It is the cardiac condition with the highest prevalence of arrhythmias [9, 10]. The natural history is extremely variable, depending upon the severity of the malformation, but prenatal diagnosis is associated with higher perinatal mortality. Current survival rates of all live births at 1 month, 1 year, and 5 years have been reported as 86%, 82%, and 80% respectively [11], a significant improvement on previous reports of 76% at 1 year and 61% at 10 years [6]. For patients surviving to adult life, the prognosis is better, with reported survival rates of 100% to age 40 years, 95% to age 50 years, and 81% to age 60 years [12].

Most cases are sporadic, with no specific known aetiology, apart from a possible association with maternal lithium [13]. Approximately 10–20% have been described in the setting of different genetic conditions such as trisomy 21, trisomy 18, chromosome 1p36 deletion, 22q11.2 duplication, chromosome 6 ring abnormality and mitochondrial complex-1 deficiency [11, 14].

The clinical features of EA vary widely from patient to patient, depending upon the overall severity, including the degree of TR, the effective RV size and function, the presence of associated lesions and the age of the patient.

Neonates with severe EA are often critically ill with severe cyanosis and may present with right heart failure and low cardiac output. Patients with prenatal cardiomegaly and hydrops often have pulmonary parenchymal hypoplasia and respiratory failure as well [6, 12, 15–17]. These babies usually have progressive improvement, as the PVR decreases during the first few weeks of life. Overall *in utero* presentation is associated with high perinatal mortality [11, 17, 18] and when the anomaly is very critical, particularly with severe lung hypoplasia, survival is unlikely and surgical options are very limited.

Infants and older children might be asymptomatic for many years, and sometimes the diagnosis is made due to an incidental finding of a cardiac murmur or arrhythmia. There is progressive development of dyspnoea, reduced exercise tolerance, and cyanosis due to a right-to-left atrial shunt within the first decades of life. In older children and adults, palpitations, pre-syncope, and syncope as manifestations of different types of arrhythmias become more prevalent [12, 15, 16]. Patients with mild EA may remain symptom-free well into adult life.

Endocarditis and paradoxical embolism are rare complications. However, sudden death is not infrequent and most often is related to arrhythmic events [6, 7, 15].

Learning point Electrocardiogram and rhythm anomalies

The typical electrocardiographic features (Figure 21.1) are right QRS mean frontal axis deviation, low QRS voltages in the right precordial leads, and signs of right atrial hypertrophy with tall P waves mainly in the inferior leads. Sometimes a superior axis can be found, frequently in association with Wolff–Parkinson–White (WPW) syndrome and features of left bundle branch block. Very commonly, there is right bundle branch block, presumably due to fibrosis of the distal conduction tissue [15]. The QRS duration has been shown to be a marker of RV dilatation and dysfunction, and QRS fragmentation seems to be associated with a higher degree of RV atrialization [19].

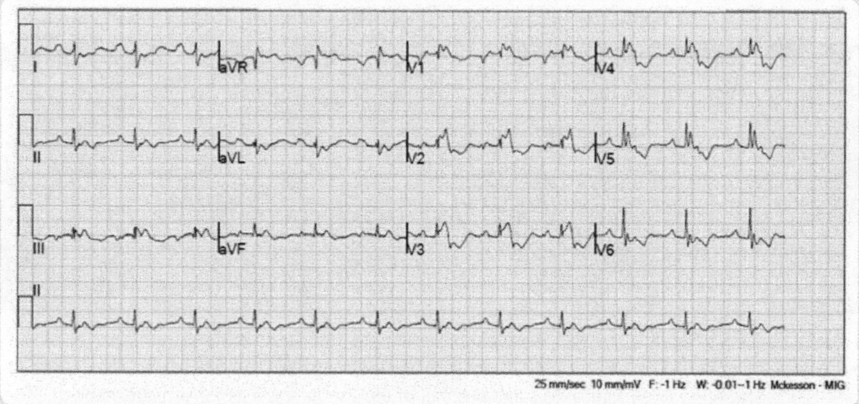

Figure 21.1 Classical 12-lead ECG showing sinus rhythm, first-degree atrioventricular block, complete right bundle branch block with QRS fragmentation, and low voltages in right precordial leads.

EA is one of the congenital heart conditions with the highest prevalence of arrhythmias. During childhood and adolescence, approximately 20% of the patients present with arrhythmias [9, 10], mainly in relation to accessory pathways. Pre-excitation and WPW syndrome (Figure 21.2) are common, with a prevalence of around 10–40% [7, 9, 20]. Not infrequently, several pathways may coexist, most of them being right-sided. The prevalence of arrhythmias in the adult population is significantly higher, varying from 35% to 80%. Atrioventricular re-entry tachycardia is common, but RA dilatation and previous surgery also predispose to atrial flutter and fibrillation. Myocardial fibrosis is, in addition, a substrate for ventricular tachycardia and atrioventricular block [7, 12, 20, 21]. Management

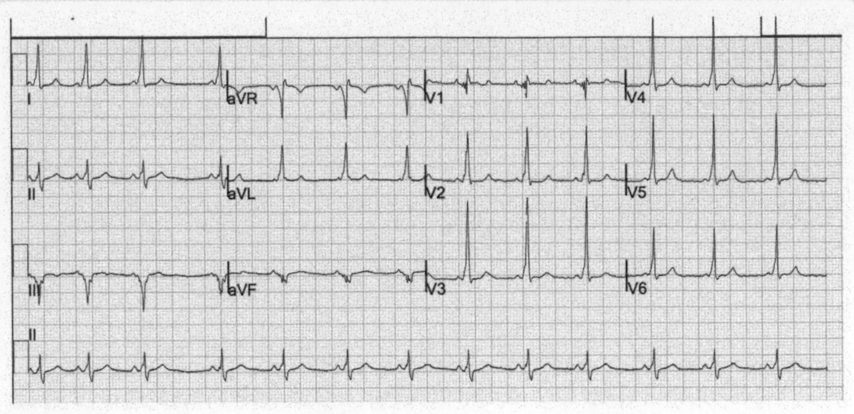

Figure 21.2 EA and WPW syndrome with the typical short PR interval and delta wave at the onset of the QRS complex.

of these patients is therefore very challenging, and multiple transcatheter or surgical ablations are often required.

Learning point Chest radiography

Chest X-ray usually shows cardiomegaly with significant RA enlargement. In severe EA, marked cardiomegaly, a globular-shaped heart, and reduced lung volumes are common. In patients with mild forms, the cardiac silhouette may have a more normal appearance and size [4, 15] (Figure 21.3).

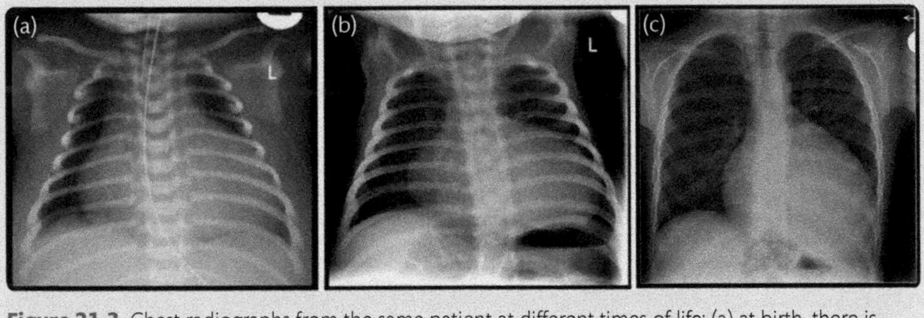

Figure 21.3 Chest radiographs from the same patient at different times of life: (a) at birth, there is severe cardiomegaly with marked RA dilatation; (b) at 1 month, the cardiothoracic ratio has decreased significantly; and (c) at 7 years, prior to surgical repair of the TV, there is a globular heart shape due to RA and RV dilatation.

Learning point Echocardiography

Echocardiography is important in the diagnosis, follow-up and surgical planning for patients with EA.

The characteristic features of EA are apical displacement of the hinge points of the septal and postero-inferior leaflets of the TV. The septal leaflet is best visualized in the apical four-chamber view (Figure 21.4). For borderline cases, the diagnosis is said to depend upon the distance between the hinge points of the septal tricuspid leaflet and the anterior mitral leaflet being >8 mm/m^2, measured in systole [22]. This is known as the displacement index and allows differentiation from the normal offsetting of the atrioventricular valves [23]. The degree of apical displacement of the postero-inferior leaflet and the position of the tricuspid orifice within the right ventricle are better assessed in the subcostal four-chamber and right oblique sections in infants (Figures 21.5 and 21.6), whereas the modified long axis view to show the RV inlet is better for older children. The presence of TV tissue close to the subpulmonary infundibulum is also indicative of severe distal displacement [2–4, 24].

Particularly important when planning surgery is the degree of tethering of the leaflets (Figure 21.7) and their mobility, especially the anterior leaflet, the presence of any fenestrations and the size of the tricuspid annulus [2–4, 24].

The RA and RV size and function and the presence of associated anomalies, such as ASD, VSD, and pulmonary stenosis, must also be assessed. The degree of anatomical severity does not necessarily correlate with functional severity. Most commonly, there is TR, typically with a central jet of regurgitation due to non-coaptation of the leaflets, but additional regurgitant jets should be defined (Figures 21.8 and 21.9). Tricuspid stenosis may be present but it is far less frequent.

Qualitative and quantitative RV and LV function should always be evaluated. Deficiency of the RV myocardium is common and best assessed by magnetic resonance imaging (MRI). It is reported that almost 20% of patients also demonstrate LV non-compaction [5], which can contribute to LV dysfunction (Figures 21.10 and 21.11).

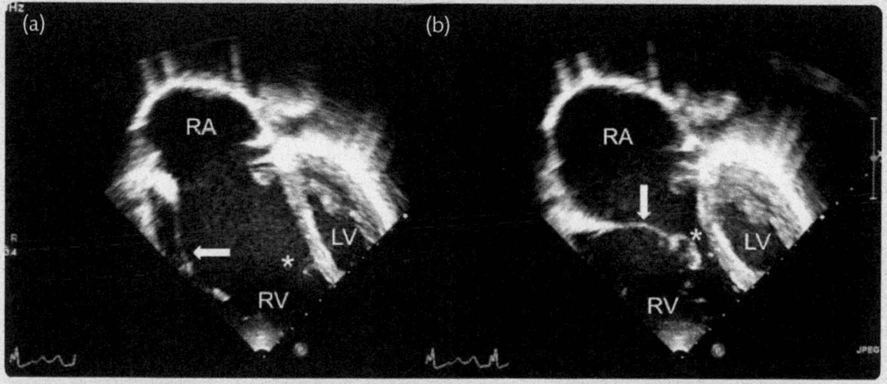

Figure 21.4 Apical four-chamber view with mild posterior angulation in diastole (a) and systole (b). The anterior leaflet (arrow) appears elongated with exaggerated 'sail-like' mobility, with no attachments to the free myocardial wall. The septal leaflet (*) appears very rudimentary and severely tethered to the ventricular septum, with an attachment point moderately displaced towards the mid-RV cavity. The right atrium and right ventricle are severely dilated and the left ventricle appears squashed.

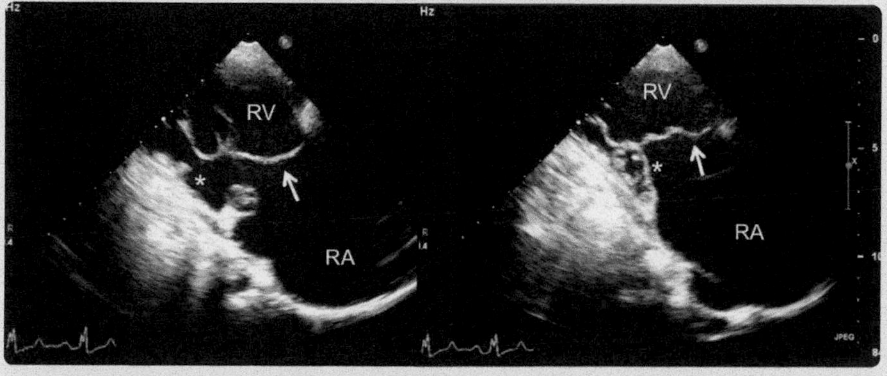

Figure 21.5 Parasternal RV inlet view during two different phases of systole. The anterior leaflet (arrow) is very elongated, and the posterior leaflet (*) is displaced and adhered to the myocardium. The mobile anterior leaflet coapts with the inferior leaflet.

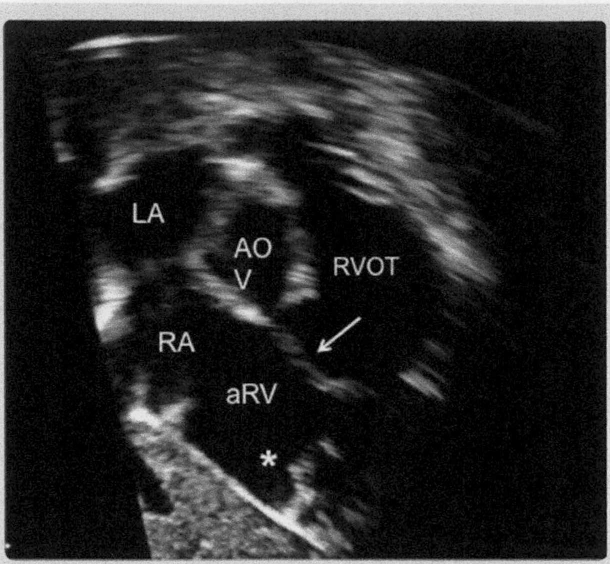

Figure 21.6 Subcostal right oblique view in which the inlet and outlet components of the right ventricle are visualized. The postero-inferior leaflet (*) is displaced into the RV cavity, and the anterior leaflet (arrow) attaches to the aorta and has good mobility, protruding into the RVOT. As a consequence, a significant portion of the right ventricle has become atrialized (aRV).

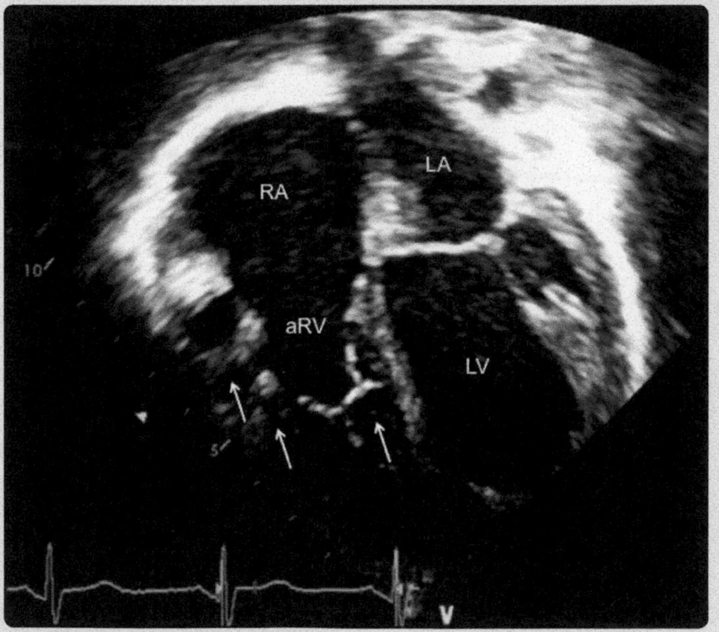

Figure 21.7 Both the anterior and septal leaflets are attached to the myocardium by muscular and fibrous tissue (arrows), limiting their mobility.

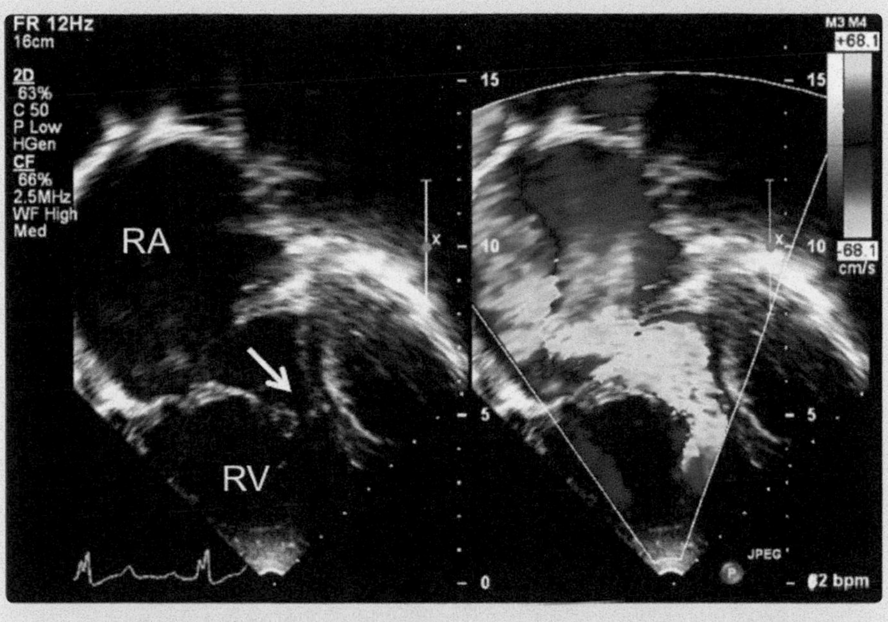

Figure 21.8 Apical four-chamber view that shows a very obvious lack of coaptation between the anterior and septal leaflets (arrow), with a broad jet of severe TR.

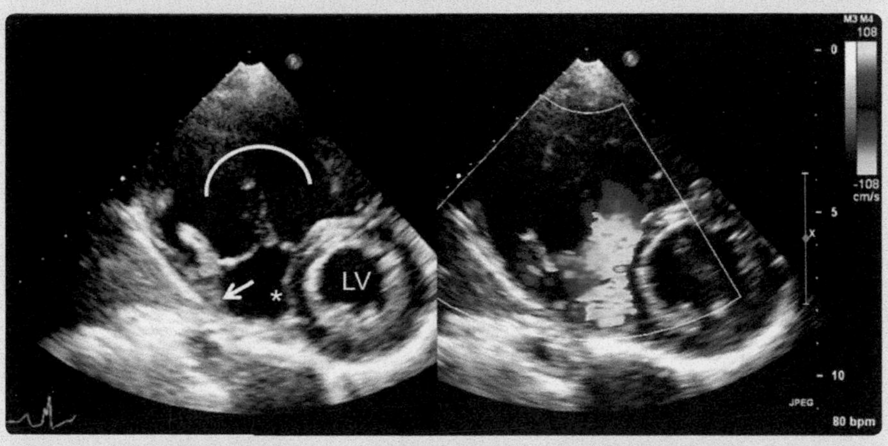

Figure 21.9 This parasternal short axis view demonstrates the tricuspid valve anatomy, with a very large anterior leaflet (curved line) and a very small posterior leaflet (arrow) tethered to the myocardium. The septal leaflet is also very adherent to the septal myocardium (*).

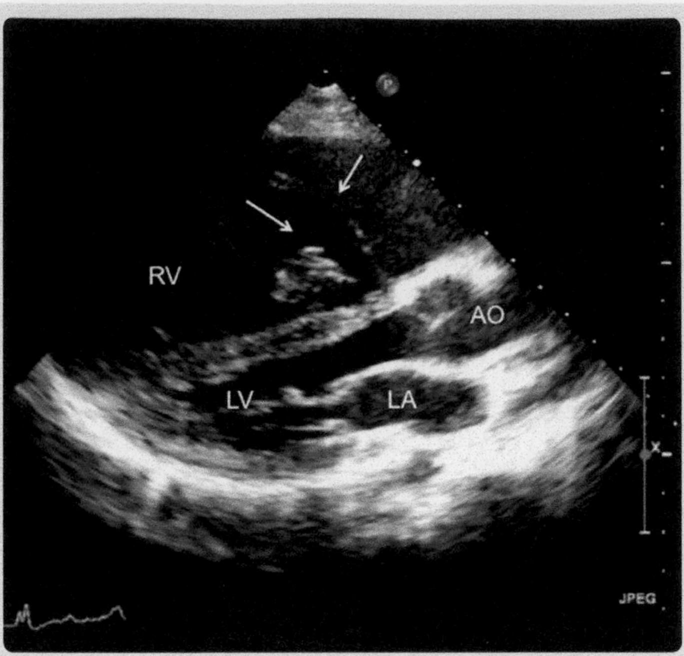

Figure 21.10 In this parasternal long axis section, there is severe RV dilatation and the left ventricle appears squashed. The anterior (long arrow) and septal (short arrow) leaflets of the TV are seen within the RV cavity towards the outlet, creating potential for RV outflow tract obstruction.

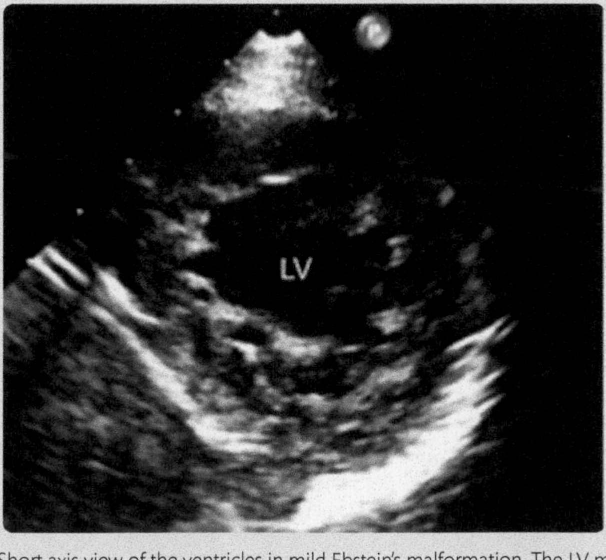

Figure 21.11 Short axis view of the ventricles in mild Ebstein's malformation. The LV myocardium has multiple trabeculations, consistent with non-compaction.

The Carpentier classification of EA [25], described in 1988, establishes four categories of severity, depending upon the degree of apical displacement of the leaflets, the mobility of the anterior leaflet, the atrialization of the right ventricle and the RV cavity size. This can be assessed by echocardiography and is useful for planning surgical intervention, although currently not employed by most modern cardiac surgeons.

The Celermajer index [6], used by some to establish the severity of the malformation and as a prognostic risk factor in neonates, is derived from the ratio of the combined area of the RA and atrialized RV to the combined area of the functional RV, left atrium, and left ventricle in a four-chamber view at end-diastole. This index establishes four categories of severity (grade 1, ratio <0.5; grade 2, 0.5–0.99; grade 3, 1–1.49; and grade 4, ≥1.5), with grades 3 and 4 associated with high perinatal morbidity and mortality.

Three-dimensional transoesophageal echocardiography is becoming an important technique as part of preoperative and intraoperative assessment.

Learning point Fetal echocardiography

Prenatal diagnosis of EA often carries a poor prognosis, having high intrauterine and neonatal mortality, with survival beyond the neonatal period ranging between 20% and 30% [17, 24, 26, 27], and 60% in a more recent cohort [11], excluding terminations of pregnancy.

Severe EA is easily diagnosed *in utero* [6, 17, 27], although mild cases can be difficult to recognize. The fetus with severe EA and significant TR frequently develops congestive heart failure, with cardiomegaly, pericardial and pleural effusions, ascites and even subcutaneous oedema. Furthermore, fetal arrhythmias may contribute to fetal hydrops and can also be diagnosed by echocardiography.

The many fetal risk factors for perinatal mortality include severe TR, low TR gradient, implying poor RV function, a cardiothoracic ratio of >90%, Celermajer index grade 3 or 4, TV annulus Z-score of >+3, reduced or absent pulmonary valve flow, retrograde arterial duct flow, gestational age at diagnosis <32 weeks, hydrops, and fetal distress [6, 25, 26]. More recently, it has been shown that the presence of pulmonary regurgitation is strongly correlated with high perinatal mortality [11, 14, 17].

He remained asymptomatic on treatment with beta-blockers for several years, with mild cyanosis and progressive development of finger clubbing. At 6 years, he presented for the first time with sustained supraventricular tachycardia (SVT) and had some additional short episodes later on. Within the next year, his exercise tolerance became significantly impaired and the arterial oxygen saturation dropped to around 80%. Echocardiogram and cardiac MRI showed moderate to severe TR and stenosis, severe RA dilatation and moderate RV enlargement with mild systolic biventricular dysfunction.

Learning point Physical examination

Patients with EA and an associated ASD usually have some degree of cyanosis at rest or on exercise. Hypoxia becomes progressively more severe with increase in age, so that finger clubbing and other signs of chronic hypoxaemia, such as polycythaemia and conjunctival hyperaemia, develop in adolescence and early adult life.

On auscultation, there are usually widely split first and second heart sounds due to delayed closure of the tricuspid and pulmonary valves. Gallop rhythm or quadruple rhythm may also be present, and frequently there is a very typical pan-systolic murmur of TR, loudest at the lower left sternal edge.

When RV failure is present, there may be hepatomegaly, peripheral oedema, and raised jugular venous pressure; the latter is difficult to recognize in infants and small children.

Learning point Cardiac magnetic resonance

Although echocardiography remains the main imaging technique for the diagnosis and continued assessment of EA, cardiac MRI is also very useful, especially for evaluation of RA and RV volumes,

Clinical tip Cardiopulmonary exercise test

Some patients with EA have a significantly reduced exercise performance, with a lower peak oxygen uptake, higher resting heart rate, lower heart rate reserve, and increased ventilatory equivalent for oxygen [30, 31]. The cardiopulmonary exercise test is a useful investigation to stratify the degree of functional compromise and helps to determine the timing of surgical repair. Surgical repair has been shown to improve the above parameters.

myocardial thickness or deficiency, ventricular function, regional contractility and the presence of myocardial non-compaction [28, 29] (Figure 21.12).

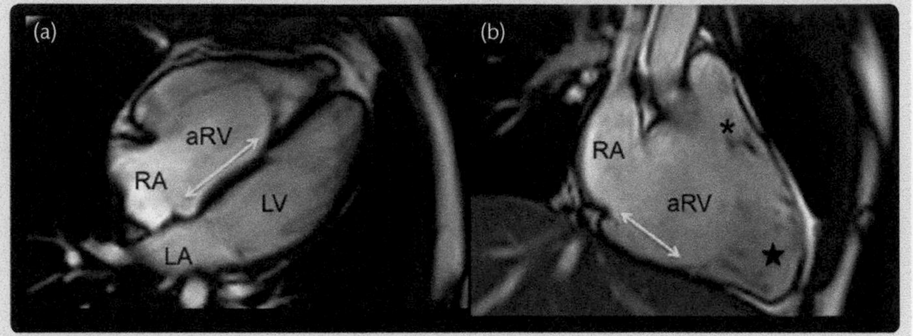

Figure 21.12 Cardiac MRI showing: (a) four-chamber view with severe displacement and adherence of the septal leaflet of the tricuspid valve (arrow) and severe RV atrialization and RV dilatation; and (b) inflow–outflow view of the right ventricle where the posterior leaflet (arrow) appears severely tethered to the myocardium and displaced into the RV cavity. The right ventricle has a uniformly thin myocardium. The RV outflow appears patent, although some attachments from the TV leaflets (*) can be seen at that level.
Images Dr S Krupickova.

He underwent a complex and prolonged electrophysiological study and two different accessory pathways were successfully identified and ablated. The procedure was complicated by atrial fibrillation requiring DC cardioversion. In addition, an antidromic atrioventricular re-entry tachycardia, together with VT, were induced, although no further attempts at ablation were made, as they were haemodynamically poorly tolerated.

Learning point Medical management

Antenatal diagnosis is important in establishing a perinatal management plan, especially in high-risk babies with poor RV function, severe TR and no forward pulmonary blood flow, as these patients will very likely be critically ill after birth. In this setting, PGE infusion may reduce neonatal hypoxia by maintaining patency of the arterial duct. In babies with severe neonatal hypoxia, mechanical ventilation and use of inhaled nitric oxide, sildenafil, or epoprostenol may improve symptoms by decreasing PVR. The consequence is an improvement in anterograde pulmonary flow, reduced severity of TR and less right-to-left atrial shunting.

Older children and adults may remain asymptomatic for years and do not necessarily require any treatment. When signs of heart failure develop, this will be managed with diuretics and afterload reduction agents such as angiotensin-converting enzyme (ACE) inhibitors. A very important part of the medical management of these patients concerns symptomatic arrhythmias and usually a combination of different drugs is necessary. Not infrequently, these tachycardias are refractory to drugs and repeat electrophysiological studies and ablation procedures are required.

Clinical tip

In neonates presenting with functional pulmonary atresia and presence of pulmonary regurgitation, it is important to be aware that patency of the arterial duct and use of vasodilators may be deleterious, as they contribute to the development and maintenance of a 'circular shunt'. Prolonged patency of the arterial duct will create a substrate for continuous steal of blood from the systemic circulation directly into the right ventricle and right atrium, with no improvement of pulmonary blood flow and, at the same time, low systemic cardiac output. In such cases, early closure of the arterial duct may be of benefit [32].

A few months later, he underwent TV repair with septal leaflet augmentation, longitudinal plication of the atrialized RV, and TV annuloplasty, together with ASD patch closure. The post-operative period was complicated by VT leading to cardiac arrest, with successful resuscitation. Despite an initially good surgical result with mild to moderate TR and mild stenosis, a month later, the insufficiency had progressed to severe, so that TV replacement with a 25-mm Mosaic bioprosthesis was required.

Immediately after TV replacement, he made very good clinical progress with significant improvement of exercise capacity, becoming practically the same as his peers. However, within the following 2 years, the tricuspid bioprosthesis developed severe regurgitation and a paravalvar leak. Furthermore, RV function deteriorated progressively and exercise capacity again became impaired. At 12 years, he underwent transcatheter implantation of a 22-mm Melody® valve in the tricuspid position and device closure of the paravalvar leak with a very satisfactory result and normal TV function.

Currently, the ventricular function is mildly impaired and mild to moderate TR has developed some 4 years following Melody® valve implantation. He remains on treatment with propranolol, flecainide and enalapril and continues to have recurrent short-lasting episodes of SVT and new evidence of pre-excitation on the ECG. Further electrophysiological studies and TV replacement will be required in the future.

Learning point Surgical management

The surgical treatment will depend upon RV size and function, the presence of associated anomalies, and the age of the patient. Surgical strategies include: (1) biventricular repair with TV repair or replacement; (2) univentricular palliation; and (3) one-and-a-half ventricular repair.

Patients with adequate RV size and function comprise the majority and will be candidates for biventricular repair, usually with closure of the ASD. Biventricular repair in the neonatal period may be feasible but carries high peri-operative mortality and is rarely performed.

TV repair is preferable to replacement at any age, but particularly in children. Various techniques have been used, most frequently those introduced by Danielson [33, 34] and Carpentier [35, 36] in the 80s. Both interventions involve the creation of a monoleaflet valve in such a way that TV coaptation is established with the ventricular septal myocardium; for these techniques to be successful, it is important that the anterior TV leaflet has adequate mobility. Inevitably, not all anatomical variations will be suitable for this approach and there is a high reported incidence of TV replacement, varying from 35% to 65%.

In 2007, da Silva described the cone reconstruction of the TV with excellent outcomes [37] and a very low incidence of TV replacement. Currently, many centres are adopting this technique. The intervention is performed through a complex process of dissection of tricuspid leaflets from the underlying myocardium, resembling an artificial delamination. The valve is then reconstructed in a cone shape, with its annulus at the atrioventricular junction and the orifice in the mid RV cavity, with the coaptation established between the valve leaflets. Da Silva described the use of a valved atrial communication allowing only right-to-left shunting. The technique can be applied to almost all anatomical variations, with excellent results—low early and late mortality rates and very low incidence of re-intervention, TV replacement, and post-operative complete heart block [37–41].

In general, when TV repair is not possible or the intraoperative echocardiogram shows a poor result, an alternative approach is TV replacement with either a bioprosthetic or a mechanical valve.

Those neonates or infants with a hypoplastic right ventricle and/or poor RV function, with associated TV stenosis or RVOT obstruction, usually present severe cyanosis and signs of heart failure at birth with a duct-dependent pulmonary circulation. When, despite medical management, severe cyanosis and congestive heart failure persist, they will generally undergo univentricular palliation with an initial Blalock–Taussig shunt or a bidirectional superior cavo-pulmonary anastomosis. When the left ventricle appears severely compressed by the right heart, the Starnes procedure [42] has been used as the initial

Clinical tip

Cardiac catheterization and angiography have limited value in the current era because echocardiography and cardiac MRI are able to provide accurate anatomical and functional information. It is used mainly for diagnostic studies prior to palliative procedures such as a bidirectional superior cavo-pulmonary connection, as part of pre-transplant assessment and, more recently, for percutaneous TV implantation.

palliation. It consists of closure of the TV with a pericardial patch and plication of the atrialized right ventricle, together with a Blalock–Taussig shunt and enlargement of the ASD.

The one-and-a-half ventricular repair in EA is another surgical option mainly used in cases of severe RV dysfunction and RV hypoplasia or as an alternative to TV replacement when there is a poor result from surgical repair with significant TR. In these cases, the TV is repaired, together with relief of RVOT obstruction, atrial septectomy and an end-to-side anastomosis of the superior vena cava to the pulmonary arteries, so that the RV preload is reduced, the pulmonary forward flow is preserved to some extent and the systemic preload is maintained.

In extreme cases, especially when biventricular dysfunction is present, cardiac transplant might be the sole and best option for some patients.

Surgical ablation or the maze procedure at the time of surgical repair was traditionally used in patients with refractory atrial arrhythmias but at present most patients undergo electrophysiological study and ablation prior to surgery, leaving surgical ablation for those cases of unsuccessful percutaneous treatment.

Historically, in asymptomatic patients without cyanosis and without significant right heart dilatation, clinical monitoring was the rule. In the current era, the excellent outcomes of cone reconstruction have resulted in a trend to early surgical repair in childhood, even in relatively asymptomatic children with moderate TR. The classical indications are still relevant and include significant symptoms of exercise intolerance, increasing cyanosis, progressive right heart dilatation and dysfunction, and poorly controlled arrhythmias.

Evidence base

In 2012, da Silva et al.'s most recent publication [38] emphasized the excellent outcomes of the cone operation for the majority of patients with Ebstein's malformation. Between 1993 and 2011, the technique was performed in 100 patients with a median age of 13.5 years. There was a hospital mortality rate of 3% related to low cardiac output or biventricular dysfunction and long-term mortality rate of 4% (endocarditis, heart failure and arrhythmia, sudden death, and accidental death). The incidence of re-repair due to recurrence of TR was 4% and only one patient developed mild tricuspid stenosis. The cone repair can therefore be applied to patients of all ages with excellent medium-term results, avoiding the need for a prosthetic TV replacement, with all the disadvantages that it carries.

Discussion

EA is a rare cardiac malformation with a wide anatomical, physiological, and clinical spectrum, with the perinatal presentation of severe EA having the worse prognosis. This case highlights the different clinical phases that patients may go through during their life and also the multiple complications that can be present and the difficulties related to both medical and surgical management.

A final word from the expert

EA is a condition in which there is extreme variability in morphology, and the challenge to clinicians, electrophysiologists, surgeons, and interventional cardiologists continues from infancy into adult life. A multidisciplinary approach to diagnosis and treatment is essential to good outcomes. The most significant contribution to the understanding of the morphology has been provided by Anderson in his wonderful description [4], whilst the cone operation described by da Silva [37, 38] has transformed the indications and outcomes of surgical management of children and adults.

References

1. Lev M, Liberthson RR, Joseph RH, et al. The pathologic anatomy of Ebstein´s disease. *Arch Path* 1970;90:334–43.
2. Zuberbuhler JR, Allwork SP, Anderson RH. The spectrum of Ebstein's anomaly of the tricuspid valve. *J Thorac Cardiovasc Surg* 1979;77:202–11.
3. Frescura C, Angelini A, Daliento L, Thiene G. Morphological aspects of Ebstein's anomaly in adults. *Thorac Cardiovasc Surg* 2000;48:203–8.
4. O'Leary PW, Dearani JA, Anderson RH. Diseases of the tricuspid valve. In: Anderson R, Baker E, Redington A, Rigby M, Penny D, Wernovsky G, editors. *Paediatric Cardiology*, 3rd edition. Philadelphia, PA: Churchill Livingstone Elsevier, 2009; pp. 713–30.
5. Attenhofer Jost CH, Connolly HM, O'Leary PW, Warnes CA, Tajik AJ, Seward JB. Left heart lesions in patients with Ebstein anomaly. *Mayo Clin Proc* 2005;80:361–8.
6. Celermajer DS, Cullen S, Sullivan ID, Spiegelhalter DJ, Wyse RK, Deanfield JE. Outcome in neonates with Ebstein's anomaly. *J Am Coll Cardiol* 1992;19:1041–6.
7. Oh JK, Holmes DR Jr, Hayes DL, Porter CB, Danielson GK. Cardiac arrhythmias in patients with surgical repair of Ebstein's anomaly. *J Am Coll Cardiol* 1985;6:1351–7.
8. Hoffman JI, Kaplan S. The incidence of congenital heart disease. *J Am Coll Cardiol* 2002;39:1890–900.
9. Delhaas T, Sarvaas GJ, Rijlaarsdam ME, et al. A multicenter, long-term study on arrhythmias in children with Ebstein anomaly. *Pediatr Cardiol* 2010;31:229–33.
10. Attenhofer Jost CH, Connolly HM, Dearani JA, Edwards WD, Danielson GK. Ebstein's anomaly. *Circulation* 2007;115:277–85.
11. Wertaschnigg D, Manlhiot C, Jaeggi M, et al. Contemporary outcomes and factors associated with mortality after a fetal or neonatal diagnosis of Ebstein anomaly and tricuspid valve disease. *Can J Cardiol* 2016;32:1500–6.
12. Luu Q, Choudhary P, Jackson D, et al. Ebstein's anomaly in those surviving to adult life—a single centre experience. *Heart Lung Circ* 2015;24:996–1001.
13. Cohen LS, Friedman JM, Jefferson JW, Johnson EM, Weiner ML. A reevaluation of risk of in utero exposure to lithium. *JAMA* 1994;271:146–50.
14. Freud LR, Escobar-Diaz MC, Kalish BT, et al. Outcomes and predictors of perinatal mortality in fetuses with Ebstein anomaly or tricuspid valve dysplasia in the current era: a multicenter study. *Circulation* 2015;132:481–9.
15. Celermajer DS, Bull C, Till JA, et al. Ebstein's anomaly: presentation and outcome from fetus to adult. *J Am Coll Cardiol* 1994;23:170–6.
16. Giuliani ER, Fuster V, Brandenburg RO, Mair DD. Ebstein's anomaly: the clinical features and natural history of Ebstein's anomaly of the tricuspid valve. *Mayo Clin Proc* 1979;54:163–73.
17. Hornberger LK, Sahn DJ, Kleinman CS, Copel JA, Reed KL. Tricuspid valve disease with significant tricuspid insufficiency in the fetus: diagnosis and outcome. *J Am Coll Cardiol* 1991;17:167–73.
18. Barre E, Durand I, Hazelzet T, David N. Ebstein's anomaly and tricuspid valve dysplasia: prognosis after diagnosis in utero. *Pediatr Cardiol* 2012;33:1391–6.
19. Egidy Assenza G, Valente AM, Geva T, et al. QRS duration and QRS fractionation on surface electrocardiogram are markers of right ventricular dysfunction and atrialization in patients with Ebstein anomaly. *Eur Heart J* 2013;34:191–200.
20. Khositseth A, Danielson GK, Dearani JA, Munger TM, Porter CJ. Supraventricular tachyarrhythmias in Ebstein anomaly: management and outcome. *J Thorac Cardiovasc Surg* 2004;128:826–33.
21. Chauvaud SM, Brancaccio G, Carpentier AF. Cardiac arrhythmia in patients undergoing surgical repair of Ebstein's anomaly. *Ann Thorac Surg* 2001;71:1547–52.

22. Edwards WD. Embryology and pathologic features of Ebstein's anomaly. *Prog Pediatr Cardiol* 1993;2:5–15.
23. Gussenhoven EJ, Stewart PA, Becker AE, Essed CE, Ligtvoet KM, De Villeneuve VH. 'Offsetting' of the septal tricuspid leaflet in normal hearts and in hearts with Ebstein's anomaly. Anatomic and echographic correlation. *Am J Cardiol* 1984;54:172–6.
24. Roberson DA, Silverman NH. Ebstein's anomaly: echocardiographic and clinical features in the fetus and neonate. *J Am Coll Cardiol* 1989;14:1300–7.
25. Carpentier A, Chauvaud S, Mace L, et al. A new reconstructive operation for Ebstein anomaly of the tricuspid valve. *J Thorac Cardiovasc Surg* 1988;96:92–101.
26. McElhinney DB, Salvin JW, Colan SD, et al. Improving outcomes in fetuses and neonates with congenital displacement (Ebstein's malformation) or dysplasia of the tricuspid valve. *Am J Cardiol* 2005;96:582–6.
27. Sharland GK, Chita SK, Allan LD. Tricuspid valve dysplasia or displacement in intrauterine life. *J Am Coll Cardiol* 1991;17:944–9.
28. Lee CM, Sheehan FH, Bouzas B, Chen SS, Gatzoulis MA, Kilner PJ. The shape and function of the right ventricle in Ebstein's anomaly. *Int J Cardiol* 2013;167:704–10.
29. Yalonetsky S, Tobler D, Greutmann M, et al. Cardiac magnetic resonance imaging and the assessment of Ebstein anomaly in adults. *Am J Cardiol* 2011;107:767–73.
30. Driscoll DJ, Mottram CD, Danielson GK. Spectrum of exercise intolerance in 45 patients with Ebstein's anomaly and observations on exercise tolerance in 11 patients after surgical repair. *J Am Coll Cardiol* 1988;11:831–6.
31. MacLellan-Tobert SG, Driscoll DJ, Mottram CD, Mahoney DW, Wollan PC, Danielson GK. Exercise tolerance in patients with Ebstein's anomaly. *J Am Coll Cardiol* 1997;29:1615–22.
32. Wald RM, Adatia I, Van Arsdell GS, Hornberger LK. Relation of limiting ductal patency to survival in neonatal Ebstein's anomaly. *Am J Cardiol* 2005;96:851–6.
33. Dearani JA, Danielson GK. Surgical management of Ebstein's anomaly in the adult. *Semin Thorac Cardiovasc Surg* 2005;17:148–54.
34. Danielson GK, Driscoll DJ, Mair DD, Warnes CA, Oliver WC Jr. Operative treatment of Ebstein anomaly. *J Thorac Cardiovasc Surg* 1992;104:1195–202.
35. Carpentier A, Chauvaud S, Mace L, et al. A new reconstructive operation for Ebstein anomaly of the tricuspid valve. *J Thorac Cardiovasc Surg* 1988;96:92–101.
36. Chauvaud S. Ebstein's malformation. surgical treatment and results. *Thorac Cardiovasc Surg* 2000;48:220–3.
37. Da Silva JP, Baumgratz JF, da Fonseca L, et al. The cone reconstruction of the tricuspid valve in Ebstein's anomaly. The operation: early and midterm results. *J Thorac Cardiovasc Surg* 2007;133:215–23.
38. da Silva JP, da Silva Lda F. Ebstein's anomaly of the tricuspid valve: the cone repair. *Semin Thorac Cardiovasc Surg Pediatr Card Surg Annu* 2012;15:38–45.
39. Lange R, Burri M, Eschenbach LK, et al. Da Silva's cone repair for Ebstein's anomaly: effect on right ventricular size and function. *Eur J Cardiothorac Surg* 2015;48:316–20.
40. Anderson HN, Dearani JA, Said SM, et al. Cone reconstruction in children with Ebstein anomaly: the Mayo Clinic experience. *Congenit Heart Dis* 2014;9:266–71.
41. Vogel M, Marx GR, Tworetzky W, et al. Ebstein's malformation of the tricuspid valve: short-term outcomes of the 'cone procedure' versus conventional surgery. *Congenit Heart Dis* 2012;7:50–8.
42. Starnes VA, Pitlick PT, Bernstein D, Griffin ML, Choy M, Shumway NE. Ebstein's anomaly appearing in the neonate. A new surgical approach. *J Thorac Cardiovasc Surg* 1991;101:1082–7.

CASE

22 Kawasaki disease

Tarek Alsaied and Justin T Tretter

Expert commentary Andrew N Redington

Case history

A 20-month-old previously healthy female presented to the emergency department with high-grade fever for 6 days. She was seen initially by the paediatrician and was started on amoxicillin for possible acute otitis media The next day, she developed a rash on her lower back which progressed to involve her legs, arms, and face, in addition to bilateral non-purulent conjunctivitis. That same evening, she developed bright red lips and swollen hands and feet. Despite being on antibiotics, she continued to have high-grade fever to 41 °C, and she became increasingly fussy and lethargic. Because of her worsening symptoms, her parents presented to the emergency department. Upon initial evaluation, she was noted to be extremely agitated, tachycardic, diaphoretic, and febrile to 41 °C. Notable findings on examination included hepatosplenomegaly, conjunctival injection, cervical lymphadenopathy, cracked red lips, diffuse maculopapular rash, and mild swelling of the hands and feet. Her cardiac examination was unremarkable, with no murmurs and no added sounds. Laboratory tests were significant for elevated inflammatory markers (C-reactive protein 8.88 mg/dl; erythrocyte sedimentation rate 68 mm/hour) and hypoalbuminaemia (2.6 g/dl). The complete blood count demonstrated leucocytosis with neutrophilia, mild anaemia, and a normal platelet count. Her liver transaminases were elevated. Urinalysis was normal. She was admitted to hospital with a working diagnosis of Kawasaki disease (KD) (Figure 22.1) (Table 22.1).

She met the diagnostic criteria for KD with persistent fever, rash, conjunctivitis, mucosal involvement, oedema of the hands and feet, and cervical lymphadenopathy. The initial echocardiogram demonstrated mild ectasia of her right and left coronary arteries, with otherwise normal cardiac structures, normal biventricular systolic function, and no pericardial effusion

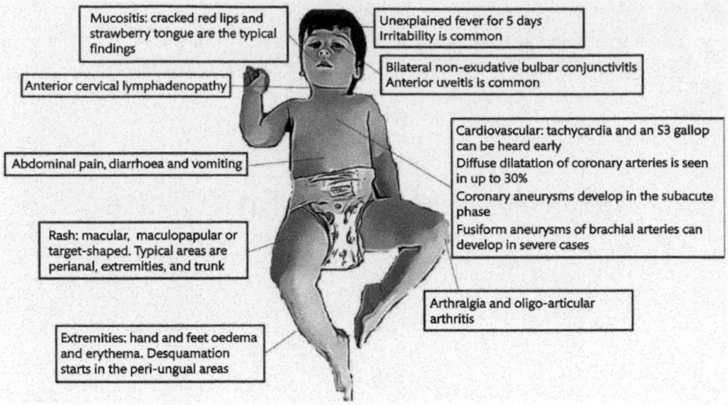

Figure 22.1 Clinical manifestations of KD.

Table 22.1 Diagnostic criteria for KD [1]*

- Bilateral bulbar conjunctival injection without purulent drainage. The erythema typically spares the limbus
- Oral mucous membrane changes, including injected or fissured lips, injected pharynx, or strawberry tongue
- Peripheral extremity changes which is usually the last manifestation to appear, including erythema of palms or soles, oedema of hands or feet (acute phase), and peri-ungual desquamation (convalescent phase)
- Skin rash usually maculopapular, morbilliform, or target-shaped. Vesicular or bullous lesions may rule out the diagnosis
- Cervical lymphadenopathy (at least one lymph node >1.5 cm in diameter)

* The diagnosis of KD requires the presence of fever for at least 5 days without any other explanation, combined with at least four of the five criteria. Of note, neither cardiac manifestations nor laboratory findings of KD are included in the diagnostic criteria for KD. These findings, however, support the diagnosis of KD in incomplete cases (Figure 22.2).
Source data from Newburger, J.W., et al., Diagnosis, treatment, and long-term management of Kawasaki disease: a statement for health professionals from the Committee on Rheumatic Fever, Endocarditis and Kawasaki Disease, Council on Cardiovascular Disease in the Young, American Heart Association. *Circulation*, 2004. 110(17): p. 2747–71.

Clinical tip Evaluation of suspected incomplete KD

- The algorithm reported in Figure 22.2 helps to standardize care in patients with potential KD. However, like most medical care algorithms, this should be recognized as a guide in clinical decision-making [1, 2].
- Sharing this algorithm with those involved in the patient's care helps to communicate and clarify the thought process behind clinical decision-making. It may be helpful to include this algorithm in the patient's clinical notes to better accomplish this.

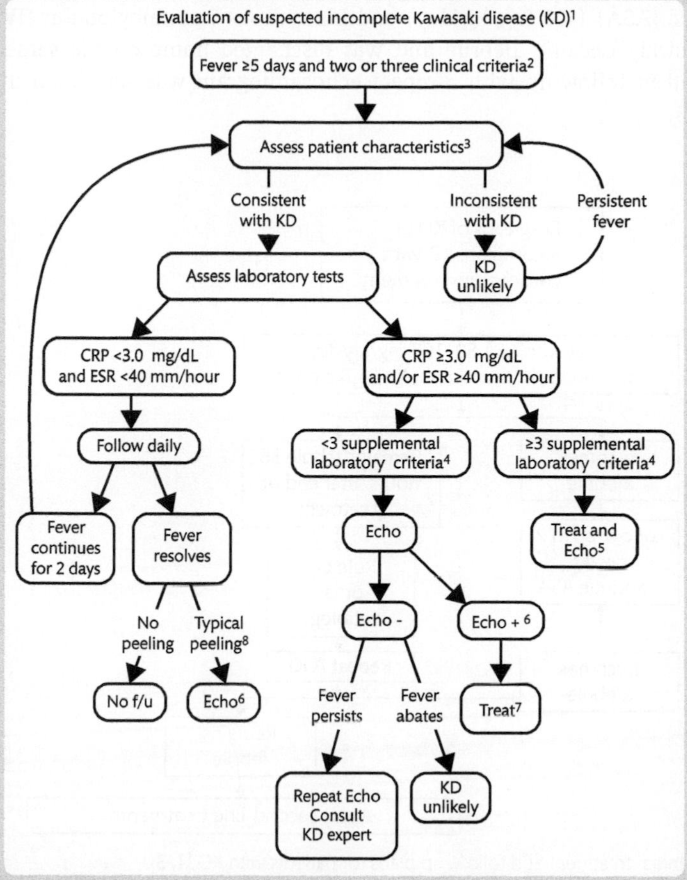

Figure 22.2 American Heart Association algorithm for the diagnosis of KD. The numerical annotation to elements of the algorithm refers to the following caveats and guidelines. (1) In the absence of a gold standard for diagnosis, this algorithm cannot be evidence-based but rather represents the informed opinion of the expert committee. Consultation with an expert should be sought anytime assistance is needed. (2) Infants ≤6 months old on day ≥7 of fever without other explanation should undergo laboratory testing and, if evidence of systemic inflammation is found, an echocardiogram, even if the infants have no clinical criteria. (3) Patient characteristics suggesting Kawasaki disease are listed in Table 22.1. Characteristics suggesting disease other than Kawasaki disease include exudative conjunctivitis, exudative pharyngitis, discrete intraoral lesions, bullous or vesicular rash, or generalized adenopathy. Consider alternative diagnoses. (4) Supplemental laboratory criteria include albumin ≤3.0 g/dl, anaemia for age, elevation of alanine aminotransferase, platelets after 7 days ≥450,000/mm^3, white blood cell count ≥15,000/mm^3, and urine ≥10 white blood cells/high-power field. (5) Can treat before performing an echocardiogram. (6) Echocardiogram is considered positive for the purposes of this algorithm if any of three conditions are met: Z-score of left anterior descending (LAD) or right coronary artery (RCA) ≥2.5; coronary arteries meet the Japanese Ministry of Health criteria for aneurysms, or ≥3 other suggestive features exist, including perivascular brightness, lack of tapering, decreased LV function, mitral regurgitation, pericardial effusion, or Z-scores in LAD or RCA of 2–2.5. (7) If the echocardiogram is positive, treatment should be given to children within 10 days of fever onset and those beyond day 10 with clinical and laboratory signs (CRP, ESR) of ongoing inflammation. (8) Typical peeling begins under the nail bed of fingers and then toes.

Reproduced from Newburger, J.W., et al., Diagnosis, treatment, and long-term management of Kawasaki disease: a statement for health professionals from the Committee on Rheumatic Fever, Endocarditis and Kawasaki Disease, Council on Cardiovascular Disease in the Young, American Heart Association. *Circulation*, 2004. 110(17): p. 2747–71 with permission from Wolters Kluwer.

Learning point Aetiology of KD

The aetiology of KD remains unknown, despite extensive research over the last 40 years. Multiple theories have been proposed, with an idiosyncratic response to infection in a genetically predisposed patient being the most widely accepted. Infectious aetiology by one or more agents is supported by the seasonal increase in KD cases and the geographic distribution in a 'wave-like' spread. However, genetic, immunologic, and environmental factors have been proposed as other potential aetiologies for this disease.

Expert comment

It remains extraordinary that the aetiology of Kawasaki disease has remained elusive, despite decades of investigation around the world. Until a diagnostic test becomes available, we will continue to rely on diagnostic algorithms for the diagnosis of typical and atypical KD, with the necessary uncertainties that go along with such an approach.

She received the standard treatment for KD, which included high-dose acetyl salicylic acid (ASA) (100 mg/kg/day) and intravenous immunoglobulin (IVIG) (2 g/kg). She quickly became afebrile and was discharged home on the same doses of ASA. Outpatient follow-up with a repeat echocardiogram was scheduled in 2 weeks (Figure 22.3).

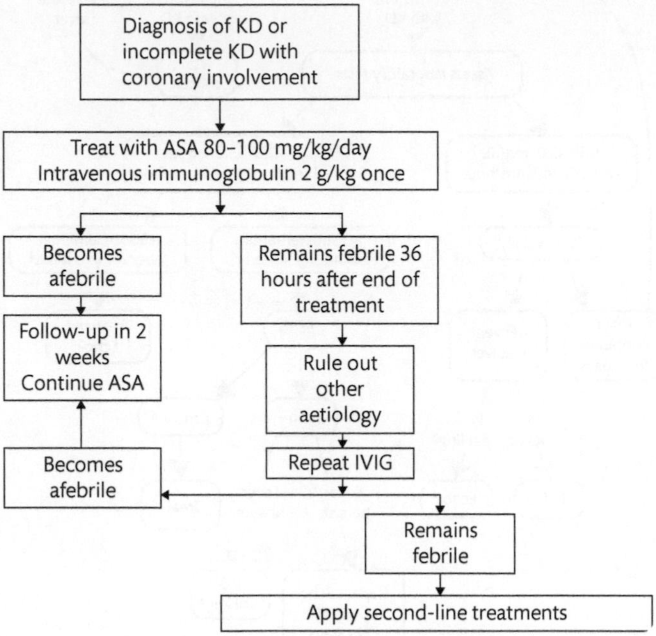

Figure 22.3 Initial treatment and follow-up plans for patients with KD [1, 3].
Source data from from Newburger, J.W., et al., Diagnosis, treatment, and long-term management of Kawasaki disease: a statement for health professionals from the Committee on Rheumatic Fever, Endocarditis and Kawasaki Disease, Council on Cardiovascular Disease in the Young, American Heart Association. Circulation, 2004. 110(17): p. 2747-71 and Newburger, J.W., M. Takahashi, and J.C. Burns, Kawasaki Disease. *J Am Coll Cardiol*, 2016. 67(14): p. 1738–49.

In clinic, she was asymptomatic and had a normal physical examination, with complete resolution of her prior signs and symptoms. Her echocardiogram demonstrated giant aneurysms of the right, left main, left anterior descending (LAD), and left circumflex (Cx) coronary arteries (Figure 22.4). There was no evidence of thrombus formation. Her electrocardiogram (ECG) showed no evidence of ischaemia. Given the new finding of multiple giant aneurysms of her coronary arteries, she was readmitted to the cardiology ward for repeated treatment with the same dose of IVIG and continued on high-dose ASA. Additionally, she was initiated on warfarin and bridged with low-molecular weight heparin until her international normalized ratio (INR) was therapeutic (INR 2–2.5). Outpatient follow-up with serial echocardiograms demonstrated an improvement in the size of all her aneurysms. Six months later, she was brought to the cardiac catheterization laboratory for coronary angiography, which demonstrated moderate aneurysmal dilatation of the left main (3 mm), proximal LAD(4.5 mm), and proximal Cx coronary arteries, with a moderate fusiform aneurysm of the proximal right coronary artery (RCA) (5.5 mm) (Figure 22.5). There was no coronary artery stenosis or evidence of thrombus formation.

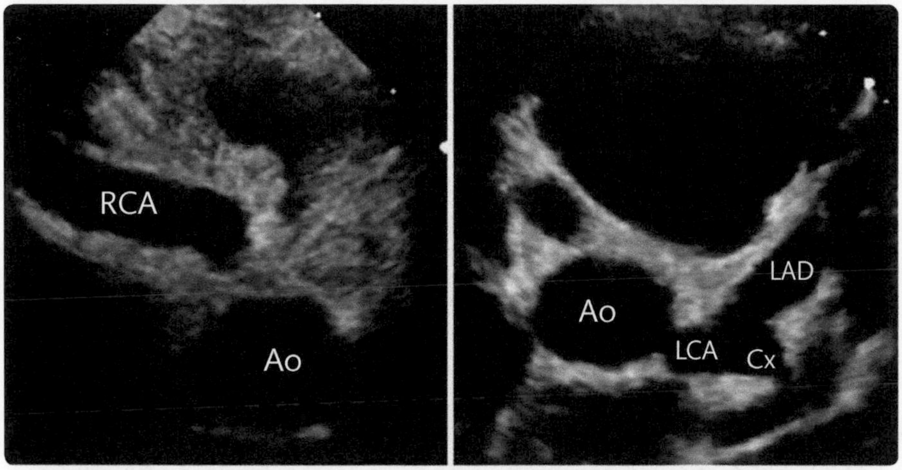

Figure 22.4 A parasternal short axis view from our patient demonstrates diffuse aneurysmal dilatation of the right coronary artery (RCA), left main coronary artery (LCA), left anterior descending (LAD), and proximal left circumflex (Cx) coronary arteries. Ao, aorta.

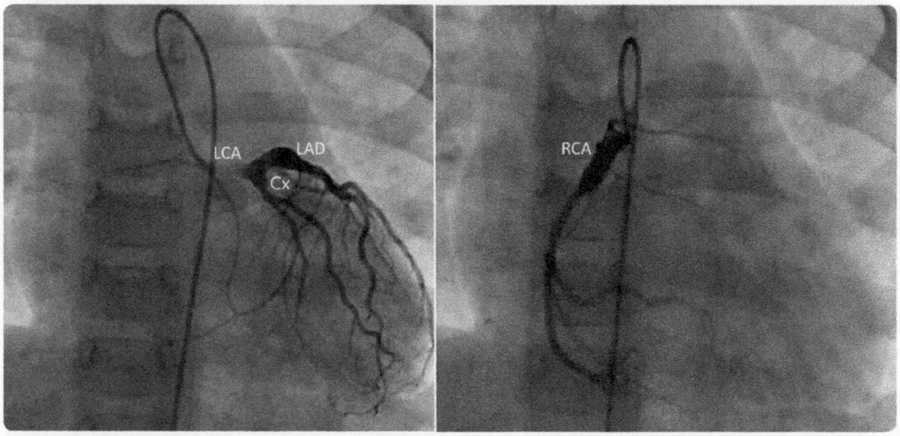

Figure 22.5 Coronary angiography (anteroposterior view). Similar to the echocardiographic images in Figure 22.4, diffuse aneurysmal dilatation of the proximal coronary arteries are demonstrated by angiography. Cx, circumflex artery; LAD, left anterior descending; LCA, left main coronary artery; RCA, right coronary artery.

Learning point Treatment for patients who develop coronary aneurysms despite initial treatment with IVIG

- A repeat dose of IVIG, either alone or in combination with steroids or infliximab [tumour necrosis factor (TNF)-α receptor antagonist], is currently the accepted practice for these patients.
- Cyclophosphamide, a cytotoxic agent, is used for rare cases of coronary disease progression despite the use of other agents.
- Other treatments currently under investigation include an interleukin-1 (IL-1) receptor antagonist (anakinra) and statin therapy [3].

Expert comment

The need for timely diagnosis and prompt initiation of treatment cannot be over-emphasized, as proper treatment has been proven to decrease the incidence of coronary artery involvement. There are now well-established treatment algorithms that serve as the mainstay for management of children presenting with suspected KD, and each institution should have a clear protocol for assessment and treatment, ideally with specialized teams overseeing its implementation.

Clinical tip Coronary artery evaluation by echocardiogram

(See Figure 22.6.)

- In most acquired and congenital paediatric cardiac diseases, evaluation of the origin of the coronary arteries is sufficient. However, in KD, it is essential to evaluate the entirety of the major coronary arteries.
- The parasternal short axis view is the main view used to evaluate the coronaries and allows measuring the left coronary artery (LCA), as well as the proximal LAD, Cx, and RCA. Artefacts pose an important problem whilst evaluating the coronaries, and careful evaluation using two-dimensional, in addition to colour Doppler, interrogation is essential to accurately identify the coronaries.
- High left parasternal views are useful to evaluate the LCA and its bifurcation.
- The parasternal long axis view can be used to evaluate the RCA origin and to evaluate the distal LAD, by angling the transducer towards the left shoulder.
- Apical and subcostal coronal views are useful to evaluate the course of the Cx and RCA in the atrioventricular groove, by angling the transducer anteriorly.
- Additionally, the LAD can be demonstrated coursing anterior to the interventricular septum from anteriorly tilted apical views.
- Measuring the coronary arteries and using Z-scores improve the sensitivity of the echocardiogram to detect coronary involvement in KD [3, 4].

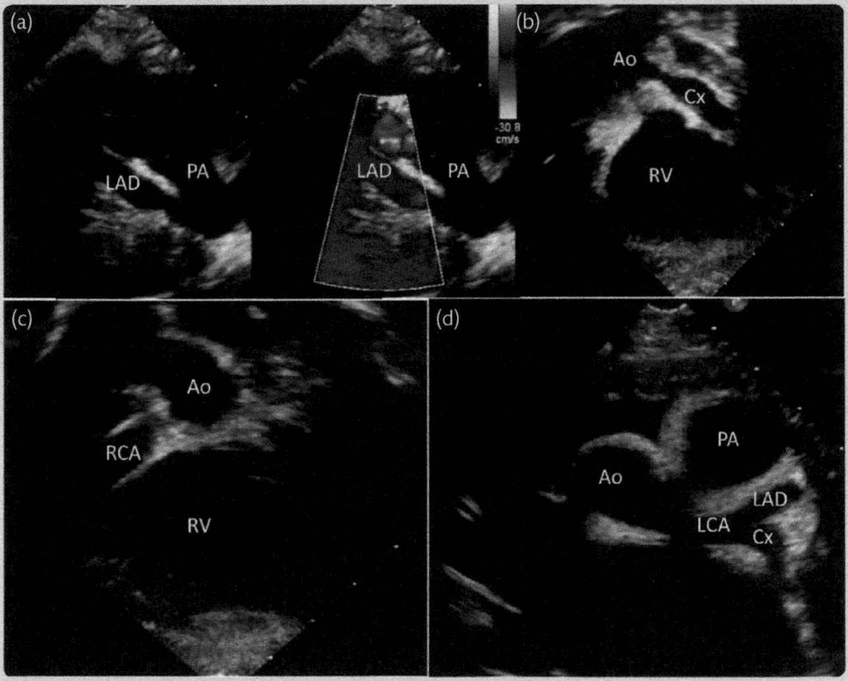

Figure 22.6 Examples of different echocardiographic views to evaluate the coronary arteries in our patient. (a) Parasternal long axis view, angling the transducer to the left shoulder to evaluate the interventricular groove. The distal left anterior descending (LAD) artery is well seen in this image. (b) Apical view with anterior tilting of the transducer showing the circumflex (Cx) artery in the atrioventricular groove. (c) Apical view with anterior tilting of the transducer shows the right coronary artery (RCA) in the atrioventricular groove. (d) A high left parasternal image showing the left coronary artery (LCA), LAD, and Cx. Ao, aorta; PA, pulmonary artery; RV, right ventricle.

Learning point Preventing coronary thrombotic complications in KD

- Treatment and follow-up investigations are tailored to the extent of the coronary artery involvement according to the risk stratification mentioned in Tables 22.2 and 22.3.
- As long-term prospective data are lacking, most recommendations are based on expert consensus.
- In general, any patient with coronary aneurysms will require long-term antiplatelet therapy at least until they resolve, with many experts suggesting lifelong treatment.
- Giant aneurysms defined as aneurysms with a diameter of >8 mm or above 10 Z-scores of normal are especially at high risk for complications and should be treated with formal anticoagulation [1–3].

Table 22.2 Risk stratification [1, 3]

Coronary risk stratification				
Z-score	Risk level	Management		
<2	1 normal coronary arteries	Antiplatelet therapy 4–6 weeks and cardiac counselling No invasive cardiac tests are warranted		
2 to <2.5	2 transient dilatation	Same as risk level 1		
≥2.5 to <5	3 small aneurysm	Low-dose aspirin beyond first 6 weeks	⊕	Lifelong surveillance tailored to conronary artery status and age: • Angiography (CT, CMR, invasive) • Stress-testing for inducible myocardial ischemia • Coronary intervention: ∘ Catheter ∘ Surgical • Counselling: ∘ Exercise recommendations ∘ Reproductive counselling ∘ Cardiovascular risk management
≥5 to <10	4 medium aneurysm	Long-term antiplatelet therapy	⊕	
≥10 or absolute dimension ≥8 mm	5 large or giant aneurysm	Long-term antiplatelet plus anticoagulation therapy ± beta blockers	⊕	

Reproduced from Newburger, J.W., M. Takahashi, and J.C. Burns, Kawasaki Disease. *J Am Coll Cardiol*, 2016. 67(14): p. 1738–49 with permission from Elseiver.

Table 22.3 Follow-up recommendations in KD

Risk level	Pharmacological therapy	Physical activity	Follow-up and diagnostic testing	Invasive testing
I (no coronary artery changes at any stage of illness)	None beyond first 6–8 weeks	No restrictions beyond first 6–8 weeks	Cardiovascular risk assessment, counselling at 5-yearly intervals	None recommended
II (transient coronary artery ectasia disappears within first 6–8 weeks)	None beyond first 6–8 weeks	No restrictions beyond first 6–8 weeks	Cardiovascular risk assessment, counselling at 3- to 5-yearly intervals	None recommended
III (one small to medium coronary artery aneurysm/major coronary artery)	Low-dose aspirin (3–5 mg/kg aspirin/day), at least until aneurysm regression documented	For patients <11-years old, no restriction beyond first 6–8 weeks; patients 11- to 20-years old, physical activity guided by biennial stress test, evaluation of myocardial perfusion scan; contact or high-impact sports discouraged for patients taking antiplatelet agents	Annual cardiology follow-up with echocardiogram + ECG, combined with cardiovascular risk assessment, counselling; biennial stress test/evaluation of myocardial perfusion scan	Angiography; if non-invasive test, suggest ischaemia
IV (≥1 large or giant coronary artery aneurysm, or multiple or complex aneurysms in same coronary artery, without obstruction)	Long-term artiplatelet therapy and warfarin (target INR 2.0–2.5) or low-molecular weight heparin (target: antifactor Xa level 0.5–1.0 U/ml) should be combined in giant aneurysms	Contact or high-impact sports should be avoided because of risk for bleeding; other physical activity recommendations guided by stress test/evaluation of myocardial perfusion scan outcome	Biannual follow-up with echocardiogram + ECG; annual stress test/evaluation of myocardial perfusion scan	First angiography at 6–12 months or sooner if clinically indicated; repeated angiography if non-invasive test, clinical, or laboratory findings suggest ischaemia; elective repeat angiography under some circumstances
V (coronary artery obstruction)	Long-term low-dose aspirin; warfarin or low-molecular weight heparin if giant aneurysm persists; consider use of beta-blockers to reduce myocardial oxygen consumption	Contact or high-impact sports should be avoided because of risk for bleeding; other physical activity recommendation guided by stress test/myocardial perfusion scan outcome	Biannual follow-up with echocardiogram and ECG; annual stress test/evaluation of myocardial perfusion scan	Angiography recommended to address therapeutic options

Reproduced from Newburger, J.W., et al., Diagnosis, treatment, and long-term management of Kawasaki disease: a statement for health professionals from the Committee on Rheumatic Fever, Endocarditis and Kawasaki Disease, Council on Cardiovascular Disease in the Young, American Heart Association. *Circulation*, 2004. 110(17): p. 2747–71 with permission from Wolters Kluwer.

A year later, her echocardiogram demonstrated a new echo-bright density within the lumen of the proximal LAD coronary, just distal to the bifurcation of the left main, concerning for thrombus formation. Her anticoagulation management had been exemplary, with minimal out-of-window recordings of her INR. However, this new finding prompted readmission and, after consultation with haematology, changing her anticoagulation regimen to low-molecular weight heparin and clopidogrel whilst being reassessed. She remained haemodynamically stable, with no ST segment changes on ECG and no elevation in serum troponin. Repeat echocardiogram demonstrated a stable size of the density, which was thought to be compatible with an organized thrombus or with localized myofibroblastic proliferation, and warfarin therapy was reinstated, in addition to her clopidigrel.

Learning point Treating coronary thrombosis in patients with KD

- Recommendations are based on treating adults with acute coronary syndromes.
- Thrombolytic treatment with streptokinase or tissue plasminogen activator is reasonable to re-establish coronary patency and rescue the areas at risk for ischaemia (level of evidence C).
- ASA and heparin or low-molecular weight heparin are also used in these patients to prevent further extension of the thrombus.
- Clopidogrel is another antiplatelet that is used in acute coronary syndrome and can be used in children with KD and coronary thrombosis [1-3].

She was followed as an outpatient for 6 more months and then underwent a repeat cardiac catheterization for coronary angiography, which showed improvement of her aneurysms, with no evidence of coronary stenosis or thrombosis. She was switched to low-dose ASA and clopidogrel, and she continued follow-up yearly with cardiology.

Clinical tip Long-term follow-up

- All patients with coronary aneurysms require lifelong follow-up.
- Regression of aneurysms is associated with luminal myofibroblastic proliferation and vascular reactivity abnormalities, whilst persistence of aneurysms carries the lifelong risk for thrombosis, stenosis, and worsening ischaemia.
- Follow-up should be tailored to the patient's clinical picture.
- Although echocardiography is the main imaging modality in children, its reliability becomes much less as the patient gets older, related to poor acoustic windows, thus limiting coronary artery interrogation. Other non-invasive imaging modalities, including computed tomographic and magnetic resonance angiography, are increasingly being used in older patients.
- Coronary angiography is recommended in patients with complex coronary involvement after the acute process resolves—6 to 12 months after the onset of illness or sooner if indicated clinically.
- Stress testing may identify patients at highest risk for coronary events.
- All patients with KD should be encouraged to avoid sedentary lifestyles. No restrictions on competitive sports should be applied to patients with normal exercise testing. Early and continuing education regarding risk factors for later atherosclerosis are an important part of ongoing follow-up.
- Surgical or percutaneous coronary revascularization is indicated in patients with angina or significant inducible ischaemia with exercise [1-3].

Discussion

KD is the most common acquired heart disease in children in developed countries. Coronary involvement is reported in 30% of patients with no treatment and decreases to 5% with IVIG treatment [3]. Risk factors for coronary involvement include male gender, higher inflammatory markers, and age below 6 months or above 8 years [5]. Failure to respond to the first dose of IVIG, which is defined as persistent fever 36 hours after the first dose, is one of the most important risk factors for the development of coronary artery aneurysms, as it may implicate that the disease process is still active [6, 7]. Repeat treatment with IVIG in these patients results in significant decrease in the risk for coronary artery aneurysms [8]. Patients who fail two doses of IVIG are at the highest risk for developing coronary artery aneurysms, and treatment options include infliximab, steroids, other cytotoxic agents, or plasmapheresis [9, 10]. Recent studies suggest that adding corticosteroids as an adjunctive therapy to the first dose of IVIG in high-risk patients may prevent the later development of coronary artery involvement [11-13]. However, until these therapies are proven to affect clinical outcomes, their routine use cannot be recommended.

Given the significant risk for coronary involvement, understanding the long-term prognosis is paramount to guide outpatient follow-up and treatment. Patients with no coronary involvement within 6 weeks of disease onset or with only mild transient coronary dilatation do not tend to have coronary manifestations later in life [3]. If aneurysms are present, they tend to increase in size in the first 2 months of the disease and generally regress within 2 years following resolution of symptoms, although progressive stenosis may develop over time. The size and number of aneurysms dictates the natural history, with those having giant aneurysms at greatest risk for complications [3]. The risk for myocardial infarction is highest in the first 2–6 weeks after the onset of fever and is usually due to mural thrombus formation [3]. In one study, long-term follow-up of patients with giant aneurysms demonstrated myocardial infarction incidence of 23%, with an 8-month median interval from the onset of KD (range 18 days to 35 years). Coronary artery bypass graft surgery was required in 36% of these patients. The median age at operation was 11 years (range 1–44 years), and the interval from the onset of KD to operation ranged from 52 days to 43 years (median 7 years) [14]. These findings highlight the importance of long-term follow-up, as dictated by coronary artery involvement. (Table 22.2).

A final word from the expert

Accurate assessment of the coronary artery anatomy is crucial to optimal treatment and follow-up of children with KD. Echocardiography is the mainstay of early evaluation, but cardiac catheterization should be performed in patients with established aneurysms and in those in whom echocardiography and/or cardiac computed tomography are suboptimal. The role of MRI, with or without perfusion imaging, is evolving and it is likely to become the modality of choice for long-term screening.

With the recent coronavirus pandemic (COVID-19) there has been reports of a multisystem inflammatory condition in children similar to KD (15). The Royal College of Paediatrics and Child Health (UK) recently released guidance on this pediatric multisystem inflammatory syndrome temporally associated with COVID-19. A number of children have been identified who develop a significant systemic inflammatory response likely secondary to COVID-19 that shares common features with other pediatric inflammatory conditions including KD. (16) This is an evolving condition which presents with its own set of challenges and early recognition by paediatricians with specialist referral including to critical care is essential.

References

1. Newburger JW et al. Diagnosis, treatment, and long-term management of Kawasaki disease: a statement for health professionals from the Committee on Rheumatic Fever, Endocarditis and Kawasaki Disease, Council on Cardiovascular Disease in the Young, American Heart Association. *Circulation* 2004;110:2747–71.
2. Newburger JW et al. Diagnosis, treatment, and long-term management of Kawasaki disease: a statement for health professionals from the Committee on Rheumatic Fever, Endocarditis, and Kawasaki Disease, Council on Cardiovascular Disease in the Young, American Heart Association. *Pediatrics* 2004;114:1708–33.
3. Newburger JW, Takahashi M, Burns JC. Kawasaki disease. *J Am Coll Cardiol* 2016;67:1738–49.
4. Margossian R et al. Predictors of coronary artery visualization in Kawasaki disease. *J Am Soc Echocardiogr* 2011;24:53–9.

5. McCrindle BW et al. Coronary artery involvement in children with Kawasaki disease: risk factors from analysis of serial normalized measurements. *Circulation* 2007;116:174–9.
6. Egami K et al. Prediction of resistance to intravenous immunoglobulin treatment in patients with Kawasaki disease. *J Pediatr* 2006;149:237–40.
7. Uehara R et al. Analysis of potential risk factors associated with nonresponse to initial intravenous immunoglobulin treatment among Kawasaki disease patients in Japan. *Pediatr Infect Dis J* 2008;27:155–60.
8. Burns JC et al. Intravenous gamma-globulin treatment and retreatment in Kawasaki disease. US/Canadian Kawasaki Syndrome Study Group. *Pediatr Infect Dis J* 1998;17:1144–8.
9. Hashino K et al. Re-treatment for immune globulin-resistant Kawasaki disease: a comparative study of additional immune globulin and steroid pulse therapy. *Pediatr Int* 2001;43:211–17.
10. Raman V et al. Response of refractory Kawasaki disease to pulse steroid and cyclosporin A therapy. *Pediatr Infect Dis J* 2001;20:635–7.
11. Chen S et al. Coronary artery complication in Kawasaki disease and the importance of early intervention: a systematic review and meta-analysis. *JAMA Pediatr* 2016;170:1156–63.
12. Kobayashi T et al. Efficacy of immunoglobulin plus prednisolone for prevention of coronary artery abnormalities in severe Kawasaki disease (RAISE study): a randomised, open-label, blinded-endpoints trial. *Lancet* 2012;379:1613–20.
13. Son MB, Newburger JW. Management of Kawasaki disease: corticosteroids revisited. *Lancet* 2012;379:1571–2.
14. Tsuda E et al. A survey of the 3-decade outcome for patients with giant aneurysms caused by Kawasaki disease. *Am Heart J* 2014;167:249–58.
15. Toniati P, Piva S, Cattalini M, Garrafa E, Regola F, Castelli F, Franceschini F, Focà E, Andreoli L, Latronico N. Tocilizumab for the treatment of severe COVID-19 pneumonia with hyperinflammatory syndrome and acute respiratory failure: A single center study of 100 patients in Brescia, Italy. *Autoimmun Rev.* 2020 May 3;102568. doi: 10.1016/j.autrev.2020.102568. [Epub ahead of print] Review.
16. Riphagen S, Gomez X, Gonzalez Martinez C, Wilkinson N, Theocharis P. Hyperinflammatory shock in children during COVID-19 Pandemic. *Lancet* 2020; DOI: https://doi.org/10.1016/S0140-6736(20)31094-1.

CASE

23 Common arterial trunk

Justin T Tretter and Tarek Alsaied

Expert commentary Andrew N Redington

Case history

A full-term 1-week-old, previously healthy infant was sent to the emergency department (ED) by his paediatrician with concern for supraventricular tachycardia. The child was brought to the paediatrician by his parents, with concern for an increased respiratory rate noted since that morning, along with diaphoresis. Upon evaluation in the ED, his vitals were significant for tachycardia with a heart rate of 215 bpm, a blood pressure of 80/32 mmHg, tachypnoea, and an oxygen saturation of 88%. His cardiac examination was notable for the following: bounding peripheral pulses and an active precordium. On auscultation, there was a normal first heart sound, followed by an ejection click, a single loud second heart sound, and no systolic murmur, but there was a grade 2/4 high-pitched diastolic murmur best heard along the left sternal border. Other significant physical examination findings included hepatomegaly. A 12-lead electrocardiogram demonstrated sinus tachycardia at the previously mentioned rate, with a normal frontal plane QRS axis, biventricular hypertrophy, and no evidence of ischaemia. A chest radiograph demonstrated moderate cardiomegaly, with increased pulmonary vascular markings and a right-sided aortic arch.

Clinical tip Common physical examination findings

- Little or no cyanosis, dependent on presence or absence of branch pulmonary artery stenosis and relative resistances of the systemic and pulmonary vascular beds
- Bounding peripheral pulses once pulmonary vascular resistance has decreased, related to diastolic run-off into the branch pulmonary arteries, even more so if associated truncal valve regurgitation
- Overactive precordium with left precordial bulge and systolic thrill along left sternal border, related to fetal ventricular volume overload when truncal regurgitation predominates
- Normal first heart sound often followed by ejection click from dysplastic truncal valve
- Loud and single second heart sound
- A 'to and fro' murmur of truncal valve stenosis and regurgitation
- Signs of heart failure if present (i.e. tachypnoea, rales, hepatomegaly) [1, 2]

An echocardiogram demonstrated common arterial trunk which was committed to the right ventricle (Figure 23.1). There was aortic dominance, with the branch pulmonary arteries arising separately from the posterior aspect of the intrapericardial common arterial trunk. The truncal valve was quadricuspid and non-stenotic, but with severe regurgitation. There was a large perimembranous outlet ventricular septal defect. The left atrium and ventricle were mildly dilated with prominent pulmonary venous and mitral valve flow. There was normal biventricular systolic function. A single coronary artery origin was demonstrated arising anteriorly from the truncal root. The aortic arch was right-sided, with mirror image branching, no evidence of coarctation, and no arterial duct.

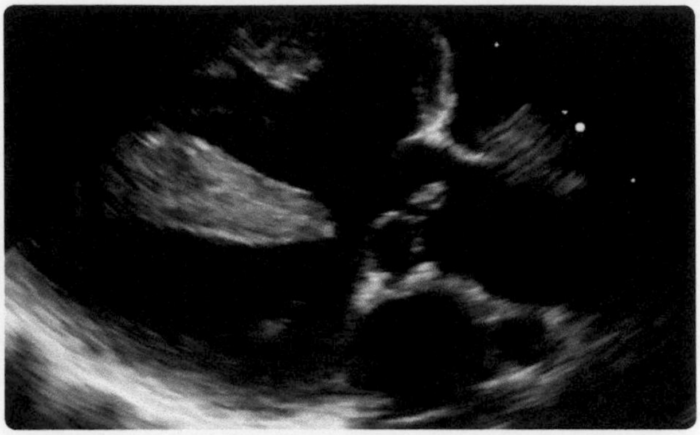

Figure 23.1 Echocardiographic parasternal long axis two-dimensional image demonstrating dominant right ventricular commitment of the truncal valve, overriding the juxta-arterial ventricular septal defect.

Learning point Morphological description

Common arterial trunk, also commonly referred to as truncus arteriosus communis, can be described according to Robert Anderson, Richard Van Praagh, or Collett and Edwards classification systems [3–6]. No matter your personal and/or institutional preference, knowledge and comfort with each system are necessary to communicate effectively with colleagues.

Anderson has coined the term common arterial trunk, preferring the use of 'American English' and emphasizing the postnatal anatomy. According to Anderson, the lesion is primarily described as being aortic dominant, pulmonary dominant, or those with balanced aortic and pulmonary pathways, followed by a description of the origins of the aortic pathway and pulmonary arteries. Pulmonary dominance is usually associated with interrupted aortic arch or coarctation (Figure 23.2). In aortic dominance, the branch pulmonary arteries usually arise together, either from a short pulmonary trunk or separately but adjacent to each other (Figure 23.3). Sometimes the pulmonary arteries arise non-adjacently, but from the trunk, and occasionally one or both of the arteries will arise from an arterial duct. Very rarely, there will be no branch pulmonary artery to one or both lungs and the pulmonary blood flow is via major aortopulmonary collateral arteries. In balanced cases, the pulmonary and aortic trunks are comparable in size and the division between the pathways extends within the pericardium [3, 4].

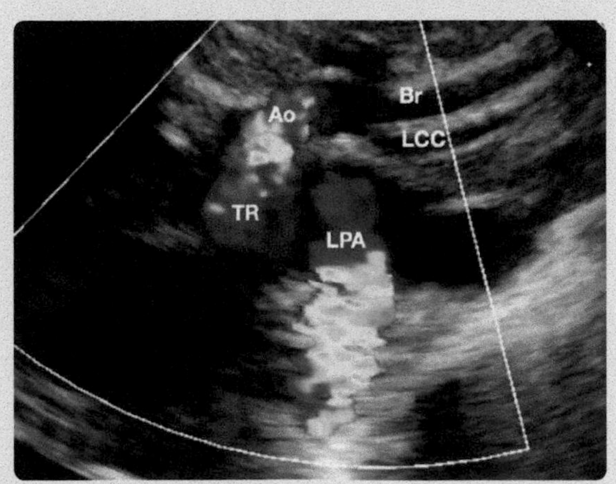

Figure 23.2 Echocardiographic suprasternal colour Doppler image demonstrating the left pulmonary artery arising from a pulmonary dominant truncal root, with interruption of the aortic arch distal to the left common carotid artery, or type B interruption. Ao, ascending aorta; Br, brachiocephalic artery; LCC, left common carotid artery; LPA, left pulmonary artery; TR, truncal root.

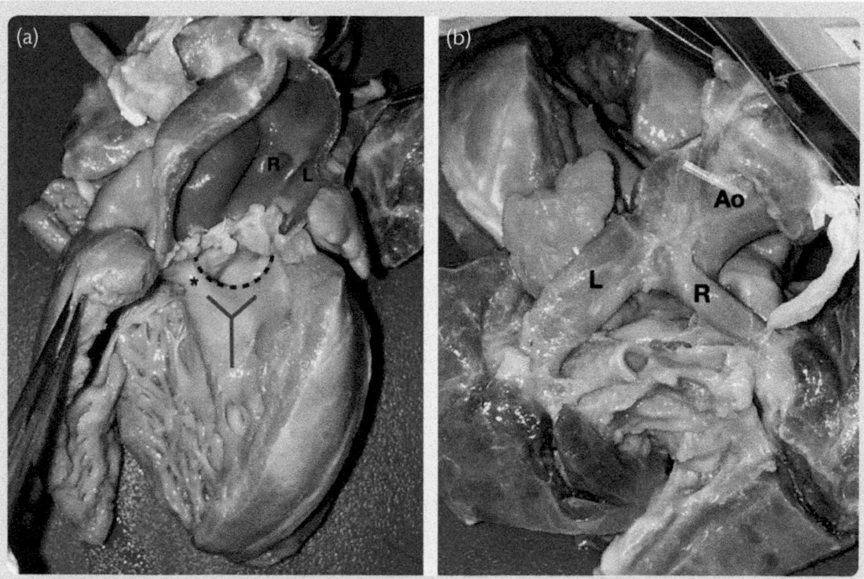

Figure 23.3 (a) The right ventricular aspect of the interventricular septum is demonstrated in a specimen with common arterial trunk with aortic dominance. The ventricular septal defect (inferior border denoted by dashed line) is cradled within the 'arms' of the septomarginal trabeculation (denoted with red 'Y'), with the thickened, nodular tricuspid truncal valve overriding the crest of the interventricular septum. The muscular portion of the postero-inferior limb of the septomarginal trabeculation (additionally denoted by an asterisk) is intact, as seen in the most common type of ventricular septal defect in common arterial trunk, the muscular outlet defect creating discontinuity between the tricuspid and truncal valves. The right (R) and left (L) branch pulmonary arteries are adjacent but arise separately from the leftward and posterior aspect of the truncal root. (b) The specimen is now viewed from the posterior aspect of the truncal root with aortic dominance, demonstrating the right (R) and left (L) branch pulmonary arteries are adjacent but arise separately from the leftward and posterior aspect of the truncal root, continuing to their respective lungs. Ao, ascending aorta.

Van Praagh's terminology describes the Latin-named truncus arteriosus communis, utilizing an alphanumeric system, initially denoted with the letter A in the more common form accompanied by a ventricular septal defect, or with the letter B in the rare form devoid of such a defect. This is followed by a number 1 through 4 to indicate the following:

- Type A1—segment of the pulmonary trunk arises from the common arterial trunk
- Type A2—branch pulmonary arteries arise directly from the common arterial trunk
- Type A3—one of the branch pulmonary arteries does not arise from the common arterial trunk and usually arises from the aorta outside the pericardium
- Type A4—associated aortic arch hypoplasia, coarctation, or interrupted aortic arch [5].

The Collett and Edwards classification system is as follows:

- Type I—analogous to Van Praagh type A1
- Type II—branch pulmonary arteries arise separately, but adjacent to each other
- Type III—branch pulmonary arteries arise separately, on opposite sides of the common arterial trunk
- Type IV—branch pulmonary arteries arise separately from an extrapericardial location. Anderson and Van Praagh do not consider this to be a form of common arterial trunk (or truncus arteriosus) [6].

Learning point Important anatomical variations and associated anomalies

- The ventricular septal defect is typically large and commonly located within the two limbs of the septomarginal trabeculation, with the truncal valve commonly overriding the crest of the interventricular septum. This is described as a muscular outlet defect (Figure 23.3a) [6]. It is perimembranous in no more than 10% of cases.
- Truncal valve morphology: tricuspid in 65–70% (Figure 23.3a), quadricuspid in 9–24%, and bicuspid in 6–23%, rarely being unicuspid or pentacuspid [7–9].
- Truncal valve origin: biventricular origin in 68–83%, right ventricular origin in 11–29%, left ventricular origin in 4–6% [6, 10].
- Some degree of truncal valve regurgitation is present in approximately 50%, with some degree of stenosis present in approximately 33% [11]. In unrepaired patients, the degree of stenosis may be overestimated due to massive over-circulation leading to falsely elevated gradients.
- A right aortic arch occurs in 21–36% [12, 13].
- An arterial duct is present in approximately half of patients, more commonly in those with pulmonary dominance [10].
- Anomalies of coronary artery origins occur in 37–49% of patients (Figure 23.4). Because the left anterior descending coronary artery is frequently small and displaced leftward, the conal branch is commonly prominent in a compensatory fashion, an important surgical consideration when constructing the right ventricular-to-pulmonary artery conduit [10, 14].

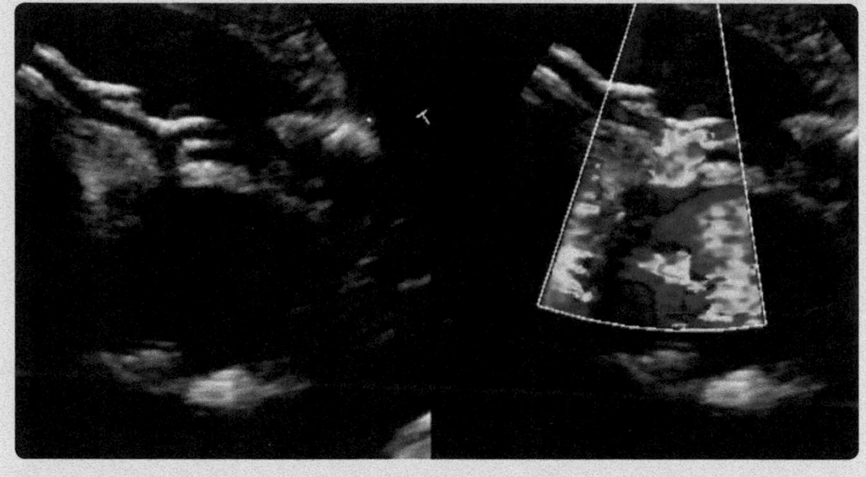

Figure 23.4 Echocardiographic parasternal short axis two-dimensional image with colour comparison, depicting a single coronary artery arising from the anterior aspect of the truncal root, bifurcating into the right and left main coronary arteries.

He was placed on 2 litres nasal cannula oxygen on room air and given one dose of furosemide 1 mg/kg intravenously. He was admitted to the cardiac intensive care unit and placed on cardiopulmonary monitoring, and continued on twice-a-day dosing of intravenous furosemide. On day 10 of life, he underwent complete surgical repair, with patch closure of the ventricular septal defect baffling the left ventricle to the truncal valve, truncal valve repair with bicuspidization and subcommissural annular reduction, removal of the branch pulmonary arteries from the truncal root with placement of an 11-mm aortic homograft conduit from the right ventricle to the branch pulmonary arteries, and primary closure of his atrial septal defect.

Clinical tip Neonatal presentation and preoperative management

- The clinical presentation can be variable but often progresses to significant pulmonary over-circulation in the first few days to weeks of life with decreasing pulmonary vascular resistance, often necessitating diuretic therapy in those presenting later than a few days of life.
- Most infants with common arterial trunk have minimal oxygen desaturation, commonly ≥90%, reflecting the large QP:QS that is often present.
- Infants with significant tachypnoea from congestive heart failure may require positive pressure ventilation in an attempt to 'stent' open the airways in the setting of interstitial pulmonary oedema, but increasing the percentage of fraction of inspired oxygen should be avoided as this will decrease pulmonary vascular resistance and further increase left-to-right shunting.
- A widened pulse pressure with low diastolic blood pressures is common, secondary to diastolic run-off into the branch pulmonary arteries and any associated truncal valve regurgitation, putting the infant at risk for mesenteric ischaemia and, if left unrepaired, chronic myocardial ischaemia due to 'coronary steal'. Enteral feeding may be inappropriate with persistently low diastolic blood pressures.
- Significant truncal valve regurgitation will expedite the onset of symptoms of congestive heart failure and can further compromise coronary blood flow.
- There is a relatively high risk for developing pulmonary hypertension if left unrepaired in the early newborn period [1, 2].

Expert comment

In the past, there was a tendency to delay repair to a few weeks or months of life. However, for all the reasons above (not least the issue of progressive coronary steal leading to ischaemic myocardial dysfunction and sudden death), most units now choose to perform complete repair within a few days of presentation.

The first post-operative night was complicated by intermittent runs of junctional ectopic tachycardia at heart rates of 170–190 bpm, with resulting hypotension, which improved following a combination of correcting hypomagnesaemia and hypocalcaemia, cooling the patient, atrial overdrive pacing utilizing temporary atrial pacing wires, and initiation of intravenous amiodarone. There were no further rhythm issues following the first post-operative night. Amiodarone was weaned off by post-operative day 3. He was weaned off the conventional ventilator by the fourth post-operative day. He was weaned off supplemental oxygen by the eighth post-operative day, and advanced to full oral feeds soon after. The patient was discharged home on the thirteenth post-operative day on twice-daily oral furosemide therapy, with a discharge echocardiogram demonstrating a good surgical result, with only mild truncal valve regurgitation, normal biventricular systolic function, and no pericardial effusion.

Clinical tip Importance of the ventricular septal defect

- Although patients with restrictive defects, or even an intact ventricular septum, have been described, common arterial trunk is most commonly associated with a large, unrestrictive juxta-arterial interventricular communication which opens into the right ventricle between the limbs of the septomarginal trabeculation and is roofed by the truncal valve leaflets (Figure 23.3a).
- There are two common types of interventricular communications:
  - Muscular outlet type—the muscular postero-inferior limb is intact, with resulting truncal and tricuspid valve fibrous discontinuity (Figures 23.3a and 23.5a)
  - Perimembranous outlet type—the postero-inferior limb is deficient, with resulting truncal and tricuspid valve fibrous continuity, as well as fibrous continuity between the atrioventricular valves (Figure 23.5b)
- Additional muscular defects should always be actively excluded, as they may significantly impact the surgical procedure [6, 15]

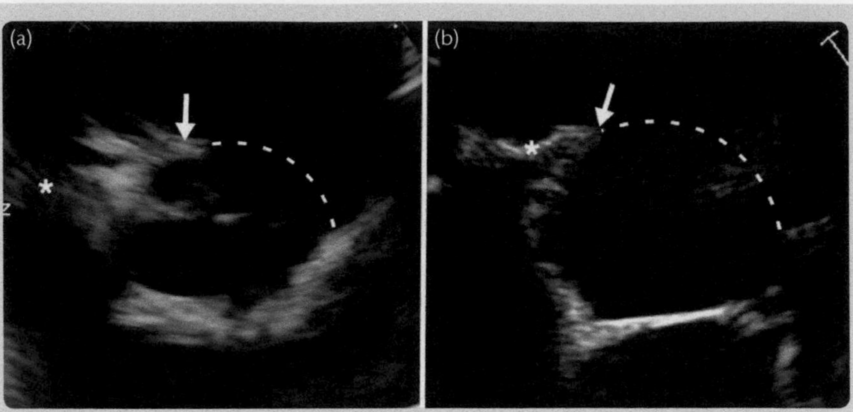

Figure 23.5 Parasternal short axis two-dimensional images of a (a) muscular-type (the white arrow points to the postero-inferior muscular rim, and the asterisk marks the septal leaflet of the tricuspid valve near its annular attachment) and a (b) perimembranous ventricular septal defect (defect denoted by white dashed line). Both defects are large and 'juxta-arterial'. However, in the muscular-type defect (a), there is fibrous discontinuity of the tricuspid (asterisk) and truncal valves caused by the interposing muscular postero-inferior limb of the septomarginal trabeculation (arrow). In the perimembranous defect (b), the communication extends into the perimembranous region of the interventricular septum, with deficiency of the postero-inferior limb of the septomarginal trabeculation, creating fibrous continuity (arrow) of the tricuspid (asterisk) and truncal valves.

Expert comment

Although this patient had a perimembranous ventricular septal defect, this is somewhat unusual. A muscular postero-inferior rim to the defect, separating the tricuspid valve from the truncal valve and creating space between the defect and the membranous septum, is seen in approximately three-quarters of patients. For this reason, post-operative complete heart block is particularly uncommon in common arterial trunk. It is speculative, but the fact that this patient had a perimembranous defect may have predisposed him to the development of post-operative junctional ectopic tachycardia [15, 16], which is frequently due to trauma and haemorrhage adjacent to the atrioventricular node which runs just posterior to the membranous septum.

The patient had a relatively uncomplicated outpatient follow-up throughout his early childhood. However, he developed progressively worsening right ventricle-to-pulmonary artery conduit stenosis and conduit regurgitation starting at around 7 years of age, with the development of worsening exertional dyspnoea. Due to severe conduit stenosis (echocardiographic mean gradient of 65 mmHg, with systemic right ventricular systolic pressure) with moderate conduit regurgitation at 9 years of age, he underwent a surgical conduit replacement. He had a good surgical result and an uncomplicated post-operative course.

Discussion

Common arterial trunk occurs in approximately 1–4% of children with congenital heart disease [5, 6, 9], thus occurring in 9–11 per 100,000 live births [17]. It is a lethal abnormality, with a mean age of death in unrepaired children of approximately 2.5 months, with the overwhelming majority dying in the first year of life [6]. DiGeorge syndrome (microdeletion 22q11.2) is identified in approximately 35–40% of patients with common arterial trunk and is even more common in those with a right aortic arch and/or an abnormal aortic arch branching pattern [18–20]. Maternal diabetes has also been implicated as a risk factor for the development of common arterial trunk [21].

Although prenatal diagnosis is becoming more common with improved obstetric ultrasound screening (Figure 23.6) [22], it is not uncommon for the diagnosis to be made postnatally. The clinical presentation is highly variable, largely dependent on the detailed combination of cardiac morphological variation. Infants with common arterial trunk sometimes go undetected in the immediate newborn period, even passing the commonly employed newborn oxygen saturation screening. In those with interruption of the aortic arch, the presentation may be that of cardiogenic shock as the arterial duct closes, compromising systemic perfusion [1, 2].

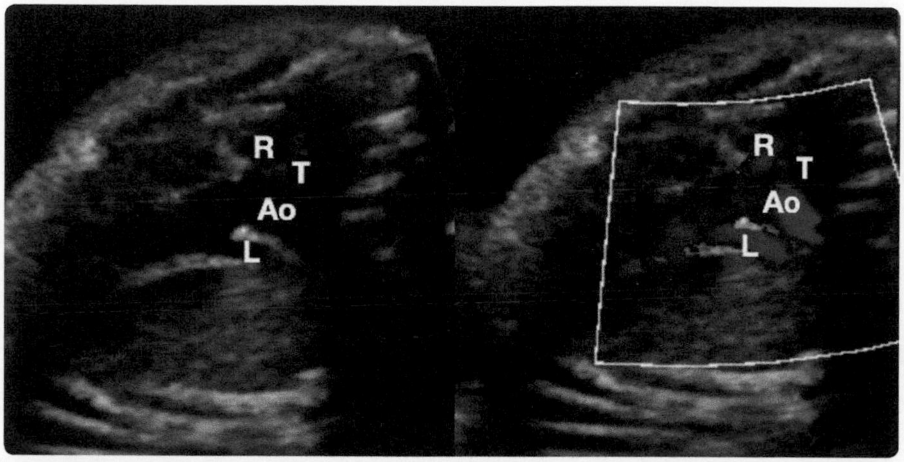

Figure 23.6 Fetal echocardiographic two-dimenstional image with colour comparison, demonstrating an aortic-dominant common arterial trunk, with the branch pulmonary arteries arising separately from opposite sides of the common arterial trunk. The aortic arch (Ao) courses leftward to the trachea (T). L, left pulmonary artery; R, right pulmonary artery.

Surgical repair within the first or second week of life is now the norm, with excellent surgical results. Although this diagnosis holds one of the higher discharge mortality rates and post-operative length of hospital stay, when compared to nine other benchmark surgeries, in a recent analysis of the Society of Thoracic Surgeons Congenital Heart Surgery database, second only to the Norwood operation, the mortality rate has fallen to < 10% (Table 23.1) [23]. Survivors of the immediate post-operative period have favourable outcomes, including good functional developmental outcomes in those with no associated chromosomal abnormalities [24]. However, lifelong cardiology follow-up is needed, with expectations of progressive right ventricle-to-pulmonary artery conduit obstruction and often significant conduit regurgitation within the first to second decades of life related to somatic growth or progressive deterioration and calcification of the conduit, necessitating eventual conduit replacement [25, 26]. Subsequent conduit replacement is also common in adults with a history of congenital heart disease and an 'adult-size' conduit, with a reported 50% occurrence of the development of severe conduit dysfunction and conduit re-intervention by 15 years of post-implant, and a 30% likelihood of undergoing conduit reoperation within the same time frame [27].

Table 23.1 The Society of Thoracic Surgeons Congenital Heart Surgery 2016 Database Aggregate Outcomes of Benchmark Operations: operative mortality and post-operative length of stay

	Off bypass coarctation	VSD	TOF	AVC	ASO	ASO + VSD	Glenn/ HemiFontan	Fontan	Common arterial trunk	Norwood
Operative mortality (%)	1	0.7	1	3.2	2.7	5.3	2.1	1.4	9.6	15.6
Post-operative average length of stay (days)	12.1	8.2	11.4	16.3	16	18.7	13.8	13.4	29.3	42.2

ASO, arterial switch operation; AVC, atrioventricular canal; TOF, tetralogy of Fallot; VSD, ventricular septal defect.
Source data from Jacobs JP, Mayer JE, Mavroudis C, O'Brien SM, Austin EH 3rd, Pasquali SK, Hill KD, He X, Overman DM, St. Louis JD, Karamlou T, Pizarro C, Hirsch-Romano JC, McDonald D, Han JM, Dokholyan RS, Tchervenkov CI, Lacour-Gayet F, Backer CL, Fraser CD, Tweddell JS, Elliott MJ, Walters H, Jonas RA, Prager RL, Shahian DM, Jacobs ML. The Society of Thoracic Surgeons Congenital Heart Surgery database: 2016 update on outcomes and quality. *Ann Thorac Surg* 2016;101:850–862.

Undoubtedly, common arterial trunk requires careful attention to detail by the diagnosing physician, as well as meticulous anatomical description in anticipation of the variable physiological derangements and guidance in surgical repair. Like many forms of congenital heart disease, this defect requires lifelong follow-up, often necessitating multiple re-interventions and reoperations.

A final word from the expert

Whilst it would be incorrect to suggest that neonatal repair of any patient with common arterial trunk is 'straightforward', the results for those with 'good anatomy' have improved remarkably over the past two decades, coinciding with a shift towards early complete repair in the neonatal period. The likelihood of a poor outcome, unsurprisingly, is much greater in very low-birthweight babies and those with severe associated haemodynamic abnormalities and non-cardiac abnormalities. Indeed, the risk for early post-operative death remains the highest in those presenting with aortic coarctation or interruption and in those requiring concomitant truncal valve surgery [28]. Furthermore, when there is associated 22q11 deletion, we can anticipate greater morbidity and prolonged hospital stays [29].

Acknowledgements

We are thankful for the help of Dr Sathish Chikkabyrappa in identifying some of the echocardiographic images for this chapter.

References

1. Marcelletti C, McGoon DC, Mair DD. The natural history of truncus arteriosus. *Circulation* 1976;54:108–11.
2. Ebert PA, Turley K, Stanger P. Surgical treatment of truncus arteriosus in the first 6 months of life. *Ann Surg* 1984;200:451–6.
3. Russell HM, Jacobs ML, Anderson RH, et al. A simplified categorization for common arterial trunk. *J Thorac Cardiovasc Surg* 2011;14:645–53.
4. Jacobs ML, Anderson RH. Rationalising the nomenclature of common arterial trunk. *Cardiol Young* 2012;22:639–46.

5. Van Praagh R, Van Praagh S. The anatomy of common aorticopulmonary trunk (truncus arteriosus communis) and its embryologic implications. A study of 57 necropsy cases. *Am J Cardiol* 1965;16:406–25.
6. Collett RW, Edwards JE. Persistent truncus arteriosus: a classification according to anatomic types. *Surg Clin North Am* 1949;29:1245–70.
7. Fuglestad SJ, Puga FJ, Danielson GK. Surgical pathology of the truncal valve: a study of 12 cases. *Am J Cardiovasc Pathol* 1988;2:39–47.
8. Crupi G, Macartney FJ, Anderson RH. Persistent truncus arteriosus. A study of 66 autopsy cases with special references to definition and morphogenesis. *Am J Cardiol* 1977;40:569–78.
9. Calder L, Van Praagh R, Van Praagh S, et al. Truncus arteriosus communis. Clinical, angiocardiographic, and pathologic findings in 100 patients. *Am Heart J* 1976;92:23–38.
10. Bharati S, McAllister HA, Rosenquist GC. The surgical anatomy of truncus arteriosus communis. *J Thorac Cardiovasc Surg* 1974;67:501–10.
11. Bengur AR. Truncus arteriosus. In: Garson A, Bricker JT, Fisher DJ, Neish SR, editors. *Science and Practice of Pediatric Cardiology*, 2nd edition. Philadelphia, PA: Lippincott Williams and Wilkins, 1998; p. 1421.
12. Butto F, Lucas RV, Edwards JE. Persistent truncus arteriosus: pathologic anatomy in 54 cases. *Pediatr Cardiol* 1986;7:95–101.
13. Marcelletti C, McGoon DC, Danielson GK. Early and late results of surgical repair of truncus arteriosus. *Circulation* 1977;55:636–41.
14. Shrivastava S, Edwards JE. Coronary arterial origin in persistent truncus arteriosus. *Circulation* 1977;55:551–4.
15. Colon M, Anderson RH, Weinberg P, Mussatto K, Bove E, Friedman AH. Anatomy, morphogenesis, diagnosis, management, and outcomes for neonates with common arterial trunk. *Cardiol Young* 2008;Suppl 3:52–62.
16. Mildh L, Hiippala A, Rautiainen P, Pettilä V, Sairanen H, Happonen JM. Junctional ectopic tachycardia after surgery for congenital heart disease: incidence, risk factors and outcome. *Eur J Cardiothorac Surg* 2011;39:75–80.
17. Hoffman JI, Kaplan S. The incidence of congenital heart disease. *J Am Coll Cardiol* 2002;39:1890–900.
18. Goldmuntz E, Clark BJ, Mitchell LE, et al. Frequency of 22q11 deletions in patients with conotruncal defects. *J Am Coll Cardiol* 1998;32:492–8.
19. Iserin L, de Lonlay P, Viot G, et al. Prevalence of the microdeletion 22q11 in newborn infants with congenital conotruncal cardiac anomalies. *Eur J Pediatr* 1998;157:881–4.
20. McElhinney DB, Driscoll DA, Emanuel BS, Goldmuntz E. Chromosome 22q11 deletion in patients with congenital conotruncal cardiac anomalies. *Pediatr Cardiol* 2003;24:569–73.
21. Lisowski LA, Verheijen PM, Copel JA, et al. Congenital heart disease in pregnancies complicated by maternal diabetes mellitus. An international clinical collaboration, literature review, and meta-analysis. *Herz* 2010;35:19–26.
22. Copel JA, Pilu G, Green J, et al. Fetal echocardiographic screening for congenital heart disease: the importance of the four-chamber view. *Am J Obstet Gynecol* 1987;157:648–55.
23. Jacobs JP, Mayer JE, Mavroudis C, et al. The Society of Thoracic Surgeons Congenital Heart Surgery database: 2016 update on outcomes and quality. *Ann Thorac Surg* 2016;101:850–62.
24. Martin BJ, Ross DB, Alton GY, et al. Clinical and functional developmental outcomes in neonates undergoing truncus arteriosus repair: a cohort study. *Ann Thorac Surg* 2016;101:1827–33.
25. Brown JW, Ruzmetov M, Okada Y, Vijay P, Turrentine MW. Truncus arteriosus repair, outcomes, risk factors, reoperation and management. *Eur J Cardiothorac Surg* 2001;20:221–7.
26. Asagai S, Inai K, Shinohara T, et al. Long-term outcomes after truncus arteriosus repair: a single-center experience for more than 40 years. *Congenit Heart Dis* 2016;11:672–7.

27. Buber J, Assenza GE, Huang A, et al. Durability of large diameter right ventricular outflow tract conduits in adults with congenital heart disease. *Int J Cardiol* 2014;175:455–63.
28. Russell HM, Pasquali SK, Jacobs JP, et al. Outcomes of repair of common arterial trunk with truncal valve surgery: a review of the society of thoracic surgeons congenital heart surgery database. *Ann Thorac Surg* 2012;93:164–9.
29. O'Byrne ML, Yang W, Mercer-Rosa L, et al. 22q11.2 Deletion syndrome is associated with increased perioperative events and more complicated postoperative course in infants undergoing infant operative correction of truncus arteriosus communis or interrupted aortic arch. *J Thorac Cardiovasc Surg* 2014;148:1597–605.

CASE

24 Pulmonary hypertension associated with congenital heart disease

Ryan Coleman and Corey Chartan

Expert commentary Nidhy Varghese

Case history

A 7-month-old female with no previously diagnosed medical conditions was transferred from an outside institution for further management. She was diagnosed with respiratory syncytial virus, rhinovirus, and enterovirus pneumonia, requiring intubation and mechanical ventilation. On the day of transfer, it was noticed that she had a number of classic phenotypic features for Down syndrome, and an echocardiogram performed revealed a preliminary diagnosis of atrioventricular septal defect (AVSD) (Table 24.1).

Table 24.1 Incidence of congenital heart disease in trisomy 21

Population-based study—Newcastle upon Tyne [10]	
Overall incidence: 42% (342 of 821) of all patients with Down syndrome	
Type of defect	**Incidence**
Complete atrioventricular septal defect (cAVSD)	125 (37%)
Ventricular septal defect (VSD)	106 (31%)
Atrial septal defect (ASD)	52 (15%)
Partial atrioventricular septal defect (pAVSD)	22 (6%)
Tetralogy of Fallot (TOF)	16 (5%)
Patent ductus arteriosus (PDA)	14 (4%)
Miscellaneous	7 (2%)
Multiple defects	80 (23%)
ASD/PDA	
Single ventricle physiology	3 (<1%)
Unbalanced cAVSD with hypoplastic right ventricle	1 (<1%)
Tricuspid atresia	1 (<1%)
Pulmonary atresia/intact ventricular septum	1 (<1%)

The study by Irving and Chaudhari represents one of the more comprehensive studies of children with Down syndrome, and because of its utilization of the Northern Congenital Abnormality Survey, it represents a comprehensive overview of likely all patients born within the 22-year period analysed.

Upon arrival to our institution, her initial vital signs were notable for saturations of 96% on an FiO_2 of 0.6, whilst being mechanically ventilated on relatively modest ventilator settings. Initial complete blood count showed a haemoglobin level of 12.3 mg/dl. Her chest radiograph revealed minor cardiomegaly, without evidence of significant congestive heart failure, and no increased pulmonary vascular markings were appreciated to suggest pulmonary over-circulation. A repeat echocardiogram was performed, which confirmed the diagnosis of AVSD and further classified it as a balanced Rastelli type C defect (Figure 24.1).

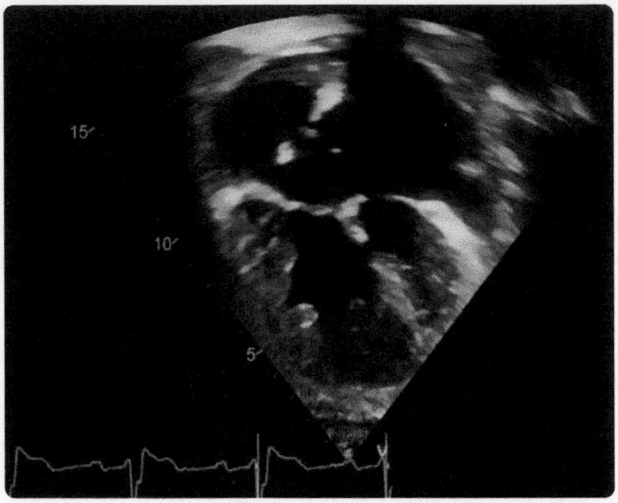

Figure 24.1 Apical four-chamber view demonstrating the atrioventricular septal defect in conjunction with significant right ventricular hypertrophy.

Learning point Pulmonary hypertension in congenital heart disease

Pulmonary hypertension (PH), particularly precapillary PH, is a frequently encountered and potentially moribund complication that can occur in patients with congenital heart disease. It is the third most common form of precapillary PH, trailing only behind idiopathic PH and PH associated with connective tissue disease [1]. In the United Kingdom, it was found that approximately 50% of cases of precapillary PH have underlying congenital heart disease or Eisenmenger syndrome [2]. Similar to idiopathic pulmonary arterial hypertension, patients with PH-CHD experience gradual changes in the structure of their pulmonary arterial bed, resulting in increased pulmonary vascular resistance. These changes initially are characterized by medial hypertrophy of the vessels, but as the disease progresses, this hypertrophy can proliferate, obliterate the lumen, and ultimately result in fibrosis and necrosis of the vasculature [3].

The type of congenital heart disease present often dictates the severity of the resultant PH. Patients with atrial-level shunts, even if large, rarely experience severe pulmonary arterial hypertension. However, patients with large conoventricular defects, large patent ductus arterioses, or truncus arteriosus experience near-universal occurrence of clinically significant PH [4–6]. It is known that left-to-right shunts can cause enough shear stress and injury to the endothelium to upregulate the production of endothelin, thus causing pulmonary arterial hypertension [7–8]. However, the reasons behind why patients without large shunts, such as those with coarctation of the aorta or seemingly insignificant atrial-level shunting, can also experience pulmonary arterial hypertension remains unclear. The presence of underlying genetic abnormalities, such as trisomy 21, only further increases the occurrence of PH-CHD [9–11].

On discussion with the patient's grandparents, who had become her primary caregivers, they stated that the patient had never been diagnosed with Down syndrome up until this point, despite seeing her paediatrician on a regular basis for routine well-child care. The grandmother stated that the mother, who was no longer involved with the patient, had a prenatal ultrasound scan suggestive of Down syndrome but declined amniocentesis. After this refusal, no further medical evaluation was undertaken to confirm this diagnosis until the current hospitalization.

The grandmother also stated that the patient would often have a cyanotic tint, particularly when crying or with feeding, but never became tachypnoeic or diaphoretic with feeds and had been gaining weight steadily, albeit slowly, since birth. Review of outside-hospital medical records also confirmed that the patient's saturations appeared to range in the low to mid 80s prior to an increase in FiO_2, which raised the saturations into the low to mid 90s.

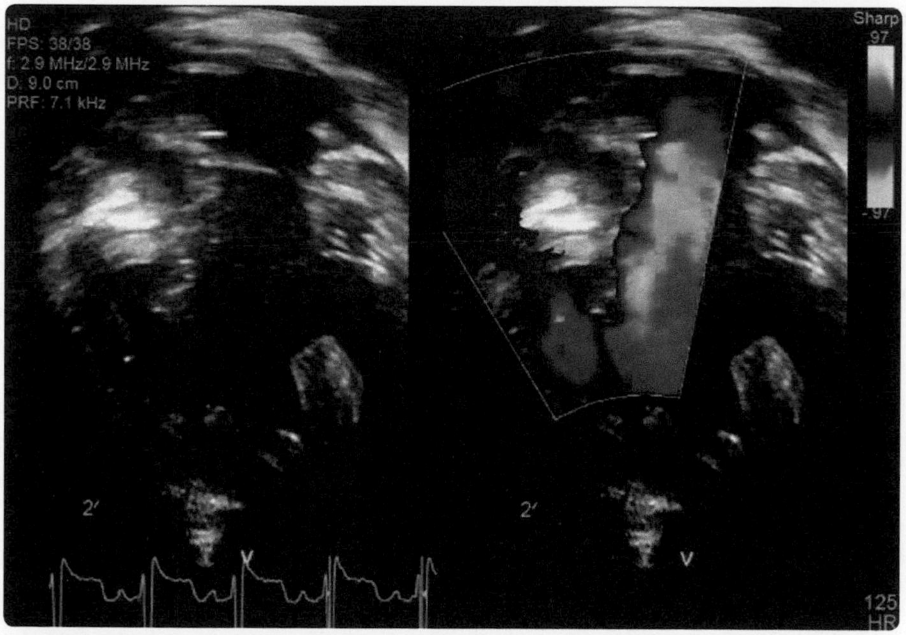

Figure 24.2 Side-by-side apical four-chamber view showing the right-to-left shunt across the ventricular septal defect demonstrating elevated right-sided pressures.

Learning point Clinical signs and symptoms associated with elevated pulmonary vascular resistance

General symptoms

- Dyspnoea with exercise—can include feeding in newborns
- Syncope/near-syncope
- Angina
- Orthopnoea/paroxysmal nocturnal dyspnoea
- Lower extremity oedema
- Abdominal distension
- Early satiety
- Poor growth or unexpected decrease in growth velocity

Specific to patients with congenital heart disease

- Cyanosis
- Lack of over-circulation symptoms—no dyspnoea, tachypnoea
- No need for diuretics to manage over-circulation symptoms
- Poor growth despite increased caloric intake

Due to her constellation of signs and symptoms suggestive of elevated pulmonary vascular resistance, the PH service was consulted for assistance with her management. Her lack of symptoms suggestive of pulmonary over-circulation and apparent baseline saturations that must have been low to account for her intermittent cyanotic appearance were suggestive of PH. Additionally, in conjunction with her chest radiograph findings and relative polycythaemia (Table 24.2), empiric sildenafil was initiated to start lowering her pulmonary vascular resistance prior to her surgical repair (see Expert comment: Important mediators of pulmonary hypertension, p. 318). Cardiac catheterization was deferred, as it was felt that it would not yield any meaningful data and would expose the patient to risks, which were not absolutely necessary (Figure 24.2).

Table 24.2 Basic mechanisms of pulmonary hypertension

	Mechanism	Common examples
Increased precapillary resistance	Constriction	Hypoxaemia *BMPR2* mutation
	Obstruction	Pulmonary embolism
	Abnormal development or destruction of vasculature	Bronchopulmonary dysplasia Connective tissue diseases
Increased post-capillary resistance	Pulmonary vein abnormalities	Pulmonary vein stenosis Pulmonary veno-occlusive disease
	Left-sided heart disease	Mitral valve stenosis Shone's complex
Increased pulmonary blood flow	Increased cardiac output	Hyperthyroidism Vein of Galen malformation
	Systemic-to-pulmonary shunts	Ventricular septal defect Atrioventricular septal defect

Learning point Medical therapy for the management of PH

Table 24.3 Medical therapy for management of PH

Drug	Class	Important points
Sildenafil PO	PDE5	Start with low dosing and gradually increase as haemodynamics tolerate
Sildenafil IV	PDE5	Start with low dosing and gradually increase as haemodynamics tolerate; tend to see hypotension approximately 30 minutes after dose given PO to IV conversion is 1 mg PO = 0.5 mg IV
Tadalafil PO	PDE5	Once-daily dosing; may improve adherence
Bosentan PO	ERA—dual ETA/ETB	Monitor liver function tests monthly; can have gastrointestinal side effects; do not use if underlying hepatic dysfunction
Ambrisentan PO	ERA—selective ET1A	Decreased hepatotoxicity compared to other ERAs
Macitentan PO	ERA—dual ET1A/ET1B	Do not use if moderate to severe hepatic dysfunction; can cause significant oedema
Epoprostenol IV	Prostanoids	Major side effects: headache, nausea/vomiting, hypotension; needs to be kept cool; half-life: 4–6 minutes
Epoprostenol IV	Prostanoids	Major side effects: headache, nausea/vomiting, hypotension; can be kept at room temperature; half-life: 4–6 minutes
Treprostinil subcutaneous	Prostanoids	Half-life: 4–5 hours; stable at room temperature
Treprostinil IV	Prostanoids	Half-life: 4–5 hours; stable at room temperature
Treprostinil inhaled	Prostanoids	6–9 inhalations/day; 1 breath = 5 mcg
Iloprost inhaled	Prostanoids	Can cause flushing/headache; can cause bronchospasm
Treprostinil PO	Prostanoids	Significant gastrointestinal side effects
Riociguat PO	Guanylyl cyclase stimulator	Do not use in combination with PDE5 inhibitors; can cause hypotension
Selexipag PO	Prostacyclin IP receptor agonist	Limited paediatric data currently available

ERA, endothelin receptor antagonist; IV, intravenous; PO, oral; PDE, phosphodiesterase; SC, subcutaneous.

Clinical tip Specific vasoactive agents for the management of acute PH

Norepinephrine

- Increases left ventricular output, systemic arterial pressure, and pulmonary blood flow.
- Decreases the pulmonary-to-systemic pressure ratio in newborns with persistent pulmonary hypertension of the newborn (PPHN) [12].

Vasopressin

- Acts via V_1 receptors on vascular smooth muscles, causing vasoconstriction via inositol-1,4,5-trisphosphate (IP_3) and Rho-kinase pathways.
- Has shown both an increase in aortic pressure and a decrease in the ratio of systolic pulmonary artery-to-aortic pressure in children with PH undergoing cardiac catheterization [13].
- Has been shown to reduce inhaled nitric oxide (NO) dose and oxygenation index and allowed for an increase in systemic arterial pressure in newborns with PPHN [14].

Milrinone

- Phosphodiesterase type 3 inhibitor that can improve cardiac contractility but can decrease both systemic and pulmonary vascular resistance.
- Has been shown to be beneficial in infants with severe PH and improve ventricular function [15].

Expert comment Important mediators of pulmonary hypertension

Upregulated or elevated mediators of PH result in pulmonary vasoconstriction that ultimately leads to increased pulmonary pressures (Table 24.4). Endothelin-1 is a classic example of a peptide produced by the endothelium that is elevated in patients with PH. It is therefore an attractive therapeutic target. Endothelin receptor antagonists have been shown to reduce pulmonary pressures in patients with PH, particularly in the setting of congenital heart disease.

Similarly, because the production of prostacyclin and NO, both common vasodilators, appears to be downregulated in patients with PH, these are also therapeutic targets. NO can be given directly via inhalation, as well as have its production augmented by either blocking phosphodiesterase-mediated degradation or stimulating its production via the prostacyclin pathway.

Table 24.4 Important mediators of pulmonary hypertension

Upregulated/elevated	Downregulated/decreased
Endothelin 1	Prostacyclin
Angiotensin II	Nitric oxide
TGF-β	Thrombomodulin
Thromboxane A_2	
von Willebrand factor	
Basic fibroblast growth factor	

Learning point Incidence of pulmonary hypertension in the setting of congenital heart disease

The chart shown in Figure 24.3 represents cohort studies from select worldwide paediatric pH centres in 2014 [16].

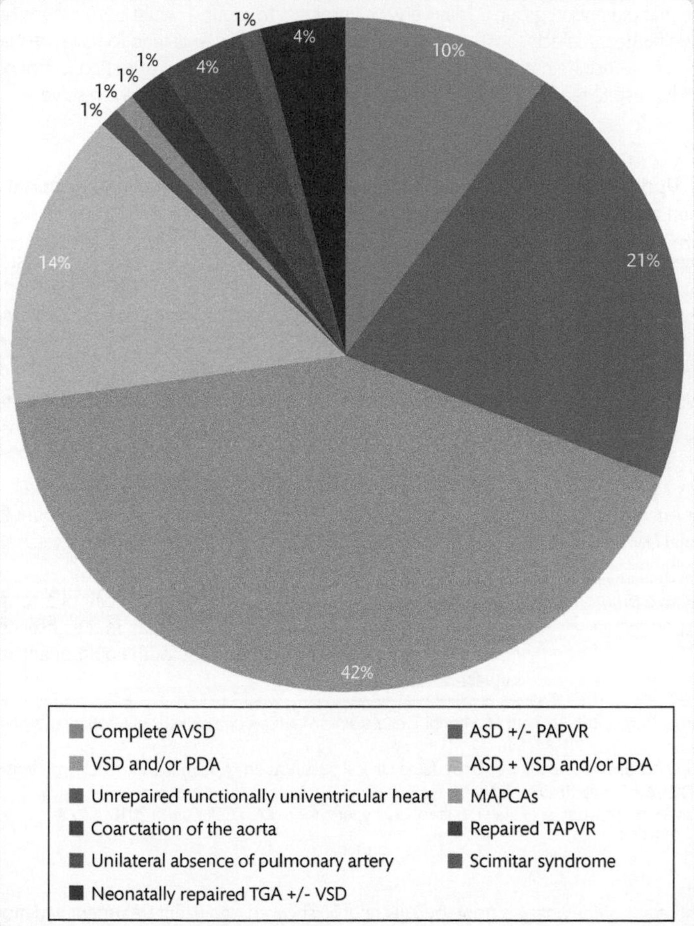

Figure 24.3 Congenital heart disease associated with pulmonary arterial hypertension. ASD, atrial septal defect; AVSD, atrioventricular septal defect; MAPCA, major aortopulmonary collateral artery; PAPVR, partial anomalous pulmonary venous return; PDA, patent ductus arteriosus; TAPVR, total anomalous pulmonary venous return; TGA, transposition of the great arteries; VSD, ventricular septal defect.

Source data from Zijlstra WMH, Douwes JM, Ploegstra MJ, et al. Clinical classification in pediatric pulmonary hypertension associated with congenital heart disease. *Pulm Circ* 2016; 6: 302–312.

Zijlstra and colleagues combined patients from three large PH referral centres (Denver, CO, USA; New York, NY, USA; and the Netherlands) who also had congenital heart disease to assess the association between congenital heart defects and PH in their cohorts. Not surprisingly, patients with ventricular septal defect (VSD) and patent ductus arteriosus (PDA), who have large left-to-right shunts, accounted for the largest population of patients. The authors then attempted to relate clinical outcomes to the Nice CHD-PH classification scheme (see Learning point: Nice classification of pulmonary arterial hypertension associated with congenital heart disease, p. 320) to assess for any relationship. However, no survival difference between the groups was observed, likely due to the significant heterogeneity of patients with congenital heart disease who have the same type of anatomical defect but have markedly different clinical manifestations of their disease.

Learning point Nice classification of pulmonary arterial hypertension associated with congenital heart disease

In 2013, at the World Symposium on Pulmonary Hypertension, held in Nice, France, a classification scheme (Table 24.5) was developed to group more accurately patients with PH associated with congenital heart disease. As this is a heterogenous patient population, challenges remain. For example, it is expected that patients in group 2 may very well progress to group 1 whilst both groups had similar congenital heart defects (post-tricuspid disease). Group 3 patients tend to have pre-tricuspid disease and seldom include patients with Down syndrome. Group 4 is the largest cohort of patients, suggesting that, despite repair of the congenital heart defect, PH does not always resolve.

Table 24.5 Updated Clinical Classification (Nice classification) for pulmonary arterial hypertension associated with congenital heart disease [17–19]

1. Eisenmenger syndrome	All large intra- and/or extracardiac defects which start as systemic-to-pulmonary shunts and ultimately lead to severely elevated pulmonary vascular resistance and ultimately reversal of shunt flow to become either bidirectional or purely pulmonary-to-systemic shunts, leading to polycythaemia, cyanosis, and other organ disease
2. Systemic-to-pulmonary shunts	Moderate to large defects: mild to moderate increases in systemic-to-pulmonary shunting without reversal of shunt flow to cause cyanosis
3. Pulmonary arterial hypertension with coincidental congenital heart disease	Dramatically elevated pulmonary vascular resistance in the presence of a congenital heart defect that does not account for elevation of pulmonary vascular resistance
4. Post-operative pulmonary arterial hypertension	Pulmonary arterial hypertension present after repair of a congenital heart defect or develops/reappears after repair in the absence of a residual shunt lesion that could account for the pulmonary arterial hypertension

Source data from Berger RM, Beghetti M, Humpl T, et al. Clinical features of paediatric pulmonary hypertension: a registry study. *Lancet* 2012; 11:537–546.
Simonneau G, Gatzoulis MA, Adatia I, et al. Updated clinical classification of pulmonary arterial hypertension. *J Am Coll Cardiol* 2013; 62(25 suppl): D34–D41.
Ivy DD, Abman SH, Barst RJ, et al. Pediatric pulmonary hypertension. *J Am Coll Cardiol* 2013; 62(25 suppl): D117–D126.

An important result of the analysis done by Zijlstra et al. showed significant treatment variation between both patients with idiopathic pulmonary arterial hypertension (IPAH) and those with PAH-CHD, as well as within the PAH-CHD subgroups. Patients with PAH-CHD often were not as aggressively managed as those with IPAH. Children in group 3 were more likely to receive triple-drug therapy (PDE5 inhibitor, endothelin receptor antagonist, and prostacyclin therapy) than any other group.

Regarding prognosis, in a 4-year follow-up, Zijlstra et al. showed that, of the total cohort, 15 patients died and one patient received lung transplantation. Ten of the patient deaths were directly related to their PH, whilst five were believed not to be directly related. Transplant-free survival at 1, 3, and 5 years was 96%, 91%, and 88%, respectively.

Approximately 2 months after arriving at our institution, the patient was taken to the operating room for repair of her defect. Her intraoperative course was notable for the finding of multiple small, unappreciated apical muscular VSDs, in addition to her AVSD, requiring multiple runs on cardiopulmonary bypass, as well as the need for re-repair of her right-sided atrioventricular valve. She also had bouts of pulmonary haemorrhage during this time and ultimately was placed in the operating room on veno-arterial extracorporeal membrane oxygenation (ECMO) with an open chest. She was placed on inhaled NO to aid her right ventricle and lower her pulmonary vascular resistance. Her sildenafil was continued via an intravenous route as well. She was brought out to the cardiac intensive care unit on epinephrine, milrinone, and sodium nitroprusside infusions (Figure 24.4).

Learning point Congenital heart defects at highest risk for post-operative pulmonary hypertensive crises

- Truncus arteriosus
- Cor triatriatum
- AVSD
- Total anomalous pulmonary venous return
- Large PDA
- D-transposition of the great arteries.

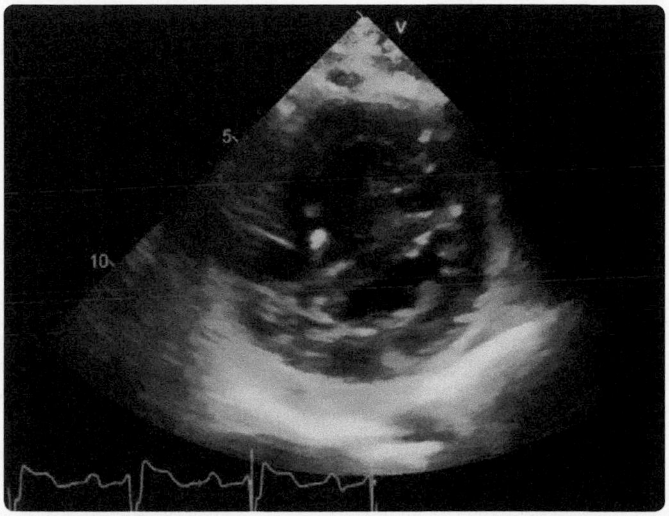

Figure 24.4 Short axis view demonstrating significant shift of the interventricular septum from right to left, creating the classic 'D-sign' seen in patients with severe pulmonary hypertension.

Learning point Key echocardiographic assessments of pulmonary hypertension in PH-CHD

Table 24.6 Key echocardiographic assessments of pulmonary hypertension in PH-CHD

Variable	Definition	Clinical use
Tricuspid regurgitation jet	Estimates the right ventricular pressure based on the velocity; can then calculate the pulmonary artery pressure by adding an estimate of the right atrial pressure	Done via use of a modified Bernoulli equation: $dP = 4 \times TRV^2$ Need full envelope to make an accurate assessment (Figure 24.5)
Tricuspid annular plane systolic excursion (TAPSE)	Directly measures displacement of the lateral annulus of the tricuspid valve during systole	Decreases as PH and right ventricular function worsen; decreased values shown to correlate with worsening survival in adults [20]; has demonstrated improvement after addition of therapy in children [21]
Right ventricular fractional area change (RVFAC)	Systolic and diastolic tracking of the ventricular endocardium	Decreased % indicates decreased function
Peak tissue velocity at tricuspid annulus (S′)	Displacement of basal free wall	Impaired S′—predicts worse right ventricular function in PH-CHD and correlates with catheterization [22–23]
Right ventricular index of myocardial performance (RIMP) or Tei index	Via tissue Doppler velocities: (isovolumic relaxation time – isovolumic contraction time)/right ventricular ejection time	Increased value implies more time in isovolumic phases and thus decreased right ventricular function [24]; will result in increased values, compared to age-matched normal; correlates well with catheterization measurements [25]
Pulmonary artery acceleration time (PAAT)	Assessment of pulmonary vascular resistance obtained by looking at interval from ejection to peak systolic flow	PAAT >120 ms suggestive of pulmonary arterial hypertension [26–27]; not as accurate if a left-to-right shunt is still present
S/D ratio	Ratio of time in systole to time in diastole as determined by tissue Doppler velocities	>1.4 inversely related to survival [28]
Right ventricular/left ventricular ratio	Measured at end-systole	>1 indicates increased risk for an adverse event and reflects compression of the left ventricle by the hypertensive right ventricle [29]
Left ventricular eccentricity index (LVEI)	Ratio of the left ventricular dimension in the minor axis parallel to the septum related to dimension perpendicular to the septum	Increase >1 in conjunction with diastolic septal flattening related to prognosis [30]

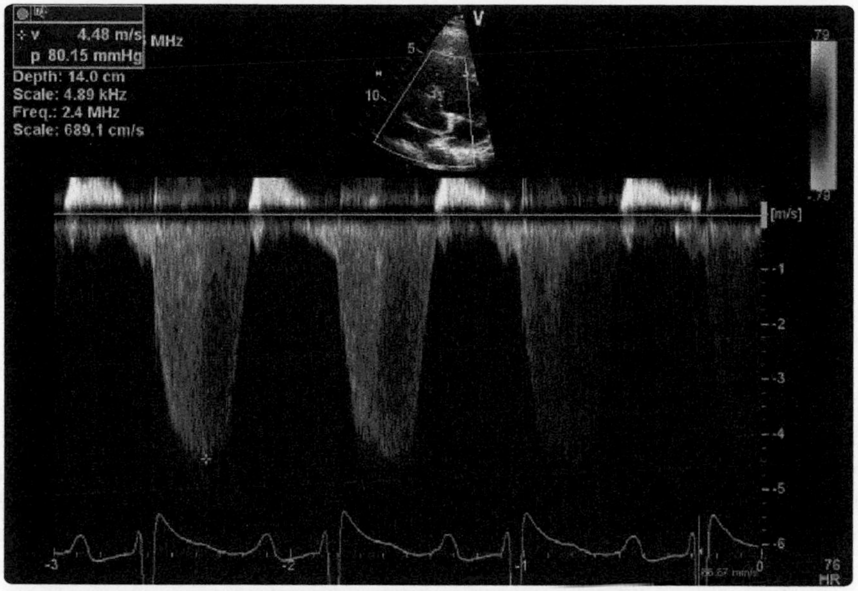

Figure 24.5 High-velocity tricuspid regurgitation jet in a 23-year-old patient with an unrepaired ventricular septal defect.

Post-operative echocardiograms were notable for mild to moderate right ventricular dysfunction and moderate right ventricular hypertrophy, with continued evidence of PH (see Learning point: Key echocardiographic assessments of pulmonary hypertension in PH-CHD, p. 322). The PH service remained actively involved in her care, whilst she was admitted to the cardiac intensive care unit, suggesting inhaled iloprost to aid in support of her struggling right ventricle and to facilitate weaning of her ECMO support (see Learning point: Mediators of pulmonary hypertension that are particularly relevant in PH-CHD, p. 323; see Expert comment: Important mediators of pulmonary hypertension, p. 318). Iloprost was considered but deferred to allow maximization of other supportive strategies, and after 6 days, she was decannulated from ECMO and her chest was then closed 2 days later.

Learning point Mediators of pulmonary hypertension that are particularly relevant in PH-CHD

Thromboxane A_2

- Produced by metabolism of arachidonic acid
- Causes vasoconstriction via phospholipase C
- Increased in children with cyanotic congenital heart disease and in children with significant left-to-right shunts [7]
- Shown to decrease after repair of a left-to-right shunt [8]
- Patients with Down syndrome are particularly prone to oversynthesis of thromboxane A_2, making them particularly prone to PH [9]

Endothelin-1

- Produced by vascular endothelial cells, causing sustained hypertension
- Effects are mediated by two distinct receptors: ET_A and ET_B

- ET_A: vasoconstricts vascular smooth muscle cells
- ET_B: vasoconstricts smooth muscle; vasodilates endothelium; clears ET-1
- Cardiopulmonary bypass: induces significant increases in ET-1, which increases both pulmonary vascular resistance and pulmonary vasoreactivity [31]

Nitric oxide

- Produced in vascular endothelium and ultimately results in vasodilation via cyclic guanosine monophosphate (cGMP) and protein kinase G, with cGMP ultimately broken down by phosphodiesterase (PDE5 in pulmonary vasculature)
- NO signalling pathways are altered by cardiopulmonary bypass and can cause decreased NO synthesis and effect, particularly pulmonary vascular endothelial dysfunction [32]

She continued to require significant ventilator support, as well as a high fraction of inspired oxygen content (see Learning point: Common triggers of post-operative PH crises, p. 324). The PH service again suggested the addition of iloprost, which was accepted this time. Therapy was initiated initially at a starting dose of 0.25 mcg/kg, inhaled every 3 hours, and titrated upward to our maximum dose of 1 mcg/kg, inhaled every 3 hours. This allowed her oxygen and inhaled NO to then be weaned. Once her post-operative acute lung injury started to resolve and her pulmonary mechanics improved, it was possible to wean off and discontinue the iloprost. Once tolerating trophic feeds, she was then started on bosentan at 1 mg/kg twice daily.

Clinical tip Management of post-operative PH

1. Ensure adequate analgesia is on board via continuous opioid and benzodiazepine infusions.
2. Use bolus doses of opioid (usually fentanyl) for any noxious stimuli—tracheal suctioning, movement, etc.—this has limited effects on haemodynamics but will often prevent a PH crisis [33].
3. Deep sedation with neuromuscular blockade as an adjunct may be necessary, particularly in the first 24–48 hours post-operatively.
4. Tight control of pCO_2, pH, and oxygen content is imperative.
5. Use of inhaled NO, if available, can significantly reduce the number of episodes that occur and it can often times ultimately be weaned off.
   a. Of note, sildenafil can be used to prevent rebound PH after weaning of inhaled NO [34].
6. Maintain adequate afterload and avoid systemic hypotension, if possible, whilst avoiding high-dose catecholamines, which can increase pulmonary vascular resistance, cause tachycardia, and increase the likelihood of post-operative arrhythmias.
7. Gentle, controlled diuresis and avoiding significant volume shifts will also reduce the risk of post-operative PH crises, as patients may be somewhat preload-dependent due to their PH.

Learning point Common triggers of post-operative PH crises

- Suboptimal ventilation strategies resulting in hypoxaemia and/or hypercarbia:
  - Inadequate tidal volumes allowing for atelectasis
  - Inappropriate intermittent mandatory ventilation rates
  - Inappropriate inspiratory times
- Significant pain and/or agitation:
  - Undersedation whilst intubated
  - Inadequate pain control during procedures (chest tube manipulation, suctioning of endotracheal tube, etc.)
- Acidosis

Learning point Pathophysiology of a PH crisis

An important part of the pathophysiology of a PH crisis is acute right ventricular failure induced by a sudden pressure load on the right ventricle (Figure 24.6). It is this sudden decompensation event that then precipitates the cascade of events resulting in low cardiac output and rapid clinical deterioration of the patient. Because of this, in patients with severe PH who are followed at our institution, we are becoming more aggressive at providing these patients with a post-tricuspid valve pressure-unloading pathway, via the creation of a Potts shunt, or stenting of the ductus arteriosus, or the creation of a VSD [41] (Figure 24.6). Though these approaches place patients at risk, it alleviates the possibility of acute right ventricular failure and assures them adequate cardiac output in the setting of an acute rise in pulmonary vascular resistance, even if the patients become deeply cyanotic.

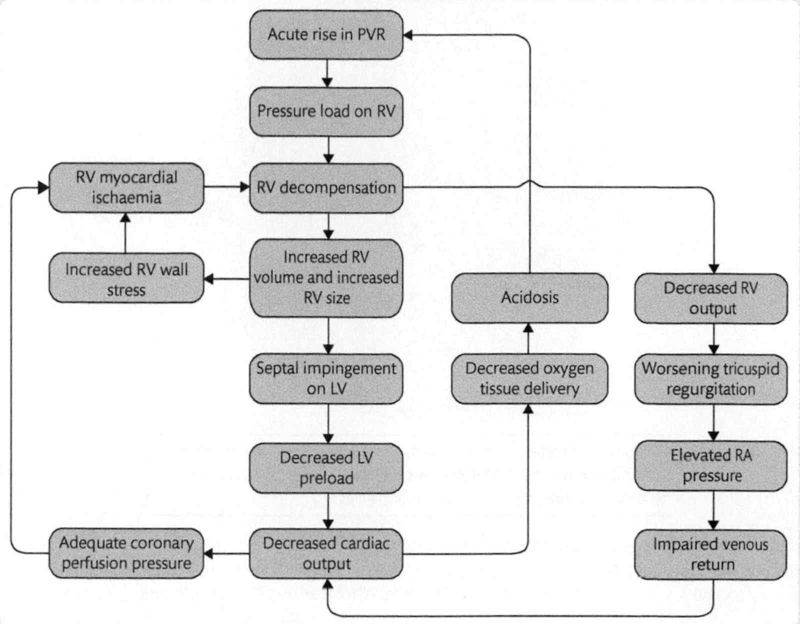

Figure 24.6 Pathophysiology of a PH crisis.

Ultimately, she was able to be extubated initially to high-flow nasal cannulae and then quickly weaned to nasal cannulae. She had a slight elevation in her liver transaminases about 1 month after the therapy was initiated, requiring a decrease in dose. Her liver function appeared stable, and she was continued on this dose of bosentan. She was discharged home approximately 2 months after her surgical repair on sildenafil and bosentan dual therapy. The patient has been doing well at home, finally gaining appropriate weight, and comes to follow-up clinic every 3 months.

Discussion

Children with Down syndrome are particularly prone to the development of PH, and it is often more severe than their counterparts (normal chromosomes) with similar congenital heart disease [35].

Zijlstra et al. nicely demonstrated (Figure 24.7) the complicated nature of PH, even within an identified subgroup such as those with PAH-CHD. Sixty patients, comprising 45% of the cohort, had clinically relevant diagnoses, in addition to their congenital heart disease. Down syndrome was the most common, identified in 50% of these patients. Some of the specific lung abnormalities included repaired congenital diaphragmatic hernia, bronchopulmonary dysplasia, and chronic lung disease. They also identified arteriovenous malformations in the lungs, glycogen storage disease, surfactant mutations, rheumatologic, haematologic, and endocrine disorders, and congenital malformation syndromes such as VACTERL (vertebral defects, anal atresia, cardiac defects, tracheo-oesophageal fistula, renal anomalies, and limb abnormalities).

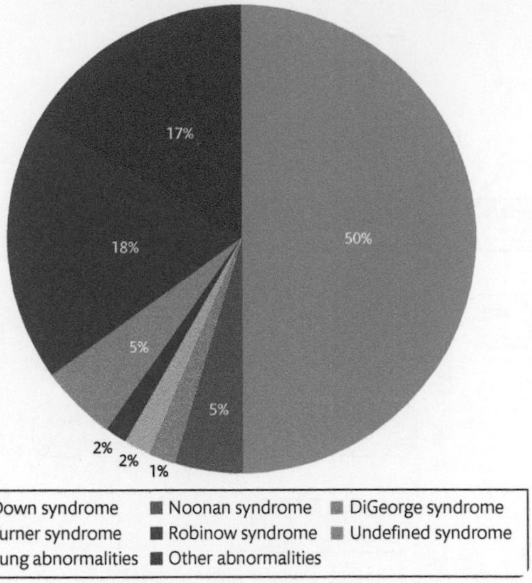

Figure 24.7 Comorbidities associated with PH-CHD [16].
Source data from Zijlstra WMH, Douwes JM, Ploegstra MJ, et al. Clinical classification in pediatric pulmonary hypertension associated with congenital heart disease. *Pulm Circ* 2016; 6: 302–312.

Zijlstra and colleagues, in 2016, published their experience (Figure 24.8) using the Nice pulmonary arterial hypertension associated with congenital heart disease (PAH-CHD) classification and its application to a combined patient cohort from Children's Hospital Colorado, USA, Columbia University Medical Center, New York, USA, and the Dutch National Referral Center for Pediatric Pulmonary Hypertension at the University Medical Center Groningen in the Netherlands. Though most patients could be grouped according to the Nice system, because of the complexity of PAH-CHD, not all children are yet able to be grouped.

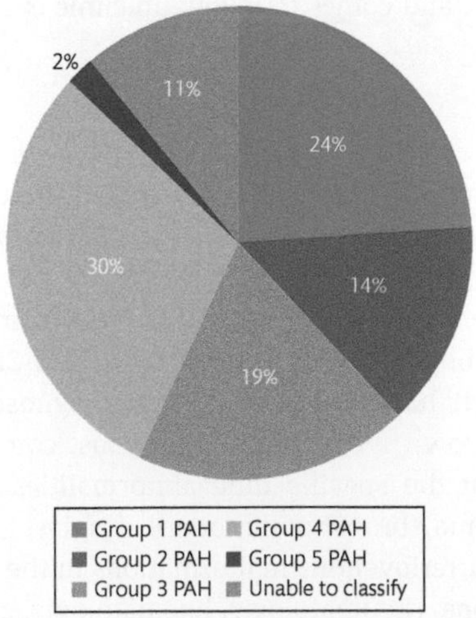

Figure 24.8 Nice clinical classification of pulmonary arterial hypertension associated with congenital heart disease (PAH-CHD) [18]. Patients with PAH-CHD (n = 134). Group 1: Eisenmenger syndrome (32 children); group 2: systemic-to-pulmonary shunt (19 children); group 3: pulmonary arterial hypertension with coincidental congenital heart disease (26 children); group 4: post-operative pulmonary arterial hypertension (40 children); group 5: multiple aortopulmonary collaterals (2 children); unable to classify (15 children).
Source data from Simonneau G, Gatzoulis MA, Adatia I, et al. Updated clinical classification of pulmonary arterial hypertension. *J Am Coll Cardiol* 2013; 62(25 suppl): D34–D41.

Expert comment

The Tracking Outcomes and Practice in Paediatric Pulmonary Hypertension (TOPP) is a global prospective study aimed at collecting data regarding diagnosis, therapy, and outcomes in paediatric patients with PH. A total of 362 patients aged 18 years or younger from 31 centres in 19 countries entered into the database between 2008 and 2010 are represented in these data. Berger et al., in 2012, reported some of the first data associated with the TOPP registry. When looking at patients in this cohort, of those with identified genetic abnormalities, Down syndrome was the most common (42 of 47 included patients). In patients with PH associated with congenital heart disease, 26 of 115 (23%) had Down syndrome.

Figure 24.9 shows the distribution of congenital heart disease associated with PH, with pulmonary arterial hypertension being the most common (APAH-CHD). This figure also nicely demonstrates a common difference between paediatric and adult patients with PH. Whereas left-sided heart disease is the most common cause of PH in adults, in paediatrics, it is a relatively rare occurrence.

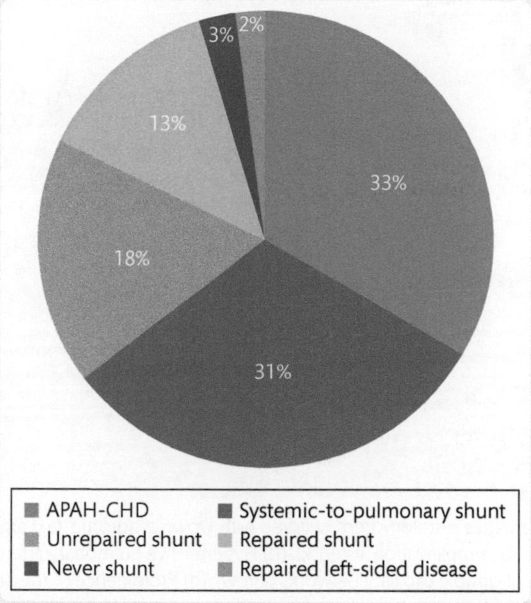

Figure 24.9 TOPP Registry Data [17].
Source data from Berger RM, Beghetti M, Humpl T, et al. Clinical features of paediatric pulmonary hypertension: a registry study. *Lancet* 2012; 11:537–546.

As listed (see Expert comment: Aetiology of pulmonary hypertension in Down syndrome, p. 329) (Figure 24.10), children with Down syndrome display a number of immature pulmonary features, both with regard to anatomical and vascular structures [36]. All of these abnormalities account for the increased frequency of PH in this specific cohort and may also explain why their PH at times seems out of proportion to what would be expected in a patient with the same congenital heart disease but without the chromosomal abnormality.

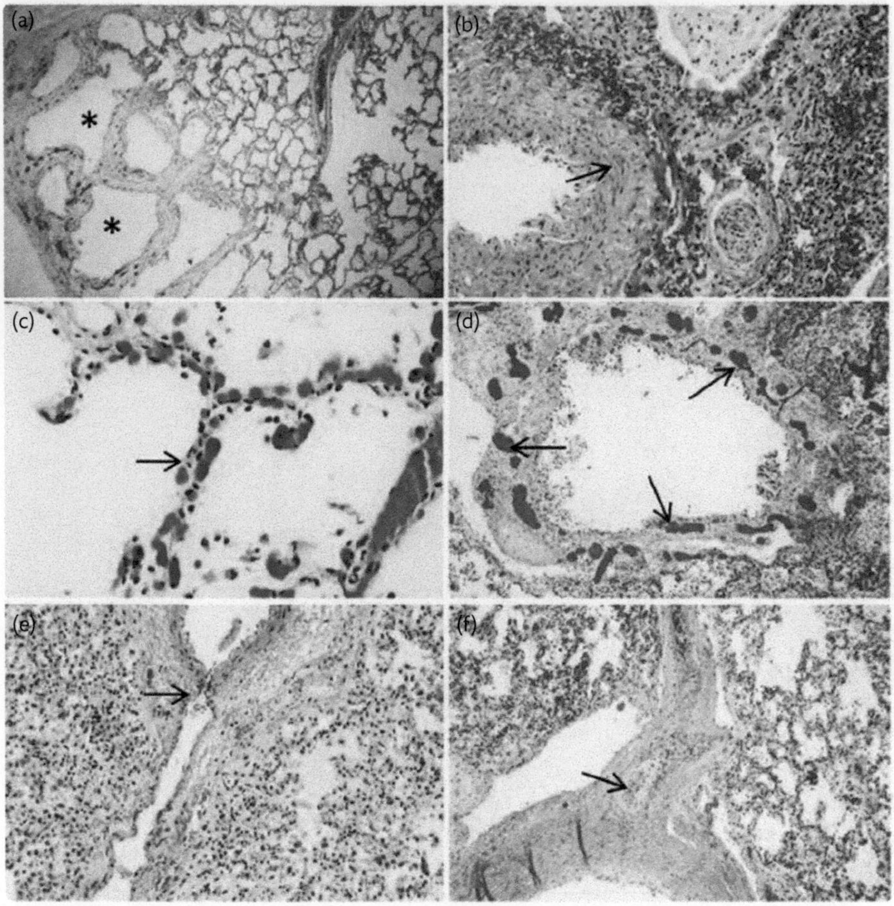

Figure 24.10 Representative histology from children with Down syndrome. (a) Large alveoli lacking secondary septae (alveolar simplification; asterisk). (b) Hypertensive pulmonary arterial remodelling (arrow). (c) Persistence of double capillary networks (arrow). (d) Prominence of the bronchial circulation (arrows). (e, f) Open intrapulmonary bronchopulmonary anastomoses (arrow).

Reproduced from Bush D, Abman SH, Galambos C. Prominent intrapulmonary bronchopulmonary anastomoses and abnormal lung development in infants and children with Down Syndrome. *J Pediatr* 2017; 180: 156–162 with permission from Elsevier.

The TOPP registry (Figure 24.9), with its international patient cohort, nicely demonstrates the relationship between PH and congenital heart disease [17]. Its strict definition of PH (requiring a PVRi > 3 WU/m^2) in the congenital heart disease population only strengthens the data and eliminates the inclusion of patients who may have elevated pulmonary pressures related to shunt flow but do not have truly elevated PVR. With patients with Down syndrome making up such a large percentage of the total cohort of patients with PH associated with congenital heart disease, it also provides important justification for aggressive screening and treatment of PH within this specific population. Of note, TOPP-2 is currently active (clinicaltrials.gov NCT02610660), with results expected in 2020.

Expert comment Aetiology of pulmonary hypertension in Down syndrome

Contributing factors to the development of PH in Down syndrome [9, 36–40] (Figure 24.10):

- Vascular immaturity:
  - Persistence of double capillary networks
  - Reduced secondary septae
  - Fewer more dilated alveoli
  - Impaired angiogenesis
- Prominent intrapulmonary bronchopulmonary anastomoses:
  - Chronic hypoxaemia from a precapillary shunt
- Increased pulmonary expression of anti-angiogenic factors:
  - Impaired vascular development can then lead to distal airspace abnormalities
- Presence of peripheral lung cysts
- Predominant biosynthesis of thromboxane A over PGI_2:
  - Increased pulmonary vasoconstriction

The group at the Pediatric Heart Lung Center in Colorado have pioneered a significant amount of this work An interesting hypothesis published by this group looked at genes controlling anti-angiogenic proteins; they found that these genes are expressed on chromosome 21 and, as a result of the trisomy, may result in overexpression of these factors (e.g. endostatin and Down syndrome critical region protein 1) and cause interruption of normal vascular development [39].

Despite knowing these differences, it remains unclear if a different treatment approach is warranted for patients with Down syndrome, as compared to those without. No formal recommendations exist at this time regarding PH-specific management of patients with Down syndrome. However, Hawkins and colleagues in 2011 proposed a management protocol to manage patients with Down syndrome that is fairly comprehensive in scope, emphasizing the importance of cardiac catheterization, repair of congenital heart disease when possible, and managing any airway obstruction that may exist [20] (Figure 24.6).

A final word from the expert

PH in the setting of congenital heart disease presents a unique management challenge, as often the potential benefits of decreasing the pulmonary vascular resistance have to be balanced against the potential effects this may have on increasing pulmonary blood flow via shunts and potentially worsening a patient's clinical status. However, not addressing the elevated pulmonary vascular resistance could complicate both their operative and post-operative courses in a very negative way. Particularly in the presence of unrepaired shunts, cardiac catheterization is frequently required to better assess and manage PH in these patients, as traditional non-invasive markers of PH obtainable via echocardiography are frequently less reliable.

References

1. Hoeper MM. Definition, classification, and epidemiology of pulmonary arterial hypertension. *Semin Respir Crit Care Med* 2009;30:369–75.
2. Haworth SG, Hislop AA. Treatment and survival in children with pulmonary arterial hypertension: the UK Pulmonary Hypertension Service for Children 2001–2006. *Heart* 2009;95:312–17.
3. Cool CD, Groshong SD, Oakley J, et al. Pulmonary hypertension: cellular and molecular mechanisms. *Chest* 2005;128(6 suppl):565S–71S.

4. Dimopoulos K, Giannakoulas G, Wort SJ, et al. Pulmonary arterial hypertension in adults with congenital heart disease: distinct differences from other causes of pulmonary arterial hypertension and management implications. *Curr Opin Cardiol* 2008;23:545–54.
5. Engelfriet PM, Duffels MG, Moller T, et al. Pulmonary arterial hypertension in adults born with a heart septal defect: the Euro Heart Survey on adult congenital heart disease. *Heart* 2007;93:682–7.
6. Engelfriet P, Boersma E, Oechslin E, et al. The spectrum of adult congenital heart disease in Europe: morbidity and mortality in a 5 year follow-up period. The Euro Heart survery on adult congenital heart disease. *Eur Heart J* 2005;26:2325–33.
7. Adatia I, Barrow SE, Stratton PD, et al. Thromboxane A2 and prostacyclin biosynthesis in children and adolescents with pulmonary vascular disease. *Circulation* 1993;88(5 Pt 1):2117–22.
8. Adatia I, Barrow SE, Stratton PD, et al. Effect of intracardiac repair on biosynthesis of thromboxane A2 and prostacyclin in children with a left to right shunt. *Br Heart J* 1994;72:452–6.
9. Fukushima H, Kosaki K, Sato R, et al. Mechanisms underlying early development of pulmonary vascular obstructive disease in Down Syndrome: an imbalance in biosynthesis of thromboxane A2 and prostacyclin. *Am J Med Genet A* 2010;152A:1919–24.
10. Irving CA, Chaudhari MP. Cardiovascular abnormalities in Down's Syndrome: spectrum, management and survival over 22 years. *Arch Dis Child* 2012;97:326–30.
11. Freeman SB, Taft LF, Dooley KJ, et al. Population-based study of congenital heart defects in Down syndrome. *Am J Med Genet* 1998;80:213–17.
12. Tourneux P, Rakza T, Bouissou A, et al. Pulmonary circulatory effects of norepinephrine in newborns with persistent pulmonary hypertension. *J Pediatr* 2008;153:345–9.
13. Siehr SL, Feinstein JA, Yang W, et al. Hemodynamic effects of phenylephrine, vasopressin and epinephrine in children ith pulmonary hypertension: a pilot study. *Pediatr Crit Care Med* 2016;17:428–37.
14. Mohamed A, Nasef N, Shah V, et al. Vasopressin as a rescue therapy for refractory pulmonary hypertension in neonates: Case series. *Pediatr Crit Care Med* 2014;15:148–54.
15. James AT, Corcoran JD, McNamara PJ, Franklin O, El-Khuffash AF. The effect of milrinone on right and left ventricular function when uased as a rescue therapy for term infants with pulmonary hypertension. *Cardiol Young* 2015;26:90–9.
16. Zijlstra WMH, Douwes JM, Ploegstra MJ, et al. Clinical classification in pediatric pulmonary hypertension associated with congenital heart disease. *Pulm Circ* 2016;6:302–12.
17. Berger RM, Beghetti M, Humpl T, et al. Clinical features of paediatric pulmonary hypertension: a registry study. *Lancet* 2012;11:537–46.
18. Simonneau G, Gatzoulis MA, Adatia I, et al. Updated clinical classification of pulmonary arterial hypertension. *J Am Coll Cardiol* 2013;62(25 suppl):D34–41.
19. Ivy DD, Abman SH, Barst RJ, et al. Pediatric pulmonary hypertension. *J Am Coll Cardiol* 2013;62(25 suppl):D117–26.
20. Hawkins A, Langton-Hewer S, Henderson J, Tulloh RM. Management of pulmonary hypertension in Down syndrome. *Eur J Pediatr* 2011;170:915–21.
21. Forfia P, Fisher M, Mathai S, et al. Tricuspid annular displacement predicts survival in pulmonary hypertension. *Am J Respir Crit Care Med* 2006;174:1034–41.
22. Bano K, Kanaan UB, Ehrlich AC, et al. Improvement in tricuspid annular plane systolic excursion with pulmonary hypertension therapy in pediatric patients. *Echocardiography* 2015;32:1228–32.
23. Koestenberger M, Nagel B, Ravekes W, et al. Tricuspid annular peak systolic velocity (S') in children and young adults with pulmonary artery hypertension secondary to congenital heart diseases, and in those with repaired Tetralogy of Fallot: echocardiography and MRI data. *J Am Soc Echocardiogr* 2012;25:1041–9.

24. Cevik A, Kula S, Olgunturk R, et al. Doppler tissue imaging provides an estimate of pulmonary arterial pressure in children ith pulmonary hypertension due to congenital intracardiac shunts. *Congenit Heart Dis* 2013;8:527–34.
25. Vonk MC, Sander MH, van den Hoogen FH, et al. Right ventricle Tei-index: a tool to increase the accuracy of non-invasive detection of pulmonary arterial hypertension in connective tissue diseases. *Eur J Echocardiogr* 2007;8:317–21.
26. Cevik A, Kula S, Olgunturk R, et al. Quantitative evaluation of right ventricle function by transthoracic echocardiography in childhood congenital heart disease patients with pulmonary hypertension. *Echocardiography* 2012;29:840–8.
27. Cevik A, Kula S, Olgunturk R, et al. Assessment of pulmonary arterial hypertension and vascular resistance by measurements of the pulmonary arterial flow velocity curve in the absence of a measured tricuspid regurgitant velocity in childhood congenital heart disease. *Pediatr Cardiol* 2013; 34:646–55.
28. Alkon J, Humpl T, Manlhiot C, et al. Usefulness of the right ventricular systolic to diastolic duration ratio to predict functional capacity and survival in children with pulmonary arterial hypertension. *Am J Cardiol* 2010;106:430–6.
29. Jone PN, Hinzman J, Wagner BD, Ivy DD, Younoszai A. Right ventricular to left ventricular diameter ratio at end-systole in evaluating outcomes in children with pulmonary hypertension. *J Am Soc Echocardiogr* 2014;27:172–8.
30. Kassem E, Humpl T, Freidberg MK. Prognostic significance of 2-dimentional, M-mode, and Doppler echo indices of right ventricular function in children with pulmonary arterial hypertension. *Am Heart J* 2013;165:1024–31.
31. Schulze-Neick I, Li J, Reader JA, et al. The endothelin antagonist BQ123 reduces pulmonary vascular resistance after surgical intervention for congenital heart disease. *J Thorac Cardiovasc Surg* 2002;124:435–41.
32. Wessel DL, Adatia I, Giglia TM, et al. Use of inhaled nitric oxide and acetylcholine in the evaluation of pulmonary hypertension and endothelial function after cardiopulmonary bypass. *Circulation* 1993;88:2128–38.
33. Hickey P, Hansen D, Wessel D, et al. Pulmonary and systemic hemodynamic responses to fentanyl in infants. *Anesth Analg* 1985;64:483–6.
34. Namachivayam P, Theilen U, Butt WW, et al. Sildenafil prevents rebound pulmonary hypertension after withdrawal of nitric oxide in children. *Am J Respir Crit Care Med* 2006;174:1042–7.
35. San T. Clinical characteristics of pulmonary arterial hypertension associated with Down Syndrome. *Pediatr Int* 2014;56:297–303.
36. Bush D, Abman SH, Galambos C. Prominent intrapulmonary bronchopulmonary anastomoses and abnormal lung development in infants and children with Down Syndrome. *J Pediatr* 2017;180:156–62.
37. Betsy L, Schloo M, Gordon F, et al. Down syndrome: patterns of disturbed lung growth. *Hum Pathol* 1990;22:919–23.
38. Cooney TP, Thurlbeck WM. Pulmonary hypoplasia in Down Syndrome. *N Engl J Med* 1982;307:1170–3.
39. Galambos C, Minic AD, Bush D, et al. Increased lung expression of anti-angiogenic factors in Down Syndrome: potential role in abnormal lung vascular growth and the risk for pulmonary hypertension. *PLoS ONE* 2016;11:e0159005.
40. Biko DM, Schwartz M, Anupindi SA, Altes TA. Subpleural lung cysts in Down syndrome: prevalence and association with coexisting diagnoses. *Pediatr Radiol* 2008;38:280–4.
41. Chartan C, Coleman R, Varghese N, Ruiz, F, Mallory, G, Justino H. *Transcatheter ventricular septal defect creation as an innovative, nonsurgical therapy for severe pulmonary hypertension with right ventricular failure*. Tenth International Conference on Neonatal and Childhood Pulmonary Vascular Disease. San Francisco, CA, 9 March 2017.

24. Coelho A, Kiess [illegible] et al. [illegible] simple, useful imaging provides an estimate of pulmonary arterial pressure [illegible] pulmonary hypertension due to [illegible] defects. Congenit Heart Dis 2013; 8: [illegible].
25. [illegible], van der [illegible] et al. [illegible] ventricle: a tool to [illegible] pulmonary hypertension in [illegible] disease. [illegible]
26. [illegible] ventricular [illegible] heart disease patients with pulmonary hypertension. [illegible] 2013; [illegible].
27. [illegible] et al. Assessment of pulmonary arterial hypertension and vascular [illegible] of the pulmonary artery [illegible] in the [illegible] congenital heart disease. [illegible] 2013; [illegible].
28. [illegible] the right ventricular [illegible] to predict [illegible] and survival in children with pulmonary arterial hypertension. [illegible] 2013; [illegible].
29. [illegible] ventricular [illegible] in children with pulmonary hypertension. [illegible] 2013; [illegible].
30. [illegible] of [illegible] in children with pulmonary arterial hypertension. [illegible] 2013; [illegible].
31. [illegible] The endothelin antagonist [illegible] reduces [illegible] in [illegible] congenital heart disease. [illegible] 2013; [illegible].
32. [illegible] and [illegible] in the [illegible] of pulmonary hypertension and [illegible]. [illegible]
33. [illegible] and systemic [illegible] responses to [illegible]. [illegible]
34. [illegible] pulmonary [illegible] 2013; [illegible].
35. [illegible] pulmonary arterial hypertension [illegible] syndrome. [illegible] 2013; [illegible].
36. [illegible] pulmonary [illegible] and abnormal lung development [illegible] children [illegible] 2013; [illegible].
37. [illegible] 2013; [illegible].
38. [illegible] Pulmonary hypertension in [illegible] syndrome. [illegible] 2013; [illegible].
39. [illegible] and [illegible] factors [illegible] pulmonary vascular growth and [illegible] risk for [illegible] 2013; [illegible].
40. [illegible] lung [illegible] 2013; [illegible].
41. [illegible] et al. [illegible] pulmonary vascular disease [illegible] International Conference of Neonatal [illegible] Pulmonary Vascular Disease, San Francisco, [illegible] March 2013.

INDEX

E

S